HEALTH TECHNOLOGY LITERACY

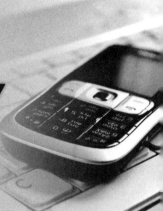

A Transdisciplinary Framework for Consumer-Oriented Practice

Maryalice Jordan-Marsh, PhD, RN, FAAN
Associate Professor
School of Social Work
University of Southern California
Los Angeles, California

D0556469

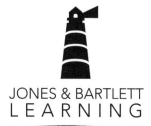

JONES & BARTLETT
LEARNING

World Headquarters

Jones & Bartlett Learning
40 Tall Pine Drive
Sudbury, MA 01776
978-443-5000
info@jblearning.com
www.jblearning.com

Jones & Bartlett Learning
Canada
6339 Ormindale Way
Mississauga, Ontario L5V 1J2
Canada

Jones & Bartlett Learning
International
Barb House, Barb Mews
London W6 7PA
United Kingdom

Jones & Bartlett Learning books and products are available through most bookstores and online booksellers. To contact Jones & Bartlett Learning directly, call 800-832-0034, fax 978-443-8000, or visit our website, www.jblearning.com.

Substantial discounts on bulk quantities of Jones & Bartlett Learning publications are available to corporations, professional associations, and other qualified organizations. For details and specific discount information, contact the special sales department at Jones & Bartlett Learning via the above contact information or send an email to specialsales@jblearning.com.

The author, editor, and publisher have made every effort to provide accurate information. However, they are not responsible for errors, omissions, or for any outcomes related to the use of the contents of this book and take no responsibility for the use of the products and procedures described. Treatments and side effects described in this book may not be applicable to all people; likewise, some people may require a dose or experience a side effect that is not described herein. Drugs and medical devices are discussed that may have limited availability controlled by the Food and Drug Administration (FDA) for use only in a research study or clinical trial. Research, clinical practice, and government regulations often change the accepted standard in this field. When consideration is being given to use of any drug in the clinical setting, the health care provider or reader is responsible for determining FDA status of the drug, reading the package insert, and reviewing prescribing information for the most up-to-date recommendations on dose, precautions, and contraindications, and determining the appropriate usage for the product. This is especially important in the case of drugs that are new or seldom used.

Production Credits

Publisher: Kevin Sullivan
Acquisitions Editor: Amy Sibley
Associate Editor: Patricia Donnelly
Editorial Assistant: Rachel Shuster
Senior Production Editor: Carolyn F. Rogers
Associate Marketing Manager: Katie Hennessy
V.P., Manufacturing and Inventory Control:
  Therese Connell

Composition: diacriTech
Cover Design: Timothy Dziewit
Cover Image: background © Chen Ping Hung/ShutterStock, Inc.;
  mobile phone on laptop © Atanas Bezov/ShutterStock, Inc.
Printing and Binding: Malloy, Inc.
Cover Printing: Malloy, Inc.

Library of Congress Cataloging-in-Publication Data

Jordan-Marsh, Maryalice.
  Health technology literacy : a transdisciplinary framework for consumer-oriented practice / Maryalice Jordan-Marsh.
    p. cm.
  Includes bibliographical references and index.
  ISBN 978-0-7637-5848-6 (pbk.)
  1. Telecommunication in medicine. 2. Medical informatics. 3. Health education. 4. Medicine, Popular. I. Title.
  [DNLM: 1. Telemedicine. 2. Consumer Participation. 3. Health Literacy. 4. Information Seeking Behavior.
    W 83.1 J82h 2011]
  R119.9.J67 2011
  610.28–dc22
                                                                                          2010016133

6048

Printed in the United States of America
14 13 12 11 10   10 9 8 7 6 5 4 3 2 1

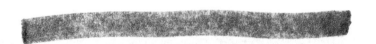

Contents

Preface

This book provides a comprehensive overview of the complex new options in health technology designed to engage consumers in their own health care. The shift in the health field to a consumer-centered model is happening at a rapid pace because of the tremendous costs of hospital care and the expectation that prevention and consumer engagement can be far more effective. Yet, many consumers have exposures to advances in health technology only through newspaper stories or lurid accounts of privacy violations. Health professionals, faculty, researchers, and consumers will require new literacies to provide leadership in this new health habitat. This book grounds participants in a socioecological framework and highlights key issues and skills for this dynamic field where the inventory has "gone viral"—multiplying exponentially in unexpected directions.

Successful use of health technology to support consumer-centered health models will depend on the connection of technology, information, social networks, and on the collaboration of health professionals and all of the stakeholders in the healthcare experience. This book offers a socioecological perspective on health technology focusing on telehealth as the key intersection between healthcare provider and the consumer. Telehealth has both *zero geography* (Hames, 2007)— it does not matter where providers are located, and a *pan geography* quality—it connects the consumer and social networks that are linked with health care, work, home, or recreation—everywhere. Telehealth as the intersection point for consumers and healthcare providers includes personal health records; online information seeking; social networking; health literacy; devices to connect, monitor, and engage; and games—the major chapter topics in this book.

The heart of the book is translating theory into literacy for professional and consumer practice. The book does this by providing a strong conceptual framework and an extensive review of research—presenting the big picture in an exciting and useable way. But the book has a translational focus—helping professionals and consumers create specific possibilities and programs with everyday considerations and implications for practice. Fortunately, new digital applications are rapidly being transferred to health care, such as games and wearable sensors. This book has a strong focus on adults—those who are coping with chronic illness, those who are experiencing age-related declines that telehealth complements, and the social network of both groups.

As baby boomers cross the threshold from full-time workers to retirees and part-time employees or to new career opportunities, they face many challenges. Many will become disconnected from their customary healthcare resources owing to shifts in coverage, separation from workplace health programs, or geographic changes in residence. They will face these challenges with the expectation of living a full life, but, in many instances they are challenged by chronic illness in themselves or in a family member. Baby boomers also expect to have control of their health care, in contrast to previous generations that relied on the physician to make decisions in the best interest of the patient. Today, of Internet-connected Americans, 80% use the Internet to seek healthcare information, many using it as their first or primary source of health information (Fox, 2010). Digital immigrants (Prensky, 2001), this older generation, are fast acquiring habits and skills of the digital natives. For digital natives—seeking health information informally occurs online on networking sites such as MySpace, during interactive virtual reality games, and on blogs and bulletin boards as well as sites endorsed by experts.

Economic and social tensions and the availability of virtual communities, Internet resources, robotics, mobile social networking, and the prospect of electronic personal health records are profoundly changing the relationship between healthcare providers and their patients. Simultaneously, healthcare costs are escalating and becoming the focus of political debates across the globe. However, learning from other countries' experience and from transdisciplinary research has been idiosyncratic and fragmented. Consumers are rarely engaged as "experts."

Now consumer/patients are going online in droves for participatory health. To date, they must cobble together their own links, usually fragmented by disease condition or health goal and function—information vs. treatment vs. social support vs. advocacy. While a myriad of online support groups exist, collaborative communities of "prosumers" (Tapscott & Williams, 2006) who participate in the creation of products and policies and treatment strategies across health needs have been slower to emerge. Engaging prosumers could speed translation of research findings, promote tailoring of applications that ensure compliance with recommendations for treatment, and jump-start new fields of inquiry and technologies. It is not clear who is ready to take the lead in a virtual culture of health where patients are partners, not simply consumers or research subjects. Are we ready to shift from "distance learning" to "mass collaboration"?

Nurses take a special responsibility for patient-centered care and are taking the lead in the area of personal health records, in particular. Nurses are ideally positioned to take the lead in bringing transdisciplinary collaboration around health technology that translates research and engineering to consumer engagement.

Despite the potential for this growing do-it-yourself health culture, online health care or eHealth has only recently come under examination by healthcare providers (Baur & Kanaan, 2006). The eHealth awareness levels and habits of older adults are even less understood, the "digital divide" being widely treated as a permanent generational barrier. The book is based on the assumption that healthcare professionals, researchers, and policy makers can no longer ignore the Internet as a factor in relations between patients/consumers and the providers of health care and health insurance. Participatory health is a fact of health care.

However, the healthcare system of today (and related research) is deeply rooted in an asymmetrical knowledge relationship between providers and patients. Similar asymmetry has developed with respect to researchers and subjects. Providers, and physicians in particular, have held power as gatekeepers not only to services but also to knowledge. Internet-based health resources threaten to level this imbalance with obvious and doubtless dramatic socioecological effect. At the same time, some consumer advocates fear that disclosing any personal health information online poses risks of identity theft and loss of insurance coverage.

Other consumer groups question whether there will be cost shifting from traditional face-to-face health services to the more impersonal Internet. This book will provide an opportunity to explore and elucidate principles that might guide how a health agency or providers can make the most of the Internet with patients and families while minimizing the disadvantages and hazards.

These shifts call for new models of assessment for practitioners and conceptual frameworks for researchers concerned with health literacy and the acquisition of and reinforcement of health behaviors and attitudes. Issues related to conducting research on health behaviors and health decisions are examined from a socioecological perspective as are new opportunities provided by existing and emerging technology.

A transdisciplinary focus where the wisdom of all the stakeholders is recognized and solutions are examined from multiple perspectives is the key to resolving what Rittel and Webber (1973) called the recurrent wicked problems of health care confronting the globe. Stakeholders are offered a socioecological framework for moving the empowerment cycle forward. The components of data, information, knowledge, and wisdom are seen as the potential for influence (change) at transition points. These components are energized by the influence or charisma (motivational power) of both people and media and limited only by the capital available (for example, economic, human, social, and sociotechnical). Being transdisciplinary and consumer centered will require a worldview that is more than the sum of knowledge of many professionals and calls for new frameworks that break down traditional boundaries (Mitchell, 2005). A socioecological framework for an empowerment cycle is presented as what Christernsen, Bohmer, and Kenagy (2001) described as a disruptive innovation in health care.

AUDIENCES

This book is designed to provide a conceptual framework for health professionals and policy makers wanting a theory- and research-based approach to the big picture. Similarly, design, engineering, and computer experts who have looked at only one segment of telehealth and want to broaden their expertise to an ecosystem focus will benefit from engaging with this material. This book is a great resource for legislators (and their staff) when they are asked to vote on policies and funding related to health technology for telehealth funding and regulation. Nurses building collaborative, coordinated care will find it complements a wide range of initiatives underway in the field of nursing. The book offers ideas to engage health professionals, technology experts, and consumers.

This book provides a springboard for groups interested in making telehealth more available, and for savvy family members wanting greater peace of mind as their parents age in some degree of isolation, whether through geographic distance or due to the supportive family member's other commitments. The book shows how monitoring aspects of telehealth and creating social engagement are critical to productive, satisfying aging in place for older adults and their loved ones.

The book, then, is very useful for consumer advocacy groups wanting to understand the benefits and risks, and to delineate which components of telehealth and telecare can be added to fully advantage adults—such as personal health records, games, and new devices. Advocates equipped with the conceptual framework and vocabulary presented here enhance their ability to participate in policy and implementation discussions.

This book is ideal as a resource for graduate students who are preparing as professionals in nursing, health, social work, engineering, computer science, psychology, gerontology, ergonomics, and interior design. The book supports the rapid shift in these newly eHealth-related professions and gives the early career professional an enduring conceptual framework and an integrated perspective, along with extensive practical tools and Web-based resources for continued use. This book is also useful for senior year undergraduates contemplating the range of fields in health technology for advanced study or career options.

OVERVIEW OF CHAPTERS

The book is organized into seven chapters describing consumer-centered aspects of health technology. The discussion is based on providing eHealth or telehealth in the home, work, or community setting (e.g., senior center, senior housing).

- Chapter 1, "Telehealth as a Fulcrum in Health Technology," introduces the empowerment cycle socioecological framework. The chapter provides an overview of the uses of the related terms, telehealth, telecare, and telemedicine, and provides a perspective on new expectations of consumers. Chapter 1 acknowledges that health care has become a wicked social problem and proposes that telehealth and new consumer engagement is a possible solution.
- Chapter 2, "Literacy for an Age of eHealth," makes a case that consumers, and to some extent, health providers need a whole new set of skills (literacies) to fully participate in new health technology. In this chapter, the elements of the socioecological framework that affect health literacy in the empowerment cycle are detailed.
- Chapter 3, "Health Information Seeking Behavior on the Web," describes the challenges of finding credible information on the Web and discusses opportunities for sharing information within one's social network. New tools for social media networking are described using the Centers for Disease Control and Prevention's list and examples. In this chapter, the complexity of the flow of data, information, and knowledge is addressed in the context of understanding consumer opportunities afforded by the Internet.
- Chapter 4, "The Personal Health Record: Building Human Capital for Health," presents details of the consumer-oriented aspect of the electronic medical record (EMR). The focus is on how the record can be designed to track and provide feedback on observations of daily living. These observations are critical to changing health behaviors for living well with a chronic illness and aging productively. The nursing leadership of Patricia Brennan under the Robert Wood Johnson Foundation initiatives is particularly pivotal.
- Chapter 5, "Devices as Adjuncts to Being Healthy at Home," introduces readers to the wide range of peripherals (devices) that can monitor, assemble information, send alerts, and make judgments about actions to take. These devices are the mechanisms by which telecare for chronic illness and telehealth for health promotion operate in the new paradigm for consumer involvement. Issues related to using these devices and suggestions for smooth incorporation into consumer-oriented settings are presented.

- Chapter 6, "Digital Games: Consumer Resources for Health Capital," introduces the "gamecare revolution." A case is made for routinely assessing the extent to which consumers are playing any kind of digital game. A proposal is made that the introduction of digital games can speed confident use of personal health records and is a potential motivator and instructional media for health behavior and attitude changes for the newly empowered consumer and their families. A case is made for assessments done by nurses and social works to include games.
- Chapter 7, "Consumer-Centric Health Technology: Wicked Problems and Deliciously Disruptive Solutions," acknowledges some of the challenges of implementing telehealth from a consumer perspective. Some interesting ethical dilemmas are posed. Then, there are a set of recommendations, new developments on the horizon—the delicious solutions. These include the emerging transdisciplinary heroes who transcend their own disciplinary boundaries to emerge with new approaches. Five heroes are named as exemplars. New partnerships among groups are presented as harbingers of the *disrupted* future. A final case is made for engaging capital and influence to engage data, information, knowledge, and wisdom at key transitions for healthy aging and living well with a chronic disease.

This book supports empowerment of all members of the healthcare team who engage on the consumer side of health technology and encourages them to implement information technology (IT). Becoming literate will enable making sense of the minute-to-minute changes, opportunities, and issues facing those who engage in health around the globe. The book is a platform for launching new initiatives, by the nature of health technology, going beyond a compendium or inventory of all possible developments. Readers are invited to a banquet of eHealth resources that has "gone viral."

REFERENCES

Baur, C., & Kanaan, S. B. (2006). Expanding the reach and impact of consumer e-health tools: Executive summary, a vision of e-health benefits for all (Electronic No. 2006). Department of Disease Prevention and Health Promotion. Retrieved December 22, 2009, from http://www.health.gov/communication/ehealth/ehealthTools/summary.htm

Christensen, C. M., Bohmer, R., & Kenagy, J. (2001). Will disruptive innovations cure health care? *Harvard Business Review, 78*(5), 102–112.

Fox, S. (2010). Crowdsourcing a survey: Health topics. *Pew Internet & American Life Project.* Retrieved July 20, 2010, from hppt://www.pewinternet.org/Commentary/2010/July/Crowdsourcing-a-Survey-Health-Topics.aspx

Hames, R. D. (2007). The five literacies of global leadership: What authentic leaders know and you need to find out. San Francisco, CA: Jossey-Bass.

Mitchell, P. H. (2005). What's in a name?: Multidisciplinary, interdisciplinary, and transdisciplinary. *Journal of Professional Nursing, 21*(6), 332–334.

Prensky, M. (2001). Digital natives, digital immigrants. *On the Horizon, 9*(5), 1–6. Retrieved December 22, 2009, from http://www.scribd.com/doc/9799/Prensky-Digital-Natives-Digital-Immigrants-Part1

Rittel, H. W. J., & Webber, M. M. (1973). Dilemmas in a general theory of planning. *Policy Sciences, 4*, 155–169.

Tapscott, D., & Williams, A. (2006). *Wikinomics: How mass collaboration changes everything.* New York: Penguin Group.

Acknowledgments

The idea of doing a book came from Dean Marilyn Flynn of the University of Southern California (USC) School of Social Work. She has supported all of my initiatives to build health technology as a new research, practice, and teaching direction. My colleagues at USC in other departments were key as we traded leadership on health technology projects, both ongoing and new: Margaret McLaughlin, Marientina Gotsis, Michàlle Morbarak, Margo Apostolos, Sarah Ingersoll, Michael Cody, and Merril Silverstein. Terry Wolff, the Director of Information Technologies, and his trusty team continually and patiently rescued me from various IT conundrums as I navigated the book and new courseware at USC.

Special thanks to Katharyn May who engaged me as a visiting professor consultant on the design and development of the *nursing intelligence* technology initiative in the University of Wisconsin School of Nursing at a critical juncture in my thinking about the book. The Robert Wood Johnson Foundation initiatives thankfully supported two of my risky innovative projects: a nursing centered project on empowerment of all members of the health team and more recently, a games for health trial.

I am truly indebted to Jae Eun Chung and Shuya Pan, who were authoritative and expert collaborators, on the games and Internet information chapters, during their doctoral studies. A great joy in designing and carrying out the book was the enthusiastic support and hard work of the following students: Penny Spector-Shleifer who did the first level of literature search support, Carol Brown who took many aspects to the next level, and Carla Lamuscio who figured out the secrets of RefWorks just at the right moment. My assistant Vivian Li was the organizer who not only worked on the book citations but kept the rest of the day-to-day logistics of my academic life in balance so I could focus.

Rachel Shuster, editorial assistant, played a vital role in the last stages by not only tracking the details but also continually being cheerful about resolving glitches. I am especially grateful to Carolyn Rogers who oversaw the copyediting and supported my preferences for style.

The book is enriched by the generosity of the copyright holders who shared their artwork and ideas without fee or minimal charges. I am grateful. Special thanks to the artist Jin DePaul, who distilled my passion for ecosystems and wisdom and social capital into the illustration that maps the major theme of the book, and who built an iconic graphic to capture the digital interactions of eHealth.

Laurel Hoa, known affectionately as "the architect of the final push," was invaluable as a sounding board, also in creating the tables and figures from notes, editing key sections, and management of logistics related to submission of the work. Michael Hoa, MD, made valuable contributions to the design and naming constructs of Figure 1.2: Ecosystem of Care Costs: A Bridge Too Far.

Family become ever more important during the long intense period of book preparation. My husband David Marsh and my daughter Myranda were lifelines. They encouraged me and rearranged their lives to suit the book schedule. David Marsh revived the book midway with his strategic organizational skills and gift for knowing how to sequence topics and opinions in chapter form—no David, no book!

CHAPTER 1

Telehealth as a Fulcrum in Health Technology

GLOBAL INTERDEPENDENCE AND THE ECOLOGY OF HEALTHCARE SYSTEMS

The human landscape is changing (Doarn et al., 2008). Across the globe we are confronted with "diminishing resources of fossil fuels, aging population, a shortage of skilled labor in healthcare…and emerging technologies for the personal space, culture, and consumer demand (Doarn et al., p. 998). The importance of framing human problems in terms of ecological perspectives is getting renewed attention in health care (Institute of medicine [IOM], 2000, 2009). Ecology is the science and art of recognizing that everything is connected to everything (Hames, 2007; Hofmeyer & Marck, 2008).

Instantaneous communication and the ability to traverse the globe in hours are factors in creating global interdependence. The technology of social media and instant access to information previously accessed only by experts is reshaping relationships between consumers and providers of service and expertise. This interdependence and flattening of previous information transfer hierarchies has implications for health care.

There is widespread recognition that we can longer assume we can go forward in the traditional manner. Experts assembled by the Institute of Medicine (IOM) examined these changes and their implications for patient provider relationships (IOM, 2009). The chief executive officer for Intel exhorts us to a new social covenant of becoming "more informed, engaged and proactive about health (Otellini, 2009, para. 4). Agencies in countries across the globe are cooperating in new ways around technology (EUnetHTA, 2008). As technology enables care that was not possible in the past, new criteria for effectiveness will be required (Currell, Urquhart, Wainwright, & Lewis, 2000).

A related assumption is that in the next decade health and health care will increasingly rely on technology to inform, support decisions, provide treatment, monitor progress, and supplement social, emotional, and physical resources. Tools will range from wikis and online support groups, to interactive programs that teach and counsel for lifestyle change and mental health, to "smart homes" and robots. Assumptions include the belief that sociotechnical capital (Resnick, 2001) is the renewable resource that drives the system. Sociotechnical capital refers "to productive combinations of social relations and information and communication technology (Resnick, 2001 [electronic version] pp. 2–3).

A shift to patient-centered care and new patient responsibilities characterize the first decade of the new millennium (IOM, 2008; Bashshur et al., 2009). In the past, the emphasis of the professional looking at the patient's perspective was on satisfaction, not engagement (Currell et al., 2000). New imperatives related to costs and reimbursements were driving calls for healthcare reform in the first year of President Obama's term.

In the United States, we have the increasing realization that we are racing toward an empty wallet with respect to Medicare. Levey (2009) in a *Los Angeles Times* article projected Medicare's expenditures for the next 10 years compared to the hospital trust fund balance (money set aside from previous contributions of employees). The expectation was that the fund would be self-renewing as new workers made new contributions. Levey highlights the potential that the fund will be out of money in 8 years (Figure 1.1). Levey makes the case that new

Figure 1.1   Growth of Healthcare Spending as Percent of GDP

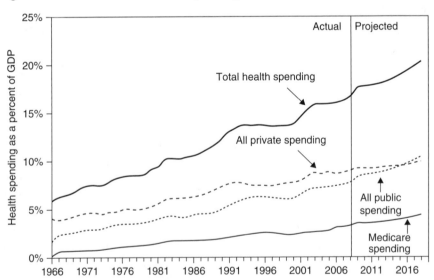

Note: GDP (gross domestic product). Total health spending is the sum of all private and public spending. Medicare spending is one component of all public spending.

Source: Medicare Payment Advisory Commission. (2009). *Healthcare spending and the Medicare program.* Retrieved February 9, 2010, from www.medpac.gov/documents/Jun09DataBookEntireReport.pdf

Figure 1.2 Bridging Costs: Coordinated Telehealth

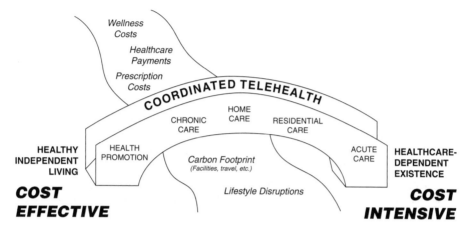

Illustration: Jin DePaul.

economics may mean bringing back "old" ideas. For example, formerly routine home visit services largely discarded as too costly, may now actually be a cost-effective solution. An examination of the relative costs associated with encounters at varying levels of healthcare (Wartena, Muskens, & Schmitt, 2009) substantiates the value of exploring new bridges. Telehealth has the potential for coordinating care by engaging all of the stakeholders in an ecosystem-aware model (Figure 1.2).

Home health care in the new millennium does not stand simply on the shoulders of people. Rather, health care at home is part of the *telehealth* vanguard as a marriage of high-tech and high-touch care; this is the focus of this chapter. First, the mess we are in is summarized and a case made for analyzing solutions in the context of the social ecology of health care and the demands for sociotechnical capital. The balance of the book examines specific domains of telecare in separate chapters: personal health records, online information, interactive devices, and games. The final chapter looks toward the future and explores the demands on health professionals in the field, researchers, and policy makers, with consequent demands for curriculum change for those in the pipeline.

The Mess We Are In

Sometimes progress requires a clear picture of the problem situation, the *mess*, from the perspective of the various stakeholders (Ackoff, 1981). Across the globe, key descriptions of contemporary healthcare challenges recur: *fragmentation of care, episodic, discontinuous, inefficiently delivered, patient role preferred over engaged consumer role.* The following have emerged across industrialized nations and developing countries. As summarized by Bashshur et al. (2009, pp. 607–608) there are seven key problems:

- Lifestyle choices and environments hostile to health promotion
- Care fragmentation: inefficient, discontinuous, episodic acute care paradigm
- Workforce structure imbalance: acute care/medical specialization vs. primary care/prevention
- Spread of chronic illness and an aging population
- Wasteful spending
- Delays in health care related to American health insurance structure
- Costs of technology imperative guided by narrow interests, not health priorities

A critical issue missing from this summary is the persistent blaming of the individual for poor lifestyle choices with inadequate attention given to analyzing and engaging social networks and environment factors as causes and resources. The consequences of these system disconnects fall particularly on those not in the American mainstream (Dentzer, 2009b).

The United States also has more people who report high out-of-pocket costs, do without care for lack of funds, and experience more medical errors than citizens of eight other industrialized countries (Shoen et al., 2008, as cited by Dentzer, 2009b). However, Shoen found healthcare delivery is still problematic in all of the industrialized countries. Unfortunately, independent of healthcare financing models, test results and records are reported as routinely missing at the time of a visit, thus requiring the duplication of tests. The implications of these problems are vast as these industrialized countries all struggle with rising rates of chronic disease. Dentzer reminds us that the World Health Organization (WHO) has declared that changes in diets, smoking, and physical inactivity could eliminate 80% of all heart disease, stroke, and type 2 diabetes worldwide. Telehealth and related tools have been showcased by the California Healthcare Foundation as promising solutions (see Sarasohn-Kahn, 2009, and other resources on the foundation's website, www.chcf.org).

Economic Boom in eHealth-Related Goods and Services

Given that older adults account for the bulk of chronic illnesses, which are extremely expensive to treat, the implications for this new worldwide "silver economy" are vast (eHealthNews.eu, 2008). Tracking data and building interventions for those at risk for chronic illness and those struggling to live well with a chronic illness will generate new careers and jobs in the production sector. Countries in the European Union believe they will have an advantage in this new market. Nistelrooij concludes Europe has moved further to implement systems and produce products that are well accepted for the growing market specific to older adults and their health. European developments can be tracked at www.eHealthNews.eu. This portal is available as an e-mail subscription and RSS feed, among other methods. Readers will note that General Electric (GE) and other American companies are actively engaged in the European market.

Putting the Consumer First: Moving to eHealth

In the eHealth paradigm, Baur and Kanaan (2006) suggested that eHealth is the "phenomenon in which consumer engagement, decision making, and tools come together to support and enhance health" (Tang & Lansky, 2005, as cited in Baur & Kanaan, 2006, p. 1). The intersection of information and communication technologies to enhance health care or improve health is tied to personal health management (Baur & Kanaan, 2006). Increasingly, this eHealth intersection involves both the Internet and an ever-increasing parade of digital devices that facilitate the connection as well as innovative software that adds structure to the information flow.

In this model, the eHealth people are the well, the newly diagnosed, and those with chronic conditions, as depicted in Figure 1.3. The needs and interests of eHealth people are highly valuable. In a truly eHealth model, thinking about living well with chronic conditions would replace treating chronic illness and include social networks. As the globe moves to a time when many people are living longer with one or more chronic conditions, our shared goal can be living well with whatever level of health challenges are confronting the consumer and his or her family and communities. The social context is important to all eHealth people, not just those with chronic challenges.

As Dentzer (2009a) concludes "It's the delivery system, stupid (p. 1216)." This creates conditions ripe for eHealth. Resurrecting Ackoff's design model (1981) might be very timely. Based on his experience, a *mess* is a system of problems that cannot be successfully fractured into parts. Dissolving the mess requires bringing in the range of stakeholders who experience the mess in different ways. Attention to both the technical and social sides of the system is deemed critical. Strategies and tools for stakeholders will be described in separate chapters. The final chapter will revisit the challenges as a whole in terms of issues and solutions.

Figure 1.3   Who Are the eHealth People?

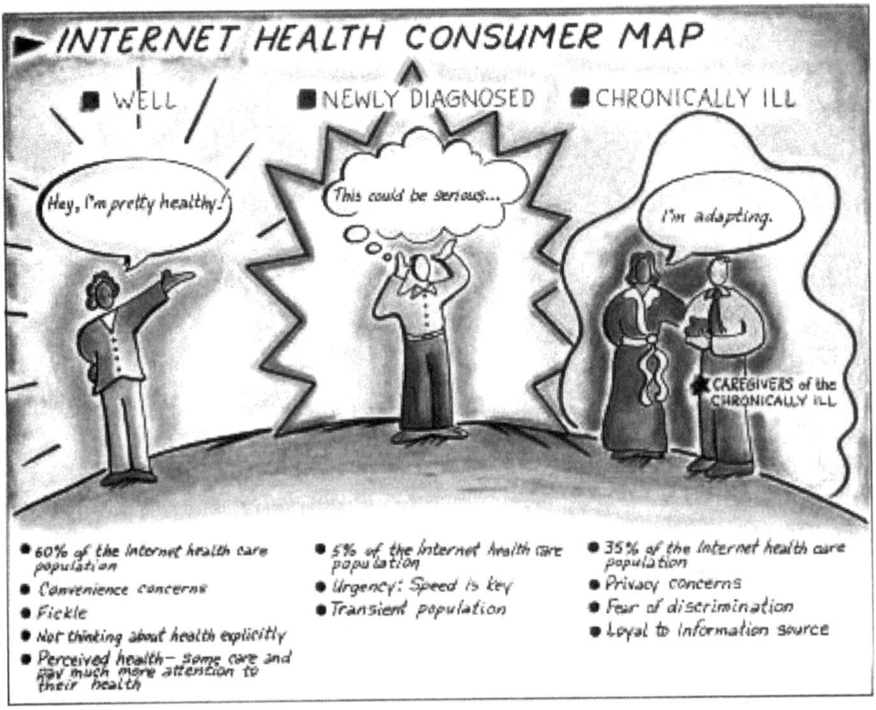

Source: Institute for the Future, 2000; artwork by The Grove Consultants International. Used with permission.

HEALTH TECHNOLOGY: THE PROMISE OF TELEHEALTH

Telehealth has been advocated as a means of improving the quality of care, creating better access for the underserved, and reducing costs (Doty, n.d.). In this book, a case is made for telehealth as a label for delivery of health technology to consumers. Table 1.1 presents types of telehealth, varieties of applications, and potential locations. This health technology approach covers a wide variety of resources for building health capital. It is also the aspect of health technology engaging consumers that has the most significant ecological impact—whether the focus is on the physical or social environment. An ecological perspective is also useful for implementing and evaluating the impact of telehealth. The case will be made in a subsequent section of this chapter.

Telehealth is not restricted by geography or provider availability. Telehealth includes social alarms, monitoring of vital signs, and daily life activity that might

Table 1.1   Types, Applications, and Uses of Telehealth: Examples

Types of Telehealth

- Telecare
- Teledermatology
- Teleradiology
- Telenursing
- Telepsychiatry
- Teledental
- Teleophthalmology
- Teleeducation (continuing education)

Types of Telehealth Applications

- Live videoconferencing
- Store-and-forward systems
- Remote patient monitoring
- E-visits and e-consultations
- Social media Health 2.0
- Telerobotics

Locations of Telehealth Practice

- Rural, remote, frontier
- Urban
- Military: Battlefield, ships
- Emergency responders
- Bioterrorism
- Ship-to-shore: Cruise ships, tankers
- Schools
- Extreme locations: Antarctic, space, underwater
- Prisons
- Hospitals

Sources: Adapted from Doty, n.d., and http://www.telehealthlawcenter.org/content/?page=18.

be linked to family or community members. Telehealth can embrace both live videoconferencing (synchronous contact) and the store-and-forward process (asynchronous engagement). Portals for patients are included. (A portal acts as an online open door with one-click access to a wide range of digital resources organized by a telecare or telehealth provider). In a telehealth arrangement, transmission of still images, remote monitoring of vital signs, and behaviors and normal life patterns all occur as needed. Call centers are also included (Johnston & Solomon, 2008).

Health management occurs in a highly mobile context for individuals with tight but geographically spread social networks. Those who are geographically and socially isolated face different "mobility" challenges. Telehealth has the potential to meet these demands. Ultimately, telehealth will flourish because adults with means to pay are busy people. The "overemployed" have to juggle personal health and needs of children and older adults, chronic illness, and a determination to promote aging in place. An evocative scenario of an intergenerational connection is provided by Mahoney (Figure 1.4). Mahoney is a gerontological nurse practitioner who has conducted multiple studies of telehealth: for working adults (Mahoney, Mutschler, Tarlow, & Liss, 2008) and adults living in independent senior housing (Mahoney, Mahoney, & Liss, 2009). Details of smart homes that are connected for telecare are described in Chapter 5.

The challenge is to definitively establish that telehealth applications are cost-effective and a good return on investment for tax payers and venture capitalists.

Figure 1.4   Everyday Telehealth Intergenerational Scenario

Ms. Stressed will turn on her unit at home as she leaves the house for work. At 10 am she will check at home to determine if Dad is up and has finished his breakfast. On the first screen she is assured by seeing the green light indicating everything she requested to be monitored is showing that those activities have occurred. She decides to pursue further and double-clicks on the screen and proceeds to the next level where she can view the activities individually. She sees that the sensor feedback reports that Dad arose at 8:30, dressed by 9, and ate his breakfast by 9:30. He is due to take 10 am medications and she watches while that turns green and is checked off. If he had not taken them by 11, she would have been notified via an e-mail notice. She exits this system and decides to get some help on how to manage Dad by sending a message to others on the Intranet e-mail support group as well as from the triage staff member at the Alzheimer's Association who is linked via her desktop system. At noon she will remotely check that he ate the sandwich she left for him. He has, and she is greatly relieved. At 2 pm she receives a call from the homemaker saying her father is not answering the door to let her in and something may be wrong. Ms. Stressed remotely checks in and sees indications of normal activity. She tells the aide she should go to the rear door and knock loudly. Ms. Stressed then checks the home sensor screen to see Dad's movements indicating that he has opened the door. One last check before she leaves work lets her know that Dad is settled and can comfortably wait until she does some errands on the way home. She comes home knowing that all is well in marked contrast to her colleague's caregiving experience. Without telecare, her colleague had to leave work several times each week to check on her mother's activities and safety.

Source: Scenario supplied by Diane Mahoney. For a report of the associated research, see: Mahoney, D. M., Mutschler, P. H., Tarlow, B., & Liss, E. (2008). Real world implementation lessons and outcomes from the worker interactive networking (WIN) project: Workplace-based online caregiver support and remote monitoring of elders at home. *Telemedicine Journal and e-Health: The Official Journal of the American Telemedicine Association, 14*(3), 224–234. doi:10.1089/tmj.2007.0046.

Otherwise, the risk is that only the rich can afford this technology. Evidence of success and the case for widening socioecological benefits is presented after explaining the basics of telehealth.

The Tangle of Terminology: *Telemedicine* to *Telehealth*

Telemedicine is a widely used term for digital resources for consumer engagement in health-related activities. Initially, some experts maintain, *telemedicine* meant that data gleaned from patients in remote locations was being reviewed by a physician. Such an engagement was either in real time or the information was stored and forwarded for review at a time convenient to the physician. Increasingly, digitally obtained data is being monitored by nurses or specially trained triage agents (Doughty et al., 2007). Digital connections are also used by patients without direct connection to a healthcare professional for monitoring their own data, learning and practicing new behaviors, and social networking around health issues. Advances in mobile phone technology make these systems even more attractive. The advantage is that a space-hungry computer workstation with broadband access is not required.

Telemedicine, as a historical term for connected health, is being complemented by *telehealth* and *telecare* and *telehealthcare* (Bashshur et al., 2009; Doughty et al., 2007; Scott, 2009; Scott et al., 2007). However, there is no apparent consensus on the choice of term at the national or international level (Martin, Kelly, Kernohan, McCreight, & Nugent, 2008). An excellent attempt at sorting out the confusions about terminology comes from the Centre for Usable Home technologies (CUHTec) Advanced Telecare Users group (Doughty et al., 2007). It proposes that we begin sorting out the discrepancies by using *telehealth* as the umbrella term. "Everyone needs their health but not everyone needs care" (Doughty et al., 2007, p. 10).

If we adopt this view, telehealth would be applications of universal potential, not tied to impairments and healthcare professionals but rather to choice. This definition would link nicely to connectivity that uses personal health records. In many instances, the connectivity goal would be pursuing health promotion or illness prevention as well as connecting for self-managed chronic conditions or to sustain an older adult living at home. This health-based application would be the contrast between having *telehealth*—a "technology that we want as part of 21st-century living and technology [*telecare*] that we need in order to maximize our quality of life and well-being" (Doughty et al., 2007, p. 10).

Telemedicine may be reserved as a name for remote monitoring or assessment that must engage a physician for reimbursement purposes. This application may be especially important in rural or urban areas where consumers are isolated from specialists, in particular by mobility and geography. Physician oversight of care for consumers in senior housing or assisted living could move to "just-in-time" care based on telecare data and consumer needs as compared to routine visits based on rigid schedules. For consumers, it is only important to appreciate that some articles and discussions of *telehealth* continue to use the term *telemedicine*, even though the application does not require real-time engagement of a physician or healthcare professional. Also, some authors will use *telecare* without attention to the independence of the consumer or engagement of the healthcare provider. With consumers in mind, the term *connected health* (see Kibbe & Kvedar, 2008) may be the most evocative and most likely to be widely adopted.

History of Telehealth

Telehealth has greatly expanded as a field of study and practice since its inception. There are varying dates in the literature. McCarty and Clancy (2002) date the first reference to telemedicine as 1948 for radiology, the 1950s for social work, and the 1970s for interactive video therapy during federally funded interactive video experiments. Others state that telemedicine began in 1959, and note the proliferation of real-time telemedicine began in the1990s (Grigsby & Sanders, 1998; Grigsby & Bennett, 2006). Certainly, the Department of Veterans Affairs health system gave telehealth a major boost by trying and developing equipment, electronic health records, and home monitoring with its vast patient group. Arnst (2006) credited these efforts as transforming the system in a comprehensive article in *Business Week* that described the potential of telehealth to whole new audiences.

Telemedicine is not a separate medical specialty. Products and services related to telemedicine are often part of a larger investment by healthcare institutions in either information technology or the delivery of clinical care. Even in the reimbursement fee structure, there is usually no distinction made between services provided on site and those provided through telemedicine, and often no separate coding is required for billing of remote services. (See *telemedicine* defined at http://www.americantelemed.org/i4a/pages/index.cfm?pageid=3333.)

Federal and commercial telehealth centers are emerging (see Table 1.2). In 2006, a process was initiated that led to the designation of six federally funded telehealth centers, one national and five regional. They each provide extensive resources and are supported by a combination of federal and nongovernmental funds. The national center focuses on addressing legal and regulatory barriers to telehealth implementation. The five other centers focus on advancing the implementation of telehealth in specific regions and communities. Every center's resources are available on each of the center's websites, and there is considerable collaboration. The Telehealth Resource Centers are supported through the Telehealth Resource Center Grant Program, which is administered by the Office for the Advancement of Telehealth in the Office of Health Information

Table 1.2   Website Resources for Telehealth

GOVERNMENTAL

The National Telehealth Resource Center (NTRC)

Funded by the Office for the Advancement of Telehealth at the Health and Resource Administration in the US Department of Health and Human Services, NTRC's mission is to advise, educate, and inform telehealth stakeholders and interested parties in the legal and regulatory issues facing telehealth. NTRC offers focused support for HRSA grantees. There are six regional centers accessible from this site as listed under their Resources Web page.

http://www.telehealthlawcenter.org

NOT FOR PROFIT

iHealthBeat

Free, daily news digest reporting on technology's impact on health care. *iHealthBeat* is part of the California HealthCare Foundation's commitment to important issues affecting healthcare policy, delivery, and financing.

http://www.ihealthbeat.org

California Healthcare Foundation Telehealth Reports and Initiatives

This nonprofit site provides news of telecare funding, research, and clinical applications across the United States. White papers on related topics are available without cost as PDFs.

http://www.chcf.org/topics/index.cfm?topic=CL707

Center for Connected Health

Center for Connected Health uses technology to deliver patient care beyond the boundaries of the hospital or doctor's office. It also promotes telehealth, remote care, and disease management initiatives. Founded by Harvard Medical School-affiliated teaching hospitals, it is a division of Partners Health Care. The center organizes an annual conference, posts relevant news, invites blogs, and advocates for telehealth.

http://www.connected-health.org

Telecare Aware

Telecare Aware provides a free news service to people interested in telecare and telehealth. It offers information about technology, products, equipment, and services aimed at helping older adults and those with disabilities retain their independence. It helps service providers and suppliers around the world keep up to date and stay in contact with each other.

http://www.telecareaware.com

Center for Aging Services Technology (CAST)

The Center for Aging Services Technology is a coalition of more than 400 technology companies, aging-services organizations, businesses, research universities, and

(continues)

Table 1.2   Website Resources for Telehealth (*continued*)

government representatives under the American Association of Homes and Services for the Aging (www.aahsa.org). It helps provide at-home services when people are in need. CAST also offers a clearinghouse designed for people to learn about new products and research in aging services technologies.

http://www.agingtech.org

CONSULTING LINKS

Continua Health Alliance

This collaboration of over 200 healthcare and technology companies focuses on chronic disease management, aging independently, and health and wellness. Assistance includes tools such as appointment scheduling, medical reminders, and consultations via e-mail or videoconferencing. The lowest level of membership is $5000, but there are publicly available resources.

http://www.continuaalliance.org

Telemedicine.com

This website is a resource for telemedicine consulting, which allows doctors to consult with patients remotely. Telemedicine.com assists with equipment installation, training, and support, and provides services such as grant writing and site assessments.

http://www.telemedicine.com

Technology, Health Resources and Services Administration, as noted on the national website.

American Telemedicine Association (ATA), an interdisciplinary professional organization, has emerged to increase innovation, improve research, and provide opportunities for collaboration. The ATA, for example, advises members about the availability of funding for telehealth applications. They note the American Recovery and Reinvestment Act. This new funding for telehealth is available through the Office of the National Coordinator for Health Information Technology (ONC), National Institutes of Health, the Health Resources and Services Administration (HRSA), US Department of Agriculture (USDA), the Department of Commerce through the National Telecommunications and Information Administration (NTIA) and the National Institute for Standards and Technology (NIST), and the Agency for Healthcare Research and Quality (AHRQ), to name just a few agencies (Rheuban, 2009).

One recently funded project is an excellent example of a creative collaboration among agencies with different consumer priorities and university centers and massive commercial entities. The partners include the Dartmouth

Institute for Security, Technology, and Society; the Dartmouth-Hitchcock Medical Center; the VA Medical Center in White River Junction, Vermont; the Dartmouth Institute for Health Policy and Clinical Practice; Google; and Intel (*Trustworthy information systems for healthcare*, 2009).

Consensus on the Benefits and Readiness of Consumers and Providers

Telehealth has four main uses: clinical, administrative, for research, and as an educational venue for patients and staff. (Center for Telehealth and e-Health Law, 2009). The clinical and educational uses are the focus of this book. Clinical services include functional support for activities of daily living; alerts and alarms where safety, security, health, or well-being are at risk; monitoring; ongoing assessment so interventions can be offered before an emergency arises; and interactive and virtual services (Doughty et al., 2007).

A well-designed telehealth program has the potential to:

- Prevent unnecessary delays in receiving treatment.
- Reduce or eliminate travel expenses.
- Reduce or eliminate the separation of families during difficult and emotional times.
- Use the services of healthcare providers in locales where the supply of physicians may be inadequate or at a surplus.
- Allow patients to spend less time in waiting rooms.
- Promote the ability to sustain living in the community rather than a residential care facility.
- Engage consumers as informed eHealth partners (Center for Telehealth and e-Health Law, 2009).

ECOSYSTEM AND SOCIOECOLOGICAL FRAMEWORK

Dissolving the mess that health care has become will require a framework that encourages taking a big perspective. Many discussions of new paradigms for improved, cost-effective quality of care are tagged with the *ecosystem* label. In a recent monograph the California HealthCare Foundation (CHCF) suggested that "telehealth alters the ecosystem" (Doty, n.d.). The "ecosystem" construct is pervasive (Adams, Grundy, Kohn, & Mounib, n.d., Carroll, Cnossen, Schnell, & Simons, 2007; IOM, 2009). Unfortunately the use of the ecosystem label in the CHCF monograph is typical in that the construct is evoked, but not defined, nor explicitly applied. Ecosystem in health has not been systematically tied to the health habitat with its social and larger environmental components (Jordan-Marsh, 2008). A habitat is where people find resources needed to survive and thrive in a difficult world. The human habitat has multiple settings for work, play, recreation, and getting expert help. Embracing an ecological focus means taking into account the social norms and networks as well as physical structures of geography and buildings and the forces of nature and industry.

Socioecology as a Frame for Promoting Telehealth

To set the stage for this discussion, an overview of socioecology theory as it applies to health is presented. First, an ecological perspective emphasizes how everything is connected to everything else (Hames, 2007). Secondly, Hofmeyer and Marck (2008) argue that "today's healthcare environments are vulnerable systems in urgent need of system ecological repairs" (p. 145). These vulnerabilities affect morbidity and mortality, workforce retention, and relationships among stakeholders. The healthcare system cannot be experienced independent of the connected social aspects and the local and larger political context. The final chapter provides a more detailed analysis of the relevance to telehealth.

Almost 10 years ago, the IOM (2000) commissioned an interdisciplinary committee to summarize the state of the art with respect to intervention strategies to promote health. The committee found "an emerging consensus" that future research and intervention should be designed in the context of an ecological model (p. 2). This was summarized as a model explained by Satariano where

> differences in levels of health and well-being are affected by a dynamic interaction between biology, behavior, and the environment, an interaction that unfolds over the life course of individuals families and communities. (p. 2)

The implications were that social and familial interactions, environmental contingencies, and persistent political, social, and economic trends balanced and challenged biological and genetic factors in shaping health and healthcare systems. The committee noted that direct and indirect influences on risks and resources (capital) included age, gender, race, ethnicity, and socioeconomic differences that should be taken into account in analyzing current conditions and planning for innovations. Health professionals have been making the case that consumer and patient relationships are a core part of the health ecosystem. In a health ecosystem, "actions, reactions, and coactions" between the healthcare providers, the healthcare client, social networks, and the environment per se become important pieces of the assessment and intervention model (Laustsen, 2006, p. 45). Consistency in messages among the members of the healthcare team about the value and limitations of telehealth are powerful in achieving successful implementation. Some strategies for fostering implementation at the provider level are discussed in the final chapter.

Habitat as Ecological Tipping Point

In the course of organizing the many frayed threads of American health care, physicians have proposed "medical homes" (Backer, 2007; Deloitte Center for Health Solutions, 2008; Soubhi, 2007). These arrangements are often organized specifically to increase the profile of the patient, nurse, and social worker on the care team—despite the "medical" label. A health habitat (Jordan-Marsh, 2008) may be a construct more apropos of the emerging patient-empowered paradigm than *medical home*. A habitat is an arrangement where conditions are good for various species to thrive surrounded by an often hostile environment. Within this arrangement, those who thrive (the *thrivers*) move from place to place. Habitat is a more encompassing model than a home. We come back to a home to live our lives, but we move about our habitat gaining the resources we need and enjoying social interaction.

If the problem is "the delivery, stupid" (Dentzer, 2009a, p. 1216), then designing systems that no longer persist in fragmenting consumer's lives could be powerful. Today's patients, clients, customers, and consumers flourish in a care model that recognizes the various settings individuals, families, and communities navigate—well beyond their "home." There is an ecological focus tied to habitat that could move policies forward to shift healthcare systems out of the fragmented medical model. An ecological perspective requires intense focus on the social environment in conjunction with physical environmental influences on health and health behaviors as well as persistent attention to local, regional, national, and global policies and politics.

Models for independence would be greatly strengthened by organizing around a *health habitat* (Jordan-Marsh, 2008). As described earlier in the chapter, in this orientation, the niche occupied by the patient, his or her physical environment, and his or her social network is seen as both opportunity and challenge in a connected, dynamic relationship. The various landscapes in the patient life path would be pivotal—home, work or school, church, social groups, shopping, and recreation as well as the healthcare geographical settings (clinic, hospital). The geography experienced by consumers and health professionals is a composite of architecture, traffic patterns, forces of nature, and the impact of industries and their by-products (e.g., pollution). Patients, providers, and social network members would collaborate to maximize available capital and join forces against a competitive and sometimes hostile world (Laustsen, 2006; Soubhi, 2007). The goal of community-based, patient-centered, ecologically designed programs is to move people from *struggling,* past *surviving* to *thriving.* Kaiser Permanente captures this spirit in its Thrive campaign. We cannot rely on systems to equilibrate and settle in the healthy direction when our observations show that ignoring interconnectedness has led to the mess we are in (Ackoff, 1981).

Telehealth Stakeholder Mapping: Who Can Play?

The range of consumers who can benefit from health resources on the Internet crosses the continuum of health and illness. Figure 1.5 provides an overview of how the Internet supports care, commerce, community, and content for the well, recently diagnosed, and the chronically ill and their caregivers. In this model drawn in 2000, telehealth monitoring and interaction about personal data is not yet highlighted as a resource for health and wellness activities for individuals and families. Newly emerging, low-cost devices, described in Chapter 6, and serious games for health, described in Chapter 5, have opened new opportunities for adults and children of all ages and health goals. Future iterations could add a whole column for telecare that complements declines in ability and mobility for older adults and those coping with disabilities, and perhaps a separate column for those in transition across what Coleman (2005) describes as the continuum of care.

Figure 1.5   Internet Healthcare Consumers: Sorting the Resources

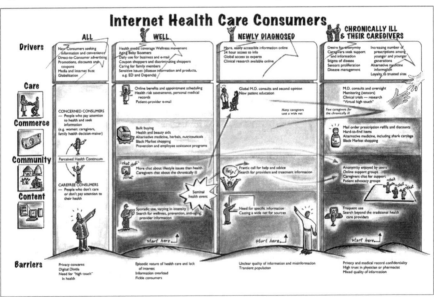

Source: Institute for the Future, 2000; artwork by The Grove Consultants International. Used with permission.

Roles and Benefits for Everybody: Stakeholder Inventory

In the digital era of telehealth, the players are not necessarily new, but their roles and centrality have changed (see Table 1.3). As discussed earlier, the patient and family are increasingly expected to take on more responsibility for their own health and care. The patient and family role in decision making is more formally acknowledged, and greater participation is expected. Sometimes the choice comes after a patient maneuvers his or her healthcare provider to decide or the patient submits to provider pressure for a particular course of action. Patients always have the last word. They react, go along, or go their own way.

Table 1.3   Benefits of Coordinated Care by Stakeholder

Stakeholder	Benefits Sought from Consumer eHealth
Consumers (e.g., patients, informal caregivers, information intermediaries)	• Private, 24/7 access to resources • Expanded choice and autonomy • New forms of social support • Possibility of better health • More efficient record management • Lower-cost healthcare services • Avoidance of duplication of services
Consumer advocacy and voluntary health organizations (e.g., AARP, American Cancer Society)	• Greater capacity for health management and education for constituents • New communication channels • More efficient service to constituents
Employers, healthcare purchasers, and third-party payers	• Healthier employees more capable of health management • Lower healthcare costs
Community-based organizations	• Constituents with greater capacity for health management and well-being • Healthier communities • Lower-cost healthcare services
Clinicians	• Greater efficiency • Better communication • More adherent and satisfied patients

(continues)

Table 1.3   Benefits of Coordinated Care by Stakeholder (*continued*)

Stakeholder	Benefits Sought from Consumer eHealth
Healthcare organizations	• More patient self-care and health management • Lower administrative costs • Improved quality and patient outcomes
Public health programs	• A healthier population more capable of self-care and less at risk for avoidable disease and trauma
eHealth developers	• Sustained use of eHealth products • New sources of support for product development and evaluation
Industry and commerce	• New advertising vehicles • Wider markets for products • Investment opportunities
Policy makers and funders (public and private)	• Effective means of implementing programs and policies • Cost-containment or cost-reduction strategies • Quality improvement strategies

Source: Adapted from Baur & Kanaan, 2006, p. 69.

Telecare and Interdisciplinary Collaboration

New constellations of professional and patient relationships are required to carry out the emerging models of telecare that are grounded in the habitat of the consumer (Jordan-Marsh, 2008). The Independence at Home Act of 2009 is a special opportunity for nurses to reinvigorate the insights of Florence Nightingale about the ecosystem. New policies and resources are possible to support known and new models to organize care. Patients and families, nurses, social workers and other specialists are empowered in new ways in these models:

• Chronic Care Model of Wagner (Wielawski, 2006)
• Care Coordination and Home Telehealth Model: VHA (Darkins et al., 2008)
• Home Based Chronic Care Model (Suter et al., 2008)
• Transitional Care Model of Naylor and colleagues (Health Workforce Solutions & Robert Wood Johnson Foundation, 2008)

- Care Transitions Intervention Model (Coleman, 2005)
- Geriatric Resources for Assessment and Care of Elders GRACE (AHRQ Innovations Exchange, 2009)
- Center for Connected Health (Kibbe & Kvedar, 2008)
- Health Guide and Quiet Care (Intel, 2009)

Attention is given to transitions, particularly in the Care Transitions Intervention Model (Coleman, 2005; and see Scott, 2009). However, current transition discussions rarely integrate the work of William Bridges (Bridges, 2003), which enriched the interdisciplinary, patient-centered model adopted by Harbor-UCLA Medical Center in their Robert Wood Johnson-funded project for systemwide change (Jordan-Marsh, Goldsmith, Siler, Sanchez, & Nazarey, 1997). Meleis has also integrated the concept of transitions in her model of nursing care building on the work of Bridges (Meleis, Sawyer, Im, Hilfinger Messias, & Schumacher, 2000). A *transition* is an intersection of opportunity and capital where potential for influence is highest in shaping decisions.

Provider-Independent eHealth Tools

Telehealth is supported by a wide range of tools that consumers can use without direct interaction with healthcare providers (Table 1.4). Baur and Kanaan (2006) did the first comprehensive overview of tools to engage consumers in eHealth. This monograph, "Expanding the reach and impact of consumer eHealth tools" is available in PDF form for free at http://www.health.gov/communication/ehealth/ehealthtools/default.htm. This report provides extensive detail about eHealth tools available as of 2006. Therefore, only a brief overview is provided here.

Table 1.4 Functions of Provider-Independent eHealth Tools

- Health information
- Behavior change
- Behavior rehearsal (games)
- Vicarious experiences: Online videos
- Decision support
- Social and emotional support
- Disease management
- Risk assessment
- Personal health data entry
- Personal health record
- Family or friend care sharing
- Care plan development
- Secure patient–provider communication

Source: Adapted from Baur & Kanaan, 2006.

Tools specific to health information, behavior change, decision support, disease management, and risk assessment are also covered in the chapter on health information. In that chapter, social support and networking are also discussed. There is a separate chapter on personal health data entry and personal health records and a detailed chapter on games as an eHealth tool for behavior rehearsal, stress management, and socioemotional support. A number of interactive computer applications have been developed to assist consumers develop new habits for health promotion or new behaviors related to self-care management (Murray, Burns, See Tai, Lai, & Nazareth, 2004). New applications are emerging to assist families to communicate around illness, such as Caring Bridge, a website where the family contact person or the patient can post updates, and everyone can leave heartening messages for the patient and the family. The resource is free.

Another health information tool that has become more extensively available is the online video. Painter (2007) describes availability on such credible sites as Mayo Clinic, WebMD, and American Cancer Society. YouTube has its own burgeoning catalog of health videos with and without credentials. YouTube and personal Web pages give consumers the opportunity to post videos they created based on their own health journeys and healthcare system experiences. Secure patient–provider communication is included in the list as it refers to links initiated by the consumer. Examples could include e-mails, Twitter, and instant messaging. These digital links are controversial in terms of confidentiality and burden on the healthcare provider in terms of time demands and liability. In general, consumers will benefit most from, and seem to prefer, a looped system where there is engagement and feedback with their healthcare team (Sarasohn-Kahn, 2009).

An additional application, thought to be the first of its kind, is an interactive care plan for cancer survivors (Hill-Kayser, Vachani, Hampshire, Jacobs, & Metz, 2009). The tool provides comprehensive information on diagnosis, treatments, prospects, and resources tailored to the needs of the inquirer. The care plan has been accessed by over 3000 consumers including survivors, health professionals, and friends or family members. The care plan applications are different than social support and information sites, such as ConnectingforCare, produced by the National Family Caregiver Association and sponsored by Intel.

Limited eHealth Research with Gender and Ethnically Diverse Groups

As with other Internet tools, most users of the interactive care plan were educated white women. A successful program engaging men who were naïve to Internet use has been reported by Watson, Bell, Kvedar, and Grant (2008). There is limited data on differences among cultural groups in using health programs (see Chapter 3).

TELEHEALTH APPLICATIONS: LEVELS OF SOCIOECOLOGICAL INFLUENCE

Environmental Level: Carbon Footprint

Telehealth has also been touted as advancing environmental goals by reducing car trips and the need for parking spaces at health facilities. Telehealth can provide savings in dedicated physical space for clinics and hospital beds. However, most current facilities are not configured for a telehealth setup. This problem exists for the healthcare agency and for consumers. The equipment does have installation and maintenance costs for both healthcare provider and the consumer. Accommodating telehealth may require giving up resources traditionally provided in clinics and hospitals.

Reducing the Carbon Footprint: Mouse Calls and Prison Telehealth

Online consultations, virtual office visits, or *mouse calls* are emerging as an option that may cut office visits by up to 10%, save 1.2% in employer-sponsored health plans, and free up time for more complex phone calls (Lowes, n.d.). Some electronic health records offer a patient portal. Practices can choose to use ordinary e-mail, which is free to the physician, or use a service that encrypts the message and forces patients to use a structured interview. Some systems provide a free text box as well. Other options that Lowes summarizes include a fee-for-service plan or a subscription plan. Three major health plans have adopted Relay-Health webVisits system (Cigna, Aetna, Blue Cross) (Lauer, 2008). These consultations do not violate the Health Insurance Portability and Accountability Act (HIPAA), Lowes asserts. There are concerns about malpractice issues and complaints that not all patients are trustworthy.

No references to the term *mouse calls* were found by other members of the healthcare team. However, Lowes (n.d.) suggests that this e-mail-based interaction is a complement to the *medical home* concept of coordinating care. In this case, nurses and social workers are likely to become triage agents as they are increasingly drawn in to formal coordinator roles in the medical home and other coordinated care interventions. The technology exists to allow certain terms or tags to signal which team member should be the first to review an e-mail. Over time, patients can learn to use the tags themselves.

If group visits become available (Clancy, Yeager, Huang, & Magruder, 2007), it might be that e-mails could be routed to the patient group with attention to confidentiality. In all cases, transparency is critical. Patients and their family members need to be aware of the limitations and risks when they sign up to use such a system, and they need to be reminded at intervals. Healthcare e-mails from a clinical practice are likely to contain a standard warning and reminder of risks

Table 1.5   Everyday Experience of Mouse Calls, the Online Consultation

- Select an e-mail address that is not work related nor shared with others.
- Discuss with your healthcare provider who will have access to your e-mails: Are they routinely reviewed by the entire team?
- Never use e-mail for urgent clinical symptoms such as chest pain or bleeding.
- Assume the provider is keeping a copy, and create your own files in a secure backup location.
- Establish a turnaround time so you know when to check on receipt.
- Consider using receipt notification on your e-mail system—it is easy to think you sent an e-mail when it is sitting on your system.
- If the provider uses a system with a structured interview, be prepared to complete all the relevant sections.
- If the e-mail is not encrypted, be cautious of the content you provide.
- Do not share passwords; do not use a password that is easily guessed.
- Avoid creating a file of passwords on your PDA, cell phone, or laptop.
- If the provider makes a recommendation that is not acceptable or not possible, advise them promptly as the e-mail of record states "patient was advised...."
- Be judicious in sending e-mails, and avoid flooding the service.
- Obtain information in writing about the charges incurred for using e-mail services.
- Recall that e-mails in this system become part of your record.
- Establish the time frame and days of week when e-mails are reviewed.

and limitations. However, it is important to build in creative ways to alert correspondents on an irregular basis as routine warnings are ignored over time. Providers and clients must agree on ground rules for having online consultations (Table 1.5).

Telehealth used at prisons reduces the need for prisoners and prison staff to travel. Remote care at the prison site minimizes escape opportunities and reduces costs of vehicles, fuel, escorts, and special accommodations at the clinical site (Johnston & Solomon, 2008). Telehealth increases the option for specialized, quality care for prisoners.

Social Fabric Influences: Family, Community, Workforce, and Workplace

Social capital is a key aspect of assessing health risks and resources. Social capital is the capacity to experience reinforcement or enforcement of group or social norms for positive health behaviors—the provision of tangible support (Kim, Subramanian, & Kawachi, 2008). There is some evidence from reviews of the literature that social capital may be especially salient for the health of residents in "highly unequal and segregated societies such as the United States" (Kim et al.,

2008, p. 183). Healthcare providers can assess the availability of social support for health in existing environments or in the habitat of the consumer. Some social capital may be accessed directly in the geographic neighborhood, some by telephone, and, increasingly, through social media provided by the Internet.

Interpersonal Level: Family

Telecare has the potential to support family relationships and other forms of social capital through convenient, no-travel access points for sharing of information. This is important for employers as travel time can be saved when employees or their family members need health services. Telehealth has tremendous potential for combating the persistent problem of *presenteeism*. This is the phenomena where employees are distracted and less engaged because of their own illness or preoccupation with life events (MacGregor, Cunningham, & Caverley, 2008). Health issues for the individual or his or her family can be significant factors. The availability of telehealth can relieve anxiety on behalf of geographically distant family members. Telehealth provides a means of monitoring family members with dependence or health issues. Telehealth can also enable a family member at work to "join" in a telemedicine consultation that his or her ill loved one is having with a healthcare provider. A pioneering study in this area is the Worker Interactive Networking (WIN) project (Mahoney et al., 2008). Workers with an elder family member at home alone during the workday were given access to an online support group and a monitoring system. This system was deployed across four states and in varying housing and business situations.

The outcomes were notable for improved worker morale and productivity and lower caregiver stress. Employers, despite initial skepticism, found no abuse of work time when participants used the system. Perhaps most propitious, workers indicated a willingness to pay for a similar service in the future. This application is particularly important because of its cost-effectiveness. Pavel, Jimison, Hayes, and Kaye (2009) describe successes and challenges of telehealth from the engineering perspective and note the risk of the technology costing more than a human caregiver. Costing should include examination of a wide range of factors. Are reliable, acceptable caregivers available—at any price? Also, family engagement is strengthened by allowing access to telehealth systems at locations and times that work around family schedules. As indicated earlier, the lowest-cost care takes place in the community and that usually requires some family investment.

Community Level: Small Community-Specific Benefits

There are potential benefits in sustaining the economy (and thus stability) of smaller communities. Kurywchak (n.d.) notes that telecare keeps dollars in the local community. He observes that routine visits by patients to care providers in large urban areas build a pattern of buying goods and services in those cities instead of local areas. However, he reports, from evaluations of telecare, that the close-knit nature of a small community can inhibit patients from seeking care for potentially embarrassing conditions and from fully sharing details. The fear is that others will see you visiting the psychiatrist or other specialist. A corresponding barrier is the concern over disclosing intimate details to someone you will see later in social or business settings. Telehealth sustains local purchases and promotes care seeking because it has a *zero-geography* structure; that is, location is not a restriction (Hames, 2007).

Organizational-Level Influences: Continuum of Care, Workforce, and Workplace

Organizational Level: Continuum of Care

Another key aspect of potential telehealth benefits is the unprecedented opportunity to shift from the American paradigm of episodic, reactive, regimented, acute care-centered model to an ecological paradigm that appreciates the impact of the environment on clinical health, social networks, and access to care. This paradigm has a *pangeographic* (everywhere quality) perspective that meets the clients where they live. Health care could become "proactive, preventive, and personalized" (Commission staff SEC, 2009, p. 3c). Choosing the location of care based on the personal preferences of key stakeholders, cost-effectiveness, and observed outcomes would be a major shift from the physical building-centric focus of today's financing system.

Organizational Level: Health Workforce Extension

The demands of a young family, caring for aging parents, and personal limits on physical capacities and preferences can mean priority shifts that limit availability to work. The usual demands of a health professional career can result in diminished work hours or withdrawal from the workforce. Extensive reviews of the literature for this topic failed to uncover this potential reason to promote telehealth: maximizing the potential of an aging workforce in health care. The aging of the health professional workforce is a major concern as chronic illness increases and the population ages. Some specialties will be more affected than others.

For example, the nursing workforce, in short supply to begin with, is characterized by high average age. Telehealth, with its revolutionary capacity for zero geography and free-form scheduling, may be an effective tool in keeping nurses and others in the workforce. Eliminating the need to drive (and park) and the expectation of a fixed-hour work schedule could be very appealing to older health professionals, to young professionals with family or back-to-school pressures, and to other health professionals who have become caretakers of their own parents. Another ecological benefit may accrue as telehealth provides a means of patients connecting with health professionals who migrated to other geographic locations as a consequence of the economic catastrophe of 2009. This presumes in-state connections until the conundrum of state licensure (local geography) that allows pangeographic access (encompasses all geographic locations) is resolved. Global reciprocity of licensure, however, is unlikely to occur until further revolutions in cultural competence occur and universal standards of health are accepted.

Organizational Level: Workplace and Intergenerational Challenges

Flexibility in the workplace of the boomer generation is ideally built around intergenerational social capital. Goals for telehealth and telecare include an intergenerational safety net and productivity multiplier (see Table 1.3).

Revolutions in the way workplaces conceptualize their role in health and health care have created new opportunities for simultaneously redesigning the way health care is carried out, coordinated, and evaluated. This opens opportunities for a social model of health in the workplace just as health research provides multiple examples of how social situations influence health problems.

Intrapersonal Factors: Reluctant Patients, Nurses, Social Workers, and Physicians

Some patients will simply be reluctant to participate in the new decision-making model (Fried, McGraw, Agostini, & Tinetti, 2008). Others will have problems juggling their multiple morbidities, and new provider conceptual frameworks will have to evolve. Providers must shift from symptom management, Fried and colleagues argue, to global, cross-disease, quality-of-life choices (Fried et al., 2008). Many older adults are reluctant to use a computer. However, once they are acclimated to computers, particularly to the Internet, they become enthusiastic users. A recent Pew update noted that "once they are connected, wired seniors are more likely to go online daily, with 69% of those 65 and older doing so, compared with 56% of all Internet users" (Coombes, 2003, para. 6). New generations of retirees will come to their senior years unwilling to give up their Internet access.

Some physicians have been reluctant to become engaged in telehealth due to the heavy burden of training, installation, and uncertain reimbursement. Mahoney (2009) reports some assisted living nurses have not been willing to use monitoring systems, insisting that only face-to-face contact suffices. Social work, initially cautious due to concerns about confidentiality, is increasingly embracing technology (Parrott & Madoc-Jones, 2008). Solutions to the intra- and interpersonal levels of influence are likely to emerge quickly once reimbursement and training issues are resolved. Some telehealth advocates believe implementation will accelerate as consumers demand the services.

Policy Level: Interoperability as the Ultimate Ecosystem

The American system of health care is highly proprietary with respect to devices, services, and operation systems. This has slowed development and implementation of telecare, which is an umbrella for device connectivity and services that will build and sustain a "personal healthcare ecosystem" (Carroll, Cnossen, Schnell, & Simons, 2007, p. 90). To build this system, Carroll et al. describe the establishment of a nonprofit collaboration of companies— Continua Health Alliance (www.continuaalliance.org). The ecological perspective means that the group focuses on setting standards for a certification and testing program that will meet standards in the United States and abroad for interoperability. All the pieces will work together. The complexity of the technical side of interoperability is illustrated in Figure 1.6. A sustainable telehealth system needs sensors that connect seamlessly to aggregate and compute data for interaction with services that will range from live contact with a healthcare provider to personal health record store-and-forward applications. Continuous or intermittent monitoring will be a core aspect, not only of implantable devices, but other noninvasive observations of vital signs and activity.

Figure 1.6   A Typical Personal Telehealth Ecosystem

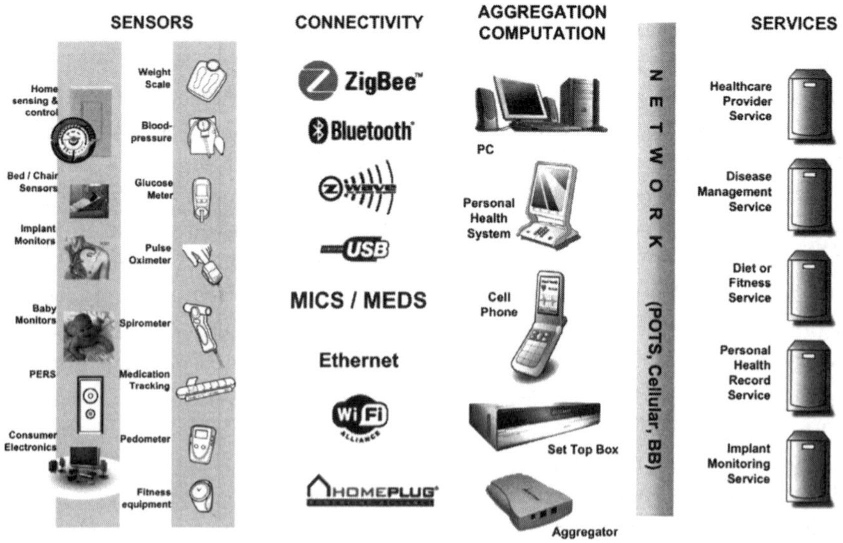

Source: Continua, 2007.

The system is ecological in the insistence that designers take into account the interlocking aspects of the devices and the services. The larger influences of the user (intrapersonal) and their social context beyond the provider is hidden in this model. It is a technical but not a socioecological view. As indicated earlier, as the US healthcare system transitions to the new paradigm, the users will often be required to assert themselves to be included in design and evaluation.

The Continua Health Alliance has invented a global community committed to interoperability enforced by setting standards and monitoring execution. Successful companies can use the Continua logo to reassure consumers. This functions similarly to the HON Code, an icon that can be displayed on a website that meets global standards for quality of health information (see Chapter 3). The technical aspects of interoperability and obtaining a Continua logo are well detailed by Carroll, Cnossen, Schnell, and Simons (2007). Such a logo could provide reassurance for healthcare entities and consumers seeking to purchase or lease a system who recognize the risk of services and technologies that cannot communicate and thus fragment care.

SOCIOTECHNICAL CAPITAL AS *THRIVAL* SKILL: BEYOND SURVIVAL

Sociotechnical Capital Collection

Assumptions relevant to telehealth implementation include the belief that sociotechnical capital is a renewable resource that drives the system (Resnick, 2001). Sociotechnical capital (STC) refers "to productive combinations of social relations and information and communication technology (Resnick, 2001, [electronic version] pp. 2–3). Kazmer (2006) summarized the key aspects. The first aspect is seen as removing barriers to interaction thus allowing engagement in places and times that otherwise would be awkward or inconvenient. STC expands one's social network through simultaneous messaging. STC allows substitute or hidden identities, thus reducing inhibitions. STC helps people structure independent and group work. STC maintains a history of interactions for shared knowledge building. Finally, STC promotes naming, which fosters development of social capital.

A related assumption is that the next decade of health and health care will be one of increasing reliance on technology to inform, support decisions, provide treatment, monitor progress and supplement social, emotional, and physical resources. Tools will range from Wikis and online support groups to interactive programs that teach and counsel for lifestyle change and mental health to smart homes and robots. Social relationships that matter will be characterized by a charisma or motivational energy. Consumers, Kazmer (2006) found, varied in their ability to disengage and to perceive relationships as dormant not disconnected after participating in an online support group. To thrive, adults of all ages will have to learn to multitask and to develop computer literacy as well as other literacies of the new millennium (see Chapter 2).

TELECARE IMPLEMENTATION: MODELS AND ROLE MODELS

Telemedicine (Barrett, 2008) uses telecommunications to provide clinical care to people at a distance. Barrett noted that there are multiple companies taking leadership in telemedicine. Her list includes ADT, Alere, Accenture Labs, Intel, Phillips, Qualcomm, RIM, General Electric (GE), and Honeywell. New groups will be moving into this area rapidly as the US economic recovery program funnels resources toward health technology. Much of the health reform literature emphasizes electronic health records. Innovative partnerships are emerging, for example, among the 200 member groups of the Continua Health Alliance and among GE, Intel, and other agencies.

Chronic Care Management Model as Springboard

Increasingly, the home is being seen as the foundation of overcoming the burden of chronic care (Darkins et al., 2008; Levey, 2009; Otellini, 2009; Suter et al., 2008). Even industry giants are concluding that we must "move beyond the centralized expert-driven medical model to distributed personal health at home" (Otellini, 2009, para. 1). Thus, across a wide range of experts, it seems home health is poised for a rebound. As Levey (2009) summarizes for the *Los Angeles Times:*

> The core idea is deceptively simple: By staying in close touch with some of their sickest patients through home visits, doctors and nurse practitioners can avoid admitting them to hospitals where costs and potential complications multiply. (p. A10)

A more apt summary is hard to imagine.

Specialists and primary care providers can collaborate with other specialists and support the chronic care manager who is on-site. This collaborative home-based paradigm is more cost-effective than the traditional requirement that forces even those patients uncomfortable with persistent symptoms and limited mobility to make their way to the physical setting of the healthcare provider.

Chronic Care Model

Many telecare applications are built around the Chronic Care Model (Wagner, 1998). The chronic care model is widely known and is the foundation for the Joint

Commission's certification for disease-specific care. The chronic care model has won an award from the National Committee for Quality Assurance, and dissemination of the model is supported by the Robert Wood Johnson Foundation. Core elements include:

- Patient safety (in the health system)
- Cultural competency (in delivery system design)
- Care coordination (in the health system and clinical information systems)
- Community policies (in community resources and policies)
- Case management (in delivery system design)

Wielawski (2006) provides an extensive discussion of the challenges of implementing the model in the community given the current reimbursement structure.

Care Coordination and Home Telehealth Models

The most extensive telehealth model in the United States is probably the Veterans Health Administration (VHA) national home telehealth program, Care Coordination/Home Telehealth (CCHT). Darkins et al. (2008) state "there is no program elsewhere in the United States of the size and complexity of VHA's national program to enable detailed comparison" (p. 1123). The model is defined by Darkins et al. (2008) as built around Wagner's Chronic Care Model and is characterized by

the use of health informatics, disease management, and home telehealth technologies to enhance and extend care and case management to facilitate access to care and improve the health of designated individuals and populations with the specific intent of providing the right care in the right place at the right time. (p. 1120)

This CCHT model is unique in that not only is a data-collection algorithm tailored to the individual, but a care coordinator has an inventory of technologies to match the veteran's needs, skills, and preferences. The range includes videophones, messaging devices, biometric devices, digital cameras, and telemonitoring devices. The messaging devices are built on disease management protocols with text-based questions for patients to answer. The Darkins et al. (2008) report does not name Health Buddy, but that device has been used by the VHA in the past. See Table 1.1 on Telecare Applications for an overview and website link. The videophones and videotelemonitors replicate face-to-face encounters through regular telephone lines. Patients at risk are prioritized every day with color-coded alerts to signal which patients need phone counseling, and which need emergency care or urgent provider assessments. Coordinators intervene to support self-management, assess biopsychosocial needs, and implement case management as appropriate. Care coordinators are reported to be predominantly social workers and nurses. However, occupational therapists, dieticians, pharmacists, and "even physicians" can lead the team. Darkins et al. (2008) provide extensive detail on variables measured. They conclude that CCHT is a "practical and cost-effective means of caring for populations of patients with chronic disease that is acceptable to both patients and clinicians" (p. 1124). Cost savings, reduced hospital admissions, and reduced bed days are significant given the demonstrated improved access and quality of care.

Home-Based Chronic Care Model

Another adaptation of the Chronic Care Model is based on a nurse home health service model. Suter and colleagues (2008) propose an adaptation to the chronic care model (as developed by Wagner, 1998). In the home-based chronic care model (HBCCM), face-to-face care is deliberately blended with telecare remote monitoring and consultations in the setting of the home.

The expanded HBCCM model is exemplary in its theory base, proactive orientation, thoughtful use of specialists, and overt link to technology. There are four major components that are highly consistent with ideal models for telecare at home: a high-touch delivery system, theory-based self-management support, specialist oversight, and technology core (Figure 1.7). Although the initial model was heavily physician oriented, the HBCCM is highly compatible with applications led by social workers or nurses. The model is notable in embedding clinical practice guidelines that can be tailored to the individual. A core feature of the model is the combination of technology with face-to-face visits.

Most visiting nurses could add to anecdotes warning that sometimes face-to-face care is critical in uncovering inexplicable clinical findings (Parchman, Romero, & Pugh, 2006). Furthermore, it may also be that initial face-to-face visits are required to establish trust, create influence, and to link data to information that can be merged with transdisciplinary expertise and client responses.

Transition-Specific Models

Transitional Care Model (TCM)

One of the earliest models to incorporate telehealth elements is associated with the work of Mary Naylor and colleagues (Health Workforce Solutions & Robert Wood Johnson Foundation, 2008). As noted on their website, the Penn research team used the Omaha system to create a web-based application that aggregated all of the assessment tools, evidence-based intervention protocols, and tracking data. This includes visits, medications, and symptoms. The TCM is particularly strong in making web-based training modules available. The case study is the framework for independent, interactive modules that promote

Figure 1.7   Home-Based Chronic Care Improvement

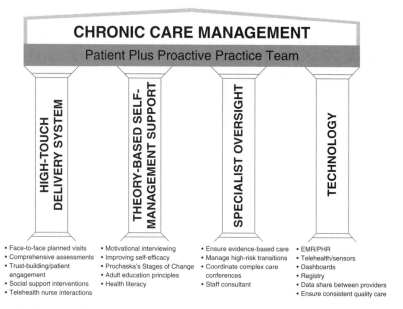

Source: Suter, Hennessey, Harrison, Norman, & Fagan, 2009.

interdisciplinary team communication. The website provides information on publications specific to this model.

Although the HBCC model does not specify attention to transitions, it is highly compatible with the care transitions interventions attributed to Naylor and colleagues (Health Workforce Solutions & Robert Wood Johnson Foundation, 2008) and those described by Coleman (2005). In these models, coaching of patients and families is seen as an activity separate from education. Coaching is a skill with specific behaviors.

Care Transitions Intervention Model

Coaching behaviors have been labeled as the "four pillars" in accomplishing transitions in care (Coleman 2005, as cited in Scott, 2009, p. 14). These are (1) attention to medication management; (2) use of a patient-centered record in which a patient can record his or her medical history, medications, and other influences; (3) timely care with a primary care physician or specialists; and (4) an understanding of "red flags" that may indicate a patient's condition is getting worse, along with how to respond. Future designs could add mobile phone technology and clothing-embedded sensors to ensure that users do not feel homebound by tethered technology.

Geriatric Resources for Assessment and Care of Elders (GRACE)

GRACE is an interdisciplinary model that features an extended interdisciplinary team led by a nurse or social worker. Details are provided at the AHRQ Innovations Exchange (2009). This model requires initial face-to-face contacts with patients and a consulting visit with the primary care provider (PCP) for the care coordinator. Individualized care plans based on protocols are developed in coordination with the PCP. Incorporation of primary care, mental health, and transition management are core components. The model uses a common electronic medical record and a longitudinal tracking system. The model explicitly follows patients across providers, conditions, and sites of care. Sensor-collected data is not described as a feature, and patient engagement in planning must be assumed, as it is not a highlight. A randomized controlled trial demonstrated that evidence-based care was delivered and emergency department visits curtailed, significant improvements in health-related quality of life were noted, and levels of satisfaction were high for physicians and patients.

Center for Connected Health

The Center for Connected Health is a collaboration of the Harvard Medical School affiliated hospitals (see Table 1.2 for website). The center provides direct patient care linked to technology. The center also provides a wide range of resources to promote dialogue, including blogs, publications, and an annual conference. This group is notable for its translational research model with consistent peer-reviewed publication of outcomes of their telehealth programs. The website notes six typical publications: three are specific to the management of diabetes, and there is one each on exercise adherence, acne, and heart failure. A recent innovation is the Smart Beat program for work sites. This could have an advantage over other disease-management options. Its technology provides real-time data, which minimizes reporting errors caused by social desirability or attention seeking. Kibbe and Kvedar (2008) provide a framework for designing a connected medical home (Table 1.6). Note the sensor and social-interaction components listed in the table. (See also the *medical home* concept [Adams et al., n.d.].)

Intel and GE Collaboration for Health Guide and Quiet Care

Two new healthcare delivery products will soon be available as telehealth and telecare models (Intel, 2009). Intel's Dishman has written extensively on new models for care. One of his early reports was an overview of the challenges of

Table 1.6   Connected Medical Home: A Cost-Effective Alternate to the Medical Home

The Center for Connected Health proposes a mix of Health 2.0 and the "patient-centered medical home" suited to a mix of health professionals.

For the patient:

- Robust and frictionless online communication with one's provider, with the medical home practice the default source of best-practice information.
- Fewer trips to the provider's office, improved prevention, and improved well-being.
- Monitoring of relevant physiologic information such as blood pressure, blood glucose, step counts, and medication adherence all fed into one's personal health record.
- A "blended" version of that record is available to one's healthcare team and one's loved ones, so that care coordination is made easier across settings of care and episodes of care.
- Access by both patients and their physicians (and other health professionals) to communities of consumers and patients with similar health challenges and goals where this personal health information would be displayed (according to the consumers' wishes) and trusted relationships with similar individuals would help move individuals to a state of more healthy behaviors and sustain them. Conceivably, a primary care provider could participate in such a community of his or her patients or subsets of his or her patients adding wisdom and coaching as the community felt it was relevant.

For the health professional:

- One might spend part of the workday caring for a few, very complicated patients, each requiring 45–60 minutes of concentrated time in the office.
- The other part of the day would be spent "surfing" various dashboards offering quality measures on one's patient populations and identifying outliers who need attention. (Note: Dashboards are a display option for viewing summary information and add convenience for users wanting a quick overview).
- Access to trended information about one's patients (blood pressures, activity levels, medication adherence, etc.) in context, fed from their private PHR and viewable at that moment in time when a complex medical decision is required.
- Patients and healthcare professionals guided by decision support would make other medical and health-related decisions. The decision support would be constantly refined, backed by self-learning software taking data from the physiologic information, the online support groups, and other data such as laboratory tests.
- One would spend some of this online time communicating with patients who have questions that need a health professional's attention.

Source: Adapted from Kibbe & Kvedar, 2008, to apply to a range of health professionals providing care.

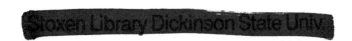

aging and the opportunities provided by technology (Barnason, Zimmerman, Nieveen, & Hertzog, 2006; Dishman, Matthews, & Dunbar-Jacob, 2004; Dishman, 2007, 2009; LaFramboise, Woster, Yager, & Yates, 2009; Zimmerman & Barnason, 2007).

The Intel Health Guide is described as a comprehensive personal health system. The features include an in-home patient device and an online interface (Intel, 2009). Features in the Health Guide system have a strong telehealth orientation with social networking features. The system will collect vital sign data, provide patient reminders and alerts, and allow videoconferencing. The press release indicates that online cognitive assessment and social interaction are included. The note does not indicate if the presence lamp and solar system display of intensity of social interaction developed at Intel and described by Morris, Lundell, Dishongh, & Needham (2009) will be included. The extent to which consumers and family members can customize the system is yet to be declared. It is not clear if this model can work through a regular telephone system or if it will be restricted to consumers with strong broadband connections.

GE Quiet Care is described as a remote passive activity and behavioral monitoring system for seniors. It partners with caregivers giving alerts to potential health issues or emergency situations (Intel, 2009). This telecare application is designed for locally monitored settings such as assisted care. No social monitoring features are described. Telemedicine connections are not presented as a feature either, although some health professional monitoring is implied.

Health Buddy as Forerunner of Telehealth Device Supports

The Health Buddy is a telehealth and telecare device tethered to a computer for providers and a tabletop device monitored by a nurse or other clinician on a standard desktop computer. (Details and photos are available at http://www.healthbuddy.com/content/language1/html/5578_ENU_XHTML.aspx.) The system is set up around daily questions about user health and well-being. The data is sent over a telephone line or Ethernet connection to a secure data center; the data is then available for review on the Web-based Health Buddy desktop. The website summarizes:

> The application is designed to quickly risk stratify and present patient results, enabling proactive providers to intervene before a patient's condition becomes acute. Patient responses are color-coded by risk level as high (red), moderate (yellow), and low (green) based on symptoms, patient behaviors, and self-care knowledge. (Health Buddy Desktop, n.d., para. 3)

A variety of peripheral devices are compatible with the Health Buddy. The website provides specific model numbers and pictures of blood glucose and blood pressure monitors, pulse oximeters, weight scales, and peak flow meters. Multiple studies have validated the success of this system in improving outcomes (Barnason et al., 2006; LaFramboise, Todero, Zimmerman, & Agrawal, 2003; LaFramboise et al., 2009; Zimmerman & Barnason, 2007). Accelerometers and pedometers to track exercise behaviors are not mentioned but seem likely partners. There is no mention of a personal health record or electronic record connection. However, this was a feature in early work with the VA system. Devices to support telehealth have proliferated and will be discussed in Chapter 5.

Neglected Social Capital Aspects of Care

All the featured models lack adequate attention to social aspects of health and health care. Social aspects include interpersonal interactions independent of healthcare provider and the social capital made available in the neighborhood through an extended network of family and friends and formal community programs. This means appreciating the social support network, the use of and potential for social media as a resource, and the prevailing norms and conditions in the surrounding community. Are there neighbors willing to knock on the door, hold a key for emergency personnel, run brief errands? Or is the individual or couple truly isolated and dependent on external services? Is there a neighbor who would hook up with the presence lamp described by Morris and colleagues (2009) and potentially a component of the new Intel/GE health guide system? Community was added as an element in the chronic care model in 2003. However, this refers to local program-level resources and policies, not consumer social capital and interactions.

Comorbidities and Self-Management Skills

In most of the care models described in the previous sections, self-management support is a call out. This is especially important with multiple comorbidities. Poor self-management is linked to poorer physical functioning (Bayliss, Ellis, & Steiner, 2007). The barriers to good self-management, they note, are embedded in financial constraints, persistent depressive symptoms, and related patient–provider communication that can be difficult, especially for seniors. On the other hand, there is emerging evidence that primary care patients with multiple illnesses are more willing to learn specific self-management skills than patients with one chronic disease (Bayliss, Ellis, & Steiner, 2007). The skills highlighted by Noel et al. (2007) are all highly amenable to a transition focus, coaching, and technology applications. The core skills include correctly following medication regimens, monitoring key symptoms, improving sleep patterns, coping with pain, and alleviating stress.

Noel et al. (2007) endorse group clinics, automated telephone management, and home visits by physician extenders. It is for the next generation of healthcare professionals to explore how these core skills and delivery strategies might be reimbursed by third-party payers and how technology may make the costs more attractive. Advance practice nurses have been recognized as having leverage in the six *D*s of outcome research (de Geest et al., 2008): death, disease, disability, discomfort, dissatisfaction, and dollars. Linking the processes of new applications in telehealth and telecare to the six *D*s will be essential to achieving widespread dissemination. Engaging communications experts in the design and evaluation of applications may be essential to full implementation of successful models of telehealth.

A critical dimension of the Independence at Home bill is moving reimbursement so that independent physicians and nurse practitioners would get a chance to share in the savings Medicare would see from home visits to patients with chronic multiple morbidities (Levey, 2009). The current disconnect in the difference between who bears the costs of installation and training and where the savings are realized has been a major factor in slowing implementation of new models of care. This is discussed extensively by Wielawski (2006) in her analysis of the chronic care model.

MANAGING THE FLOW IN HEALTHCARE TECHNOLOGY: A SOCIOECOLOGICAL MODEL

Technology provides ways to encompass and document the progression of factors that lead to behavior and behavior change. Nelson (2002) reported she built on a commonly used definition developed by Blum in 1986. Three types of healthcare computing applications were identified: data, information, and knowledge. Nelson and Joos (1989, as cited in Nelson, 2002) had expanded this definition for nursing informatics to include wisdom. Nelson made the case that when humans engage in learning, they act as "open systems that take in data, information, knowledge, and wisdom" (p. 15). This extended framework has been adopted by the American Nurses Association (2008) as part of the scope and standards of nursing informatics. However, it has relevance for all of the disciplines engaged in the design, engineering, and implementation of telehealth. The wealth of data newly available will call for data-mining expertise using a theoretical exploratory analysis and pattern of discovery and new inter-disciplinary hypothesis testing (Mucke, 2009).

As the healthcare team newly recognizes the importance of all of the members (the patient and social workers in particular), extensions of observations and intervention points are required. In this book, the emphasis is on operating in the ecosystem. This means reframing how technology and health can empower individuals and groups in the healthcare system. First, increasing attention is given to transitions as opportunities for decisions and new actions in the health habitat. The habitat idea comes from ecology and recognizes that patients and professionals live and interact in a wide range of environments that affect their health and ability to become or stay healthy. Relationships in an ecological model are in a continuous, connected cycle that is energized or stymied by available capital and the influence or charisma of individuals, groups, and media that attract consumers (and professionals) to proposed actions and attitudes. A new model is proposed to capture this socioecological process (Figure 1.8). It is detailed in subsequent chapters.

Figure 1.8   The Socioecology of Health Literacy: The Empowerment Cycle

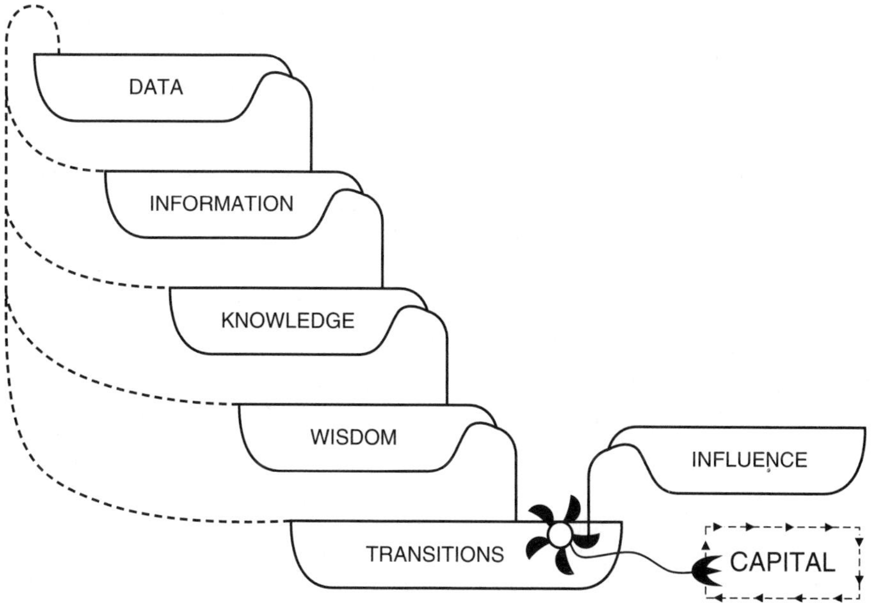

Illustration: Jin DePaul.

In the next chapters, elements of telecare that become *capital* if sufficiently *influential* or charismatic are detailed. These elements are health literacy, online health information, personal health records, devices specific to telehealth, and games. The final chapter will review the state of the science, spell out persistent barriers to accomplishing patient-centered, cost-effective care, and make recommendations for the next round of studies and for preparing the current and future generations to lead and sustain socioecological, patient-centered health technology.

REFERENCES

Ackoff, R. L. (1981). The art and science of mess management. *Interfaces, 11*(1), 20–26.

Adams, J., Grundy, P., Kohn, M. S., & Mounib, E. L. (n.d.). *Patient centered medical home*. Somers, NY: IBM Global Business Services. Retrieved August 11, 2010, from http://ibm.com/healthcare/medicalhome

AHRQ Innovations Exchange. (2009, October). Team-developed care plan and ongoing care management by social workers and nurse practitioners result in better outcomes and fewer emergency department visits for low-income seniors. [Innovation profile update] http://www.innovations.ahrq.gov/content.aspx?id=2066.

American Nurses Association. (2008). *Nursing informatics: Scope and standards of practice*. Silver Spring, MD: Author.

Arnst, C. (2006, July 17). The best medical care in the US: How Veterans Affairs transformed itself—and what it means for the rest of us. *Business Week*, 50–56.

Backer, L. A. (2007). The medical home: An idea whose time has come...again. *Family Practice Management, 14*(8), 38–41.

Barnason, S., Zimmerman, L., Nieveen, J., & Hertzog, M. (2006). Impact of a telehealth intervention to augment home health care on functional and recovery outcomes of elderly patients undergoing coronary artery bypass grafting. *Heart & Lung, 35*(4), 225–233.

Barrett, L. (2008). *Healthy@home: Using technology to remain independent. A literature review*. Washington, DC: AARP Foundation.

Bashshur, R. L., Shannon, G. W., Krupinski, E. A., Grigsby, J., Kvedar, J. C., Weinstein, R. S., et al. (2009). National telemedicine initiatives: Essential to healthcare reform. *Telemedicine and E-Health, 15*(6), 600–610.

Baur, C., & Kanaan, S. B. (2006). *Expanding the reach and impact of consumer e-health tools: Executive summary, a vision of e-health benefits for all* (Electronic No. 2006) U. S. Department of Health and Human Services, Office of Disease Prevention and Health Promotion. Retrieved February 9, 2010, from http://www.health.gov/communication/ehealth/ehealthTools/summary.htm

Bayliss, E. A., Ellis, J. L., & Steiner, J. F. (2007). Barriers to self-management and quality-of-life outcomes in seniors with multimorbidities. *Annals of Family Medicine, 5*(5), 395–402.

Bridges, W. (2003). *Managing transitions: Making the most of change* (2nd ed.). Cambridge, MA: Da Capo Press.

Carroll, R., Cnossen, R., Schnell, M., & Simons, D. (2007). Continua: An interoperable personal health care ecosystem. *IEEE Pervasive Computing, 4*(6), 90–94.

Center for Telehealth and e-Health Law. (2009). Retrieved October 16, 2009, from http://www.telehealthlawcenter.org/content/?page=18

Clancy, D. E., Yeager, D. E., Huang, P., & Magruder, K. M. (2007). Further evaluating the acceptability of group visits in an uninsured or inadequately insured patient population with uncontrolled type 2 diabetes. *Diabetes Educator, 33*(2), 309–314.

Coleman, J. (2005). Case management imbedded into disease management: The formula for effective disease management in HMOs and IDSs. *Case Manager, 16*(6), 40–42.

Commission Staff SEC. (2009). *Telemedicine for the benefit of patients, healthcare systems and society* (SEC [2009] 943 final ed.) Retrieved February 9, 2010, from http://ec.europa.eu/information_society/activities/health/policy/telemedicine/index_en.htm

Coombes, A. (2003, November 23). *Older Americans ramp up Internet use—MarketWatch.* Retrieved November 6, 2009, from http://www.marketwatch.com/story/older-americans-ramp-up-internet-use

Currell, R., Urquhart, C., Wainwright, P., & Lewis, R. (2000). Telemedicine versus face to face patient care: Effects on professional practice and health care outcomes. *Cochrane Database of Systematic Reviews, 2.* Art. No.: CD002098. doi: 10.1002/14651858.CD002098.

Darkins, A., Ryan, P., Kobb, R., Foster, L., Edmonson, E., Wakefield, B., et al. (2008). Care coordination/home telehealth: The systematic implementation of health informatics, home telehealth, and disease management to support the care of veteran patients with chronic conditions. *Telemedicine Journal & E-Health, 14*(10), 1118–1126.

de Geest, S., Moons, P., Callens, B., Gut, C., Lindpainter, L., & Spirig, R. (2008). Introducing advanced practice nurses/nurse practitioners in health care systems: A framework for reflection and analysis. *Swiss Medical Weekly, 138,* 621–628.

Deloitte Center for Health Solutions. (2008). *The medical home: Disruptive innovation for a new primary care model* (No. 8010). Washington, DC: Author.

Dentzer, S. (2009a). Health information technology: On the fast track at last? *Health Affairs, 28*(2), 320–321.

Dentzer, S. (2009b). Reform chronic illness care? Yes, we can. *Health Affairs, 28*(1), 12–13.

Dishman, E. (2007). *Health technology and innovation at Intel.* Retrieved June 24, 2009, from http://hitanalyst.files.wordpress.com/2008/07/day1_1100_dishman21.pdf

Dishman, E. (2009). Searching for health reform in all the wrong places. *Health Care Reform | Health Commentary,* Retrieved April 22, 2010, from http://healthcommentary.org/public/blog/177922

Dishman, E., Matthews, J. T., & Dunbar-Jacob, J. (2004). Everyday health: Technology for adaptive aging. In R. Pew & S. Van Hemel (Eds.), *Technology for adaptive aging: Workshop report and papers* (pp. 179–208). Washington, DC: National Academies Press. Retrieved February 9, 2010, from http://www.nap.edu/books/0309091160/html/179.html

Doarn, C. R., Yellowlees, P., Jeffries, D. A., Lordan, D., Davis, S., Hammack, G., et al. (2008). Societal drivers in the applications of telehealth. *Telemedicine Journal & E-Health, 14*(9), 998–1002.

Doty, C. (n.d.) *Delivering care anytime, anywhere: Telehealth alters the medical ecosystem-CHCF.org.* Retrieved August 22, 2009, from http://www.chcf.org/topics/view.cfm?itemID=133787

Doughty, K., Monk, A., Bayliss, C., Brown, S., Dewsbury, L., Dunk, B., et al. (2007). Telecare, telehealth, and assistive technologies, do we know what we're talking about? *Journal of Assistive Technologies, 1*(2), 6–10.

eHealthNews.eu. (2008, January 28). *New ICTs for elderly must respect dignity.* Retrieved September 6, 2009, from http://www.ehealthnews.eu/research/962-new-icts-for-elderly-must-respect-dignity

EUnetHTA. (2008). *EUnetHTA—European network for HTA.* Retrieved September 1, 2009, from http://www.eunethta.net/upload/Fact_sheet/June162008EUnetHTAFactsheet.pdf

Fried, T. R., McGraw, S., Agostini, J. V., & Tinetti, M. E. (2008). Views of older persons with multiple morbidities on competing outcomes and clinical decision-making. *Journal of the American Geriatrics Society, 56*(10), 1839–1844.

Grigsby, J., & Bennett, R. E. (2006). Alternatives to randomized controlled trials in telemedicine. *Journal of Telemedicine & Telecare, 12*(Suppl 2), S77–S84.

Grigsby, J., & Sanders, J. H. (1998). Telemedicine: Where it is and where it's going. *Annals of Internal Medicine, 129*(2), 123–127.

Hames, R. D. (2007). *The five literacies of global leadership: What authentic leaders know and you need to find out.* San Francisco: Jossey-Bass.

Health Buddy Desktop. (n.d.). Retrieved April 22, 2010, from http://www.healthbuddy.com/content/language1/html/5656_ENU_XHTML.aspx

Health Workforce Solutions & Robert Wood Johnson Foundation. (2008). *Transitional care model: key elements.* Retrieved July 27, 2010, from http://www.innovativecaremodels.com/care_models/21/key_elements

Hill-Kayser, C. E., Vachani, C., Hampshire, M. K., Jacobs, L. A., & Metz, J. M. (2009). An Internet tool for creation of cancer survivorship care plans for survivors and health care providers: Design, implementation, use and user satisfaction. *Hill-Kayser Journal of Medical Internet Research.* Retrieved September 4, 2009, from http://www.jmir.org/2009/3/e39

Hofmeyer, A., & Marck, P. B. (2008). Building social capital in healthcare organizations: Thinking ecologically for safer care. *Nursing Outlook, 56*(4), 145–151.

Institute of Medicine. (2000). In B. D. Smedley & S. L. Syme (Eds.), *Promoting health: Intervention strategies from social and behavioral research.* Washington DC: National Academies Press.

Institute of Medicine. (2008). *Knowing what works in health care: A roadmap for the nation.* Washington DC: National Academies Press.

Institute of Medicine. (2009). *Health literacy, eHealth, and communication: Putting the consumer first: Workshop summary.* Washington, DC: National Academies Press.

Intel. (2009). GE and Intel to form healthcare alliance. Retrieved October 16, 2009, from http://www.intel.com/pressroom/archive/releases/20090402corp.htm

Johnston, B., & Solomon, N. A. (2008). *Telemedicine in California: Progress, challenges, and opportunities.* Oakland, CA: California HealthCare Foundation. Retrieved April 22, 2010, from http://www.chcf.org/topics/view.cfm?itemid=133682

Jordan-Marsh, M. (2008). Health habitat aspects of software as a service (SAAS/WEB2.0) reinforcing diabetic self-confidence: The PHRddBRASIL case. *DESAFIO International Symposium: Diabetes, Health Education and Guided Physical Activities* (pp. 39–42).

Jordan-Marsh, M., Goldsmith, S. R., Siler, P., Sanchez, E., & Nazarey, P. (1997). Structural innovations and transitions for the nurse executive in the change agent role. In S. Beyers (Ed.), *The executive nurse: Leadership for new health care transitions* (pp. 84–85). Albany, NY: Delmar.

Kazmer, M. M. (2006). Creation and loss of sociotechnical capital among information professionals educated online. *Library & Information Science Research, 28*(2), 172–191.

Kibbe, D., & Kvedar, J. C. (2008, December 22). The health care blog: The connected medical home: Health 2.0 says "hello" to the medical home model. Retrieved February 9, 2010, from http://www.thehealthcareblog.com/the_health_care_blog/2008/12/the-connected-m.html

Kim, D., Subramanian, S. V., & Kawachi, I. (2008). Social capital and physical health: A systematic review of the literature. In I. Kawachi, S. V. Subramanian, & D. Kim (Eds.), *Social capital and health* (pp. 139–190). New York: Springer.

Kurywchak, D. A. (n.d.). *Telemedicine.com, inc.—Frequently asked questions.* Retrieved August 23, 2009, from http://www.telemedicine.com/faqs.html#Q13

LaFramboise, L. M., Todero, C. M., Zimmerman, L., & Agrawal, S. (2003). Comparison of Health Buddy with traditional approaches to heart failure management. *Family & Community Health, 26*(4), 275–288.

LaFramboise, L. M., Woster, J., Yager, A., & Yates, B. C. (2009). A technological life buoy: Patient perceptions of the Health Buddy. *Journal of Cardiovascular Nursing, 24*(3), 216–224.

Lauer, G. (2008, April 18). Virtual visits moving into medical mainstream. *iHealthBeat.* Retrieved October 16, 2009, from http://www.ihealthbeat.org/Features/2008/Virtual-Visits-Moving-Into-Medical-Mainstream.aspx

Laustsen, G. (2006). Environment, ecosystems, and ecological behavior: A dialogue toward developing nursing ecological theory. *Advances in Nursing Science, 29*(1), 43–54.

Levey, N. N. (2009, August 25). Getting cheaper, better healthcare at home? *Los Angeles Times.* Retrieved August 25, 2009, from http://www.latimes.com/news/nationworld/nation/healthcare/la-na-healthcare-housecalls25-2009aug25,0,1019530.story

Lowes, R. (n.d.). *Getting paid for mouse calls.* Retrieved August 29, 2009, from http://www.physicianspractice.com/index/fuseaction/articles.details/articleID/1309.htm

MacGregor, J. N., Cunningham, J. B., & Caverley, N. (2008). Factors in absenteeism and presenteeism: Life events and health events. *Management Research News, 31*(8), 607–615.

Mahoney, D. F., Mahoney, E. L., & Liss, E. (2009). AT EASE: Automated technology for elder assessment, safety, and environmental monitoring. *Gerontechnology, 8*(1), 11–25.

Mahoney, D. M., Mutschler, P. H., Tarlow, B., & Liss, E. (2008). Real-world implementation lessons and outcomes from the worker interactive networking (WIN) project: Workplace-based online caregiver support and remote monitoring of elders at home. *Telemedicine Journal and e-Health, 14*(3), 224–234.

Martin, S., Kelly, G., Kernohan, W. G., McCreight, B., & Nugent, C. (2008). Smart home technologies for health and social care support. *Cochrane Database of Systematic Reviews, 4.* Art. No.: CD006412. doi: 10.1002/14651858.CD006412.pub2.

McCarty, D., & Clancy, C. (2002). Telehealth: Implications for social work practice. *Social Work, 47*(2), 153–161.

Meleis, A. I., Sawyer, L. M., Im, E. O., Hilfinger Messias, D. K., & Schumacher, K. (2000). Experiencing transitions: An emerging middle-range theory. *Advances in Nursing Science, 23*(1), 12–28.

Morris, M. E., Lundell, J., Dishongh, T., & Needham, B. (2009). Fostering social engagement and self-efficacy in later life: Studies with ubiquitous computing. In P. Markopoulos, B. De Ruyter, & W. Mackay (Eds.), *Awareness systems: Advances in theory, methodology, and design* (pp. 335–349). London: Springer.

Mucke, H. A. (2009). Making sense of data. *Bio IT World, 8*(5), 10.

Murray, E., Burns, J., See Tai, S., Lai, R., & Nazareth, I. (2004). Interactive health communication applications for people with chronic disease. *Cochrane Database of Systematic Reviews, 4.* Art. No.: CD004274. doi: 10.1002/14651858.CD004274.pub4.

Nelson, R. (2002). Major theories supporting health care informatics. In S. P. Englebart & R. Nelson (Eds.), *Health care informatics: An interdisciplinary approach* (pp. 3–27). St. Louis, MO: Mosby.

Noel, P. H., Parchman, M. L., Williams, J. W., Jr., Cornell, J. E., Shuko, L., Zeber, J. E., et al. (2007). The challenges of multimorbidity from the patient perspective. *Journal of General Internal Medicine, 22*(Suppl. 3), 419–424.

Otellini, P. (2009, July 27). We need a personal health reformation. *Politico.* Retrieved February 9, 2010, from http://www.politico.com/news/stories/0709/25395.html

Painter, K. (2007, October 21). *Medicine on demand.* Retrieved September 6, 2009, from http://www.usatoday.com/news/health/painter/2007-10-21-your-health_N.htm

Parchman, M. L., Romero, R. L., & Pugh, J. A. (2006). Encounters by patients with type 2 diabetes—Complex and demanding: An observational study. *Annals of Family Medicine, 4*(1), 40–45.

Parrott, L., & Madoc-Jones, I. (2008). Reclaiming information and communication technologies for empowering social work practice. *Journal of Social Work, 8*(2), 181–197. doi: 10.1177/1468017307084739.

Pavel, M., Jimison, H., Hayes, T., & Kaye, J. (2009). Technology in support of successful aging. *The Bridge, 39*(1), 5–12. Retrieved February 9, 2010, from http://www.nae.edu/File.aspx?id=12500

Resnick, P. (2001). Beyond bowling together: SocioTechnical capital in human–computer interaction in the new millennium. In J. M. Carroll (Ed.), *Human–computer interaction in the new millennium* (pp. 647–672). Boston: Addison-Wesley. Retrieved February 9, 2010, from http://www.si.umich.edu/presnick/papers/stk/ResnickSTK.pdf

Rheuban, K. (2009). *American Telemedicine Association 2009 Presidential Address. Telemedicine and e-Health, 15*(6): 614–615. doi:10.1089/tmj.2009.9957.

Sarasohn-Kahn, J. (2009). *Participatory health: Online and mobile tools help chronically ill manage their care.* Sacramento, CA: California Healthcare Foundation. Retrieved October 30, 2009, from http://www.chcf.org/documents/chronicdisease/ParticipatoryHealthTools.pdf

Scott, R. (2009). Augmenting transitions: A unique and effective approach to securing fluid transitions. *Collaborative Practice Supplement,* 13–14.

Scott, R. E., McCarthy, F. G., Jennett, P. A., Perverseff, T., Lorenzetti, D., Saeed, A., et al. (2007). Telehealth outcomes: A synthesis of the literature and recommendations for outcome indicators. *Journal of Telemedicine & Telecare, 13*(2), 1–38.

Soubhi, H. (2007). Toward an ecosystemic approach to chronic care design and practice in primary care. *Annals of Family Medicine, 5*(3), 263–269.

Suter, P., Hennessey, B., Harrison, G., Fagan, M., Norman, B., & Suter, W. N. (2008). Home-based chronic care: An expanded integrative model for home health professionals. *Home Healthcare Nurse, 26*(4), 222–229.

Trustworthy information systems for healthcare. (2009). Retrieved August 17, 2009, from http://www.ists.dartmouth.edu/projects/tish.html

Wagner, E. H. (1998). Chronic disease management: What will it take to improve care for chronic illness? *Effective Clinical Practice, 1*(1), 2–4.

Wartena, F., Muskens, J., & Schmitt, L. (2009). Continua: The impact of a personal telehealth ecosystem. *International Conference on eHealth, Telemedecine, and Social Medicine, 1,* 13–18. doi: 10.1109/eTELEMED.2009.8.

Watson, A. J., Bell, A. G., Kvedar, J. C., & Grant, R. W. (2008). Reevaluating the digital divide: Current lack of Internet use is not a barrier to adoption of novel health information technology. *Diabetes Care, 31*(3), 433–435.

Wielawski, I. M. (2006). Improving chronic illness care. *Robert Wood Johnson Foundation Anthology: To Improve Health and Health Care, 10,* 1–17.

Zimmerman, L., & Barnason, S. (2007). Use of a telehealth device to deliver a symptom management intervention to cardiac surgical patients. *Journal of Cardiovascular Nursing, 22*(1), 32–37.

CHAPTER 2

Literacy for an Age of eHealth

SOCIOECOLOGY OF HEALTH LITERACY

In this digital age, consumers, health professionals, and all of the stake-holders in the healthcare enterprise encounter opportunities and challenges for which they have not been systematically prepared. The Internet and digital technology have combined to create a health habitat where thriving requires new skills and resources. The first chapter provided an overview of the new context of health care. In this chapter, the confluence of resources and energy in the form of capital for literacy is the focus.

Much of the development of the healthcare system around the globe, but particularly in the United States, has evolved around an architecture model of dividing humans into parts. Today we have cardiac specialists, gastrointestinal specialists, mental health specialists, and so on. The environment is reemerging as a core component of understanding human health and health behaviors. Environment is physical in terms of ambience of the space where the person lives, works, and plays; it is physical in terms of air quality, architecture of space, and availability of tangible resources for survival (capital). However, equally important forms of capital in the human environment are social factors—the skills and abilities of the individual and the members of his or her social network and related resources. Socioecology as a framework was presented in the opening chapter. To navigate the newly emerging "health habitat" (Jordan-Marsh, 2008) in the globally challenged economy requires multiple literacies to sustain and build capital. These are basics for the consumer empowerment that has become an expectation in the domain of eHealth.

Human capital is the mix of values and capacities built on attitudes, skills, and knowledge that an individual draws on to accomplish life goals. This capital is accumulated through formal education and life experience. Health capital is a mix of capacities as well. Chief among these is literacy. The challenge of literacy with respect to health technology is that it is a skill with, at minimum, cognitive, psychomotor, and technical components. A case might be made that to thrive in the new millennium requires a new host of literacies. Thriving in the new world of eHealth means the consumer must take full advantage of personal health capital and create sociotechnical capital (see Chapter 1, Overview). Sociotechnical capital refers to values and abilities required to interact in a digital world.

To maximize sociotechnical capital around health literacy, a socioecological perspective on the confluence of resources provides an organizing framework. As depicted in Figure 2.1, health behaviors, attitudes, and decisions are influenced by new access to data, which can be aggregated as information that can be interpreted as knowledge. This accumulation of knowledge can be analyzed on the basis of personal experience and insight (wisdom) and shared with others in one's social network to access the wisdom of peers, family, and health professionals. The extent to which individuals (families and communities) have access to comprehensive, real-time and stored data, have assistance in aggregating data, make sense of information, build knowledge, and seek and share wisdom is a reflection of available capital. The potential for influencing health is limited or extended by this capital. The confluence of these resources at times of transition (decision points) is also heavily affected by sources of influence (charisma—the motivational power of individuals and of media). The World Health Organization (2010) called for recognition of the power (influence)

Figure 2.1   The Socioecology of Health Literacy: The Empowerment Cycle

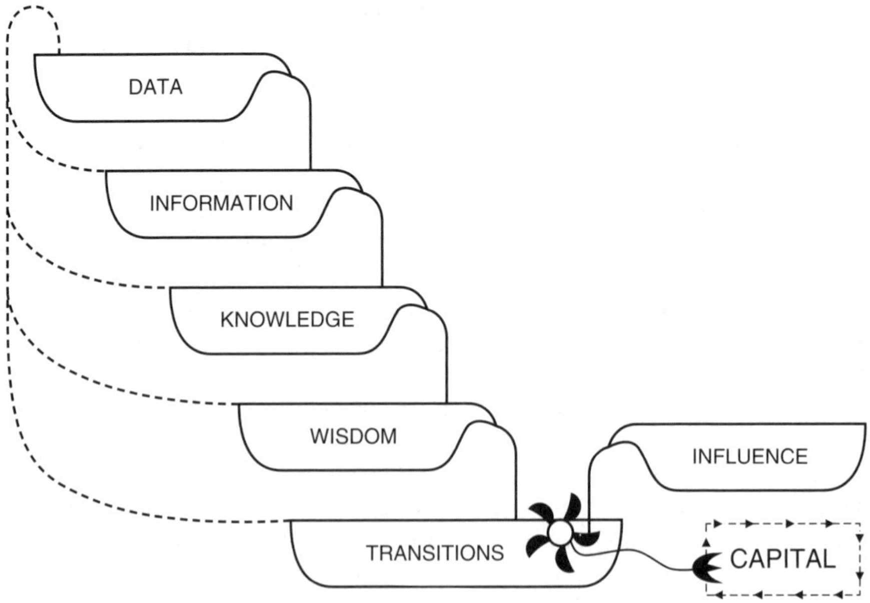

Illustration: Jin DePaul.

dimension of health literacy. Influence, WHO noted, relates both to control over information and to empowerment of individuals and communities in their quest for development of social capital.

Literacy requires not only skill in accessing resources but in evaluating resources. The entire team (from professional to patient and family and any caregivers) can be dazzled and distracted by the charisma of websites, games, and other applications designed to sell a product or a point of view. *Charisma* is that elusive but obvious quality that draws us to others and persuades us the person could be important in our lives. Consumers are used to weighing the charisma of individuals as they seek experts and partners in accomplishing their health agendas in face-to-face encounters. It is equally important to be aware of the charisma/compelling influence of well-designed websites and other digital resources. (Commercial advertising, for example, has deliberate and sophisticated charisma.) Experts and large sums of money will increasingly be engaged in building desirability and "drawing power" for websites, digital services, and products as the market for health technology grows.

Data, information, knowledge, and various forms of wisdom are all available on the Internet and through digital devices. The task of contemporary consumers, their advocates, and health professionals is to develop literacy so that these resources are well understood and the consumer is not overwhelmed but empowered. As consumers face transitions in their healthcare goals, they are subject to a variety of influences and strengthened or constrained by the capital available to them. Well-designed, credible websites are an important potential source of capital for gathering information and becoming knowledgeable prior to making transition decisions related to health.

Developments Advancing eHealth

The emerging phenomenon of eHealth was discussed in detail in the previous chapter. In a recent workshop, the Institute of Medicine (IOM) described it as "the use of emerging interactive health information technologies" (Institute of Medicine [IOM], 2009, p. 1). eHealth is expected to improve the healthcare system and increase tailoring care to individual consumers. These features are anticipated to improve access especially for underserved populations. As discussed in the Chapter 1 overview, there are major shifts in electronic aspects of American health care specific to the American Recovery and Reinvestment Act of 2009. Title IV of the Health Information Technology for Economic and Clinical Health Act (HITECH Act) calls for massive funding for electronic health records. These records will be the foundation of moving eHealth into the forefront of public and private healthcare resources.

Furthermore, the framework for *Healthy People 2020* has three priorities: prevention, preparedness, and health information technology (HIT) (Harris & Friedman, 2009). Harris and Friedman describe the foundational element of the new strategic plan as a combination of health literacy, health information technology, and health communications for personal and population health. These are components that might be labeled *sociotechnical capital for health*.

Sociotechnical Capital and Health

For health, *sociotechnical capital* (Resnik, 2001) means using digital resources (e.g., online sites and peripheral devices) for wellness activities, management of chronic illnesses, and recovery from trauma. Whether analyses are done by application providers such as WebMd or pollsters, there seems to be a consensus that the nature of health care in the United States is changing. Consumers are asking different questions and have different expectations of the patient–doctor encounter (Harris Poll, 2009). Froude (interviewed in Ackerman, 2009) explains that consumers are going online for more efficient ways to navigate the healthcare system. Simultaneously, experiences with other consumer services online have raised new expectations of efficiency and convenience when seeking healthcare information and support.

As with all aspects of capital, values, attitudes, skills, supportive resources, and opportunities combine to create an environment that makes productive engagement possible. Digital literacy for engaged health is a necessary, but not sufficient, source of capital. Health literacy is the critical cornerstone. In a digital age, health literacy requires connecting with the Internet as a means of obtaining information, engaging in decision making, communicating with healthcare providers and sources of social support, and monitoring relevant data for evaluation and collaboration.

Health Technology for Collaborative Communication

Collaboration will take on new meaning in health care as data on observations specific to daily living and home-based monitoring are collected and posted to websites. These website communications can be shared with healthcare professionals, home-based caregivers, or geographically separated family and friends wanting to participate in health activities. Running partners already share data and can adjust plans based on information posted online. Remote family members with access to data on changes in social activity of parents may plan more frequent visits or phone calls. Primary care health professionals may link in a specialist to comment on unexpected changes in blood glucose and weight. In subsequent chapters on personal health records, games, and telehealth, other areas of collaboration will become clear.

Digital literacy requires Internet interaction, but it also calls on the ability to use mobile devices, handheld appliances, CDs, DVDs, and "smart home" technology components. Combining Internet resources and digital devices is the foundation of eHealth. Increasingly, there are virtual and physical "gadgets" that bridge applications and create opportunities for truly tailoring care to the lives and preferences of individuals. These adjuncts to the Internet are discussed in detail in the chapter on devices. In this chapter, the focus is on the attitudes, values, skills, and resources required to engage or interact with health-specific digital technology—literacies for sociotechnical capital (Resnick, 2001).

Developmental Considerations in Technology Adaptation

Building literacy for sociotechnical capital therefore requires a shift from worrying about the digital divide to promoting digital inclusion; such could be accomplished by tackling barriers to access that exist (Harrgitai, 2002). One approach to understanding different patterns of use would be examining opportunities and expectations in a developmental framework. First, van Bronswijk et al. (2009) argue that we can think of the onset of aging a transition similiar to the onset of puberty. This perspective probably frames the digital divide nicely in terms of the skills of adults compared to those of children in the new millennium. Personal experience and developmentally predictable limitations in function create a wide range of variation in differences in both ability to cope and the rate at which the ability to cope changes. Culture will have an impact on willingness to engage with the digital world and styles of interaction. This normative influence will be especially important with respect to the delivery of telehealth—see Chapter 7.

There are some phases of human development that may be close to universal for assessing individuals in terms of their "technology generation." van Bronswijk and colleagues (2009) propose four technology-relevant ages (p. 6):

1. Formative age
2. Main working for income and family formation phase
3. Active retirement
4. Frailty and dependence with rapid senescence

These stages are useful, they propose, for focusing research. From a practice perspective, it may also be useful to think of the context of technology encounters and priorities. van Bronswijk et al.'s (2009) observations are most relevant to industrialized countries. Individuals in the formative age will be engaging with technology first within the setting of the family, school, or other social settings. Priorities may be entertainment, family connections and communication, coordination, and school achievement. The importance of these activities will vary with the age of the child. The particular needs and risks experienced by adolescents engaging with technology deserve special attention and will not be covered here. Adults in the income and family formation phase will be looking for technology that increases their productivity and facilitates communication and social support. Workplace technology may be the dominant context. The remaining phases can be greatly enhanced by overt programs to support engaged aging for those in active retirement. Those in active retirement may be dependent on community resources such as libraries and community centers to obtain access to the Internet, although the Pew American Life and Internet Project suggests that broadband access continues to grow in American homes (Horrigan, 2009). Family members and health professionals who work with adults characterized by frailty and dependence are increasingly looking to technology to provide unobtrusive monitoring and support. Access here may be in the home (a smart home being the most inclusive application) or in senior housing and nursing homes. The chapter on devices is of particular value on this topic.

The New Literacy Paradigm

A major shift in our understanding of learning has come with the digital age. The 3 *R*s (reading, 'riting, 'rithmetic) have become the 4 *E*s (exposing knowledge, employing information, expressing ideas compellingly, and ethics—right and wrong on the information highway) notes Armstrong and Warlick (2004). What consumers know is not so important as what they "know to do." The 4 *E*s model means that we must all give up the model where first we "learn to read" and then "read to learn." Consumers must have the ability to "read to do." Armstrong and Warlick, as cited by Wien-Peckham (n.d.), note that a major problem is that globally, systems on the digital highway are proceeding as though this matrix of skills and attitudes was already in place. However, Wien-Peckham warns that given current literacy levels, catastrophe is ahead. As the United States hurtles toward electronic health records with the expectation that consumers will be active and informed, the cost savings promised may fail to materialize.

Values in Digital Literacy Capital: Balancing Expert and Normative Power

Building digital literacy capital for the new era of health reform requires valuing interdependence. Interdependence is an achievement of the "working for income and family formation" phase of development. Interdependence requires an acknowledgment that collaborating with experts and sources of social support is a means of empowerment for self-care. Implicit in the emerging models is the expectation of personal, social, and civic responsibility. This model of interdependence is consistent with the Chronic Care Model (Wagner, 1998), which is receiving increasing interest (over 500 citations for the original article; see Improving Chronic Illness Care, n.d.). The Chronic Care Model is notable in its clear emphasis on an informed and active patient engaging with an interdisciplinary practice team (Wagner, 1998). Studies using a randomized controlled trial design have validated the effectiveness of the model in multiple contexts (Coleman, Austin, Brach, & Wagner, 2009).

The informed and active adult weighs personal preferences with expert knowledge of available options, services, and devices. Wisdom comes from drawing on these insights and recognition of what is normative (usual) and what is possible. Empowerment comes from understanding how the possibilities made clear by experts might be achieved given the individual's sources of capital. Individuals who are fiercely independent and unable to seek or accept assistance or advice are poor candidates for digital literacy. In the new world of eHealth, paternalistic approaches where the health professional carries the bulk of the conversation are giving way to approaches that empower consumers (Bickmore & Giorgino, 2006). Embracing eHealth calls for valuing expert professional power but balancing it with a recognition of the power inherent in a consumer's own life experiences, skills, motivations, and preferences (his or her capital).

Equally great in value is the ability to learn new things, and the wisdom to take advantage of available capital for successful transitions. Digital literacy requires psychomotor skills and the ability to navigate in unfamiliar territory. This can be quite challenging. Valuing new learning can moderate the frequently frustrating experiences on the path to acquiring the ability to use digital technology. Healthcare providers can reinforce this value as an important aspect of engaged aging across the life span.

Attitudes and Anticipatory Guidance

Anticipatory guidance is the skill of helping someone and his or her family to cope with developmental challenges. However, it is rarely proposed as a strategy for building health or digital literacy. Health professionals may meaningfully inform consumers of the difficulties ahead in building sociotechnical capital and developing health literacy. Providers can also strengthen consumer resolve by sharing their own jagged journey to digital expertise (exercising normative power). Related attitudes that sustain engagement during the learning curve include tolerance for making mistakes and the ability to learn from peers, the younger generation, and designated experts. Once engaged with health-related technology, a tolerance for lack of stability in performance of applications and devices is critical. As adults are introduced to technology that is newly available or simply new to them, sharing experiences and the normality of glitches and breakdowns may help. Encouraging older adults to reminisce about other learning challenges they have had to surmount may be powerful in overcoming resistance to new technology.

DIGITAL INCLUSION

For many adults, digital technology for health represents a true paradigm shift, not only in assumptions about self-care, but in the behaviors, skills, and attitudes required to engage. As Hargittai (2002) points out, the dilemma of the digital divide is no longer a binary problem of access—yes or no. Many people have a means of access, but among adults there is tremendous variation in their skill levels and willingness to participate. As the world moves toward the ever-increasing use of technology for health, commerce, and government interactions, a more focused understanding of the barriers to Internet access for adults is required.

Barriers to Digital Inclusion

DiMaggio and Hargittai (2001, as cited in Hargittai, 2002) suggested five dimensions along which divides may exist, as shown in Table 2.1.

To broaden digital inclusion, the first barrier to overcome is whether the consumer has the *technical means*. Does the individual or group have the necessary hardware, software, and connectivity? Horrigan (2007) inventories these as assets and includes cell phones and other devices that connect to the Internet and facilitate electronic communication and participation. Broadband access is increasingly available in the United States (Horrigan, 2009). This Pew Internet

---

Table 2.1   Barriers to Digital Inclusion

1. Technical means
2. Autonomy of use
3. Use patterns
4. Social support networks
5. Literacies and skills

Source: Adapted from DiMaggio & Hargittai, 2001.

study suggests that 65% of Americans have access. Older adults and households with less than $30,000 annual income showed growth in Internet usage over the past year. This increase in access has occurred despite the current recession. Respondents were more likely to cut back on cable TV or cell phone services (not cell phone access) than broadband access.

Another dimension of broadening digital inclusion is expanding autonomy in use. Some Internet users have access only at school, work, or public spaces such as the library, community center, or Internet cafés. For some individuals this limits the time of day they can go online. E. Rice (personal communication, July 12, 2009) notes that for homeless teens, they have access to the Internet mostly through teen centers that close on weekends and evenings. The consequence is that when family members would have the freedom and time to respond, the estranged teen is not available online. For some people, leaving home for Internet access in the evening is risky.

Another aspect of analyzing digital inclusion is *autonomy within Internet framework*—some users may be restricted in which websites they can visit. This can be due to firewalls that may have been installed to restrict access to pornographic material or online purchase sites. Additionally, employers may have policies prohibiting use of work site resources for personal purposes. Furthermore, individuals may be reluctant to visit certain sites for fear of having their activity observed. They may also be concerned their employer, agency, or family may be tracking their searches. Some communities are working to provide free wireless access within their geographic boundaries. This will enhance digital inclusion. Health professionals might play a role in assisting advocacy groups to make a strong case for providing broadband access for free.

Another potential barrier to digital inclusion is *use patterns*. Some individuals may lack the literacy to take full advantage of Internet resources. The Pew Internet and American Life Project website provides an interactive quiz for self-assessment (see Pew Internet and American Life Project, n.d.). Horrigan (2007) has developed a typology of users of technology. His results suggest that there are 10 types of users, summarized in Table 2.2.

The 10 types can be grouped roughly into *elite users* who have the most information technology, engage with user-generated content, and are highly satisfied with their experience. The second level is *middle of the road users*; these people are task oriented rather than self-expressionists. They vary on whether technology is beneficial or problematic. The final level is those with few *technology assets*. Technology is on the edge of their lives, and some are truly "off the network" using neither cell phones nor Internet. Although Horrigan provides proportions of the population by level, it is not clear what the current breakdown would be given 2009 data on increases in broadband access (Horrigan, 2009). Health professionals making plans for individual consumers or designing programs for patient groups may find the Pew Internet quiz useful

Table 2.2   Types of Technology Users by Percentage and Key Aspects

	Group Name	% of Adult Population	What You Need to Know About Them
Elite tech users (31% of American adults)	Omnivores	8	They have the most information gadgets and services, which they use voraciously to participate in cyberspace and express themselves online, and do a range of Web 2.0 activities such as blogging or managing their own Web pages.
	Connectors	7	Between feature-packed cell phones and frequent online use, they connect to people and manage digital content using ICTs—all with high levels of satisfaction about how ICTs let them work with community groups and pursue hobbies.
	Lackluster veterans	8	They are frequent users of the Internet and less avid about cell phones. They are not thrilled with ICT-enabled connectivity.
	Productivity enhancers	8	They have strongly positive views about how technology lets them keep up with others, do their jobs, and learn new things.
Middle-of-the-road tech users (20%)	Mobile centrics	10	They fully embrace the functionality of their cell phones. They use the Internet, but not often, and like how ICTs connect them to others.
	Connected but hassled	10	They have invested in a lot of technology, but they find the connectivity intrusive and information something of a burden.

Table 2.2   Types of Technology Users by Percentage and Key Aspects (*continued*)

	Group Name	% of Adult Population	What You Need to Know About Them
Few tech assets (49%)	Inexperienced experimenters	8	They occasionally take advantage of interactivity, but if they had more experience, they might do more with ICTs.
	Light but satisfied	15	They have some technology, but it does not play a central role in their daily lives. They are satisfied with what ICTs do for them.
	Indifferents	11	Despite having either cell phones or online access, these users use ICTs only intermittently and find connectivity annoying.
	Off the network	15	Those with neither cell phones nor Internet connectivity tend to be older adults who are content with old media.

Note: ICT = Information and communication technologies.

Source: Horrigan, 2007, p. 5. Used with permission.

in planning for specific consumer groups. The various literacies required for effective use of health resources in the digital age are discussed in this chapter in some detail.

Digital inclusion can be greatly affected by *social support networks*. This is the extent to which an individual or group can call on others for assistance. Gaining assistance with minimal financial, time, or socioemotional cost is important. Equally important is the size of the social network and whether it encourages patterns of engagement across the network using technology. The healthcare community is increasingly a critical part of the social network for consumers who are becoming partners in their health planning. Finally, Hargittai (2002) reminds us that *skill* in using technology is a critical fulcrum in minimizing the digital divide. To skill can be added the prerequisite of *literacy*.

In the remainder of the chapter, the literacies needed for developing health capital are described (Figure 2.2). These are a composite of a dramatically new paradigm of expectations of consumers and health professionals. Although the literacies in the figure were initially phrased as requirements for academic achievement in the 21st century, "digital literacy, inventive thinking, effective communication, and high productivity" are clearly called for in the philosophy behind health reform efforts in the United States (see especially the Institute of Medicine [2009] workshop summary on eHealth).

Scope of the Challenge: Prevalence of Literacy and Technology Issues

Progress in Technology Access

Before we can ask how effectively consumers can use health-related technology, it is important to understand their technology assets, attitudes, and

Figure 2.2   21st Century Learning: Consumer Health Technology Interface

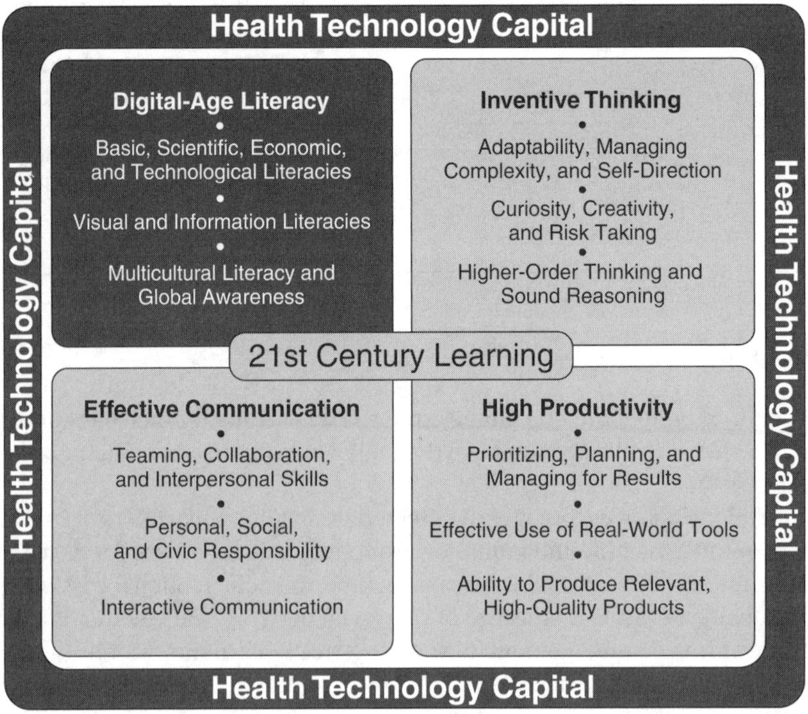

Source: Modified from North Central Regional Education Laboratory (2003). Reprinted with permission of Learning Point Associates.

behavior patterns. While the various Pew studies of American Internet-related behaviors show some progress (Horrigan, 2009), there are still some groups that are not engaging in technology beyond watching television and using land-line telephones. Older adults tend to use less technology. Also, Horrigan noted that African Americans experienced their second year of slower than average growth in broadband access.

In 2007 Horrigan reported that 20% of the American population is very aware of and has access to information and communication technology but is dissatisfied. Two-thirds acknowledged that they needed help to set up new devices. Surprisingly, 66% of Americans with cell phones or Internet access do not find themselves more productive. Horrigan argues that limitations in usability and usefulness are major factors in the slow adoption of information and communication technologies. He concludes that some Americans are uninterested or "collectively hostile" to cyberspace. So, there is both hope for the general population and concern for those who remain isolated from what is becoming the technology mainstream. Remaining technologically isolated has the potential to exacerbate health disparities among this population. The risk is that current global economic constraints on governments and healthcare agencies and health professional expectations of connectedness may combine to create indifference or prejudice. At the provider level, as health professionals become more skilled in and habituated to providing eHealth, they may become contemptuous and impatient with those who lack access or choose not to learn. At the policy level, the voices of those who are not technologically connected may become muted and easily ignored. Consumer advocates and health professionals ideally will continue to assess healthcare resources in terms of access for the full range of consumer (and provider) skills.

Constraints of General Literacy Levels

In the IOM report on health literacy, Norman (2009) cites a variety of resources to make the case that only 6 out of 10 Americans and Canadians have adequate literacy, making it difficult for them to function in everyday society. Contemporary health interventions are increasingly online, thus largely text based, which means that 4 out of every 10 people who might benefit from an online intervention may be left out. There is limited data on numeracy. Miller et al. (2007, as cited in Norman) found that 25% had very limited mathematical literacy (Norman, 2009). This means that the eHealth tasks that require consumers to do simple calculations, read charts, and apply age-related guidelines will be difficult or impossible for one-quarter of the population to complete without assistance.

Literacy as a Continuum of Complexity

Consumers and those in their social network who embrace the new expectations for engagement in decisions about health take on dramatic new responsibilities. In the past, consumers held the role of patients and were primarily responsible for providing data or allowing data to be collected about them. Now consumers are called on to traverse the continuum of *data, information, knowledge,* and *wisdom* to make or participate in key decisions about their health and health care. This creates new expectations for healthcare providers as well. This progression or continuum represents the dynamic tension of eHealth opportunity. This progression has been added to the ecological framework (see Figure 2.1), based on the work of Nelson (1989, 2002) and was incorporated in the informatics standards of the American Nurses Association (2008).

Consumers increasingly will interact in new ways around data as electronic health records (EHRs) include a personal health record (PHR) component. Consumers will need to name their symptoms and responses using the taxonomy of their EHR/PHR. Consumers will collect data such as blood glucose, blood pressure, and activity levels and organize it by uploading it to websites with personally selected information categories. The consumer will organize information about his or her daily routines and create variables to track data of personal interest. Using various gadgets and software programs combined with feedback from healthcare providers, consumers will be called on to use the knowledge generated to make wise decisions about their lifestyle, medications, and interface with technology. Over time, consumers will not only develop wisdom about their health and self-care, but they will increasingly share that wisdom in their own social network and in online interactions.

Challenges Posed by Low Levels of Health Literacy

Health literacy data is even more grim than general literacy data. The National Assessment of Adult Literacy (NAAL) team (White, 2008) found limited health literacy for adults (Table 2.3). Less than 15% of adults were assessed as attaining full proficiency in health literacy. (The tasks required for attaining the designated levels are presented in a subsequent section.)

The proportion of literate adults continued to decrease with age (Federal Interagency Forum on Aging-Related Statistics, 2008). Thirty-nine percent of people age 75 and over had below basic health literacy, compared with 23% of people ages 65 to 74, and 13% of people ages 50 to 64. Among older Americans, the average level of health literacy—the extent to which people can obtain, process, and understand basic health information and services—was lower than that of any other age group.

Table 2.3   Health Literacy Levels by Task and US Population Proficiencies

Health Literacy Level	Task Examples	Percentage
Proficient	Using a table, calculate an employee's share of health insurance costs for a year.	12%
Intermediate	Read instructions on a prescription label, and determine what time a person can take the medication.	53%
Basic	Read a pamphlet, and give two reasons a person with no symptoms should be tested for a disease.	21%
Below basic	Read a set of short instructions, and identify what is permissible to drink before a medical test.	14%

Source: Office of Disease Prevention and Health Promotion, 2008.

DIGITAL LITERACY: COMPOSITE OF LITERACIES AND OVERLAPPING SKILLS

Prior to embarking on eHealth-related tasks, a person must have basic literacies and skills that taken together form a composite of digital literacies. Digital literacies for health technology interactions include the expectation that consumers will be able to (1) read, comprehend, and use available information to make judgments; (2) choose among tools and be able to use them; and (3) act to convey information and related decisions to healthcare providers and family (Hargittai, 2002). Meeting these expectations requires a set of interlocking attitudes and skills (Eshet, 2002).

Managing Digital Flexibility in Analyzing Information Resources

Information literacy in the digital age begins with awareness of the flexibility afforded by the Internet as a media context. An information-literate person knows "how knowledge is organized, how to find information, and how to use information in a way that others can learn from them" (American Library

Association Presidential Committee on Information Literacy, 1989, as cited by Norman, 2009, p. 12). Perhaps the most critical aspect of information literacy is filtering. This strategy protects consumers from unknowingly being influenced by Web-based resources. Eshkat-Alkali and Amichai-Hamburger (2004) describe the filtering as first identifying "erroneous, irrelevant, falsified, or biased information" and then preventing its infiltration into "the learner's system of considerations" (p. 423). This filtering extends not only to what the consumer accesses, but what consumers provide as they engage online.

Socioemotional Literacy: The Awareness of Influence

Socioemotional literacy required for cyberspace is infrequently mentioned in the digital literacy body of work. However, given the emerging centrality of social networking, it is critical that consumers are aware of the norms of sharing online and recognize affective dimensions (Barak, Bonel-Nissim, & Suler, 2008). Socioemotionally literate consumers are "willing to share their own data and knowledge with others, capable of evaluating data, possessing an abstract thinking, and able to design knowledge through virtual collaboration" (Eshet-Alkali & Amichai-Hamburger, 2004, p. 423). This practice creates both opportunities and risks. A habit of filtering one's own contributions is a safeguard. Socioemotional filtering is a strategy for avoiding cybertraps where digitally available personal information can be distorted or manipulated to maximize potentially compelling *influences* on attitudes or choices more congruent with someone else's agenda.

The skills of socioemotional literacy are closely tied to what is sometimes called *media literacy* (Norman, 2009). This refers to the skills necessary to think critically and to act based on information from media-based messages. Norman argues that media literacy places information in a social and political context and considers issues such as the marketplace, audience relations, and the role of the medium in the message. To some extent, these are socioemotional dimensions as the participants seek to play on feelings and beliefs to make their point with cyberaudiences. Those with low media literacy lack awareness of bias or perspective in media pronouncements, both in terms of what is presented and what is not presented.

Socioemotional media literacy requires anticipating that there are explicit and implicit messages in media presentation that require filtering through personal value systems. These dual meanings must be discerned and analyzed to use the information effectively. Consumers of technology are literate when they appreciate that everyone has an agenda, and that sometimes that agenda will validate your own beliefs and move your own priorities along. Whether that is beneficial depends on the outcome and who is evaluating the results.

Diminishing Digital Fatigue

Given the demands of filtering and the complexity of how information is provided in the digital world, the evidence that online reading creates higher cognitive load than reading from printed text is not surprising. The pages full of seemingly unrelated photos, stories, headlines, and links can create severe disorientation (Eshet-Alkalai & Geri, 2007). Eshet-Alkalai and Amichai-Hamburger (2004) suggest the result is diminished ownership by readers, limited engagement, and lessened willingness to learn.

Based on a series of studies, Eshet-Alkalai and colleagues (Eshet-Alkalai & Amichai-Hamburger, 2004; Eshet-Alkalai & Geri, 2007) propose literacies that will enable consumers to participate effectively in a digital world. These include *photovisual literacy*, which is learning to read from pictures and icons as though they were text. *Reproduction literacy* refers to the ability to make something new and original from preexisting materials. This parallels an emerging expectation of being engaged in the sharing and production of user-cenered knowledge, which will be important in eHealth engagement. Reproduction literacy is an expectation new to many adults—they may be puzzled by the call to participate in the "copy and paste" culture of creativity and ingenuity. Other authors have combined related skills under the term *visual literacy* (Metros, 2008b). A detailed discussion of visual literacy is presented later in this chapter. Reproduction skills are closely related to *lateral* or *branching literacy* as described by Eshet-Alkalai and Amichai-Hamburger (2004). The ability to branch out and create knowledge by using associative thinking and synthesis skills builds from lateral rather than linear learning. Branching literacy uses the power of the hypertext format. The average website is a mosaic of images, sound bytes, essays, and links. Not only is the overall impression fragmented, but the user can leap from item to item—branching. Internet-based information providers can promote jumping from topic to topic with hyperlinks; they can also falsify information in ways difficult to detect. Given this potential for inappropriate influence, the core aspect of information literacy is to have a critical thinking filter—to "trust nobody" (Eshet-Alkalai & Amichai-Hamburger, 2004). This connotes a habit of vigilance with respect to the quality and credibility of information.

However, the hyperlink is useful when a consumer needs a definition or reference to better understand a point. It is important to be able to make connections across sources—with people whose opinion is trusted, with printed text, and with websites—and more recently with blogs, knols, wikis, and tweets. Consumers with poor information literacy may be unaware of the power of triangulating impressions across sources (and links) to fully grasp the information needed to make basic decisions (Norman, 2009).

Risks of Digital Flexibility for the Consumer

Digital technology has enabled easy access to information without the guiding analytical skills of a librarian. Digital technology has made it fairly simple to present a professional and credible appearance. However, just because a website has an authoritative demeanor does not mean that the information it contains is accurate or complete.

Mash Ups: Recreated Capital

Ownership of online material is an important aspect of literacy, whether it falls under information or computer literacy. This is an area that requires new understandings of copyright and has been a topic of intense controversy with respect to music and video files. The author's undergraduate students, for example, have very different beliefs about the morality of using ("copying") parts of products accessed online. Similarly, although it is becoming clearer to them that music and video must be acquired and shared in a legal format, PDFs, especially of books, have not come under that umbrella. As the healthcare community increases the call to engage consumers in production of materials and resources to share, these issues will become more critical.

Almost anyone can manipulate widely available visual images, music, interactive applications and text from original materials to make a point or build a prejudicial case. These composites, called *mash ups*, are a form of user-generated content that pulls material from the Web for new purposes (see Wikipedia citation in Shih & Kagal, 2009). Transparency in crediting sources is important, but can be complex (Shih & Kagal, 2009). As health professionals and consumer groups exercise creativity in eHealth applications, tools like the PIPES resource developed by Shih and Kagal will become critical in ensuring that copyrights are not violated. Failure to fairly attribute content could side track or delay innovation in digital health applications.

Finally, information searching and reading is no longer lateral, which is a mixed blessing. The average website is a mosaic of images, sound bytes, essays, and links. Not only is the overall impression fragmented, but the user can leap from item to item. Internet-based information providers can promote jumping from topic to topic with hyperlinks; they can also falsify information in ways difficult to detect. The hyperlink is useful when a consumer needs a definition or reference to better understand a point. It is important to be able to make connections across sources—with people whose opinion is trusted, with printed text, and with websites—and more recently with blogs, knols, wikis, and tweets. Consumers with poor information literacy may be unaware of the power of triangulating impressions across sources to fully grasp the information needed to make basic decisions (Norman, 2009). Branching literacy, successful use of hyperlinks without getting confused, becomes critical.

Science and the Mask of Respectability

Science literacy is a specific subset of information literacy. Norman (2009, citing Laugskh, 2000) summarizes *science literacy* as an "understanding of the nature, aims, methods, applications, limitations, and politics of creating knowledge" (p. 13). Norman observes that 83% of Americans are considered unable to understand basic science—in particular its cumulative nature. It is easy for consumers to conclude that simply because a prestigious journal prints a study with seemingly clear conclusions, they must leap to action. Ioannidis (2005) has studied highly cited articles and concluded that almost a third of the highly cited studies in medical research turn out to be refuted or weakened by subsequent studies. In most instances, he argues that this is the scientific process, and consumers need to be aware of the tendency of journals to publish only positive findings. He affirms that most of the time, findings are confirmed. However, in a later study of persistent citing of refuted studies, Ioannidis and colleagues concluded, "it can be difficult to discern whether perpetuated beliefs are based on careful consideration of all evidence and differential interpretation, inappropriate entrenchment of old information, lack of dissemination of newer data, or purposeful silencing of their existence" (Tatsioni, Bonitsis, & Ioannidis, 2007, p. 2525). Interestingly, they did not dwell on how the nature of the Web, in addition to the habits of journal editors, makes it easy to scoop up multiple citations and conclude that the bulk of the evidence is in favor of a particular point of view. Google offers its Google scholar feature that can tell the user how often an article has been cited, but a careful search must be done to see if these citations support or refute a point of view. Many scholars and consumers forget the importance of triangulation—inspecting a variety of sources rather than relying on one.

In addition, despite the move to evidence-based practice, citing systematic reviews of the literature, such as those provided by the Cochrane Collaboration, is still not a threshold criteria for publishing study reports or policy papers. Even systematic reviews must be subjected to triangulation as the case of the "click and get sick" fiasco shows (Eysenbach & Kummervold, 2005). In this case, a systematic review of the literature insisted that people who used health information on the Internet got sicker. The study was eventually withdrawn and error acknowledged. However, perhaps thanks to a story in *Newsweek* magazine, and magnified by the catchy headline in a time when Internet information was suspect, the story persisted. Many sources swiftly cited the original study and the newsy article, but few picked up the acknowledgment of error. This illustrates the importance of traingulation. Secondary citations, such as the news reports above, can create a mask of respectability. Literate consumers will have an attitude of skepticism and a habit of critical analysis. Pew Internet studies suggest that Americans are developing a healthy critical attitude to health information found on the Web (e.g., Fox & Jones, 2009).

Socioemotional literacy required for cyberspace is infrequently mentioned in the digital literacy body of work. However, given the emerging centrality of social networking, it is critical that consumers are aware of the norms of sharing online and recognize affective dimensions (Barak, Boniel-Nissim & Suler, 2008). This literacy requires skill in avoiding cybertraps. Socioemotionally literate consumers are "willing to share their own data and knowledge with others, capable of evaluating data, possessing an abstract thinking, and able to design knowledge through virtual collaboration" (Eshet-Alkali & Amichai-Hamburger, 2004, p. 423). The skills of socioemotional literacy are closely tied to what is sometimes called *media literacy* (Norman, 2009). This refers to the skills necessary to think critically and to act based on information from media-based messages. Norman argues that media literacy places information in a social and political context and considers issues such as the marketplace, audience relations, and the role of the medium in the message. To some extent, these are socioemotional dimensions as the participants seek to play on feelings and beliefs to make their point with cyberaudiences. Those with low media literacy lack awareness of bias or perspective in media pronouncements, both in terms of what is presented and what is not presented. Media literacy requires anticipating that there are explicit and implicit messages in media presentations. These dual meanings must be discerned and analyzed to use the information effectively. Consumers of technology are literate when they appreciate that everyone has an agenda, and that sometimes that agenda will validate your own beliefs and move your own priorities along. Whether that is beneficial depends on the outcome and who is evaluating the results.

Platforms to Access the Internet

Digital literacy requires the ability to navigate the Internet through at least one platform: a computer workstation, handheld device, or a mobile device. Some adults will be called on to participate in telehealth and use a wide range of Internet applications and complementary devices. These applications and devices are adjuncts to a variety of health-related activities. Details of telehealth, Internet applications, and related devices are discussed in separate chapters. This discussion focuses on the skills necessary to access health information and health behavior change resources. These are the skills that build health capital.

Some experts argue that the consumer of the eHealth era must acquire multiple skills to be truly fluent in the media of health exchanges. One model of these core literacies has been summarized by Metros and colleagues (SETDA, 2007) (Table 2.4).

Table 2.5 was prepared to assist educators in understanding core elements of a curriculum for building competencies needed for the digital age. It is more comprehensive than what is needed by the ordinary consumer. However, reading across the columns gives the health professional a sweeping view of the wide range of new expectations for consumer-level skills. For purposes of this book, digital literacy will be an overarching framework that encompasses all of these, albeit in slightly different categories.

The literacies of computer, information, and security will be addressed. Health literacy will be presented as a particular form of information literacy that includes health content, technology, visual media, and numeracy skills.

Core Literacies for Sociotechnical Capital of Health

Basic among these skills are computer literacy, security literacy, information and science literacy, and health literacy. Computer literacy refers to the ability to operate in computer-supported environments, and includes both technical competence and an understanding of how information is presented electronically. Security literacy is knowing the risks of providing personal information, accessing certain files, and protecting one's self from phishing and infectious attacks. Information literacy is knowing how knowledge is organized and includes how to find and use information (American Library Association Committee, 1989, as cited in Norman, 2009). Health literacy has been defined as "the degree to which individuals have the capacity to obtain, process, and understand basic health information and services needed to make appropriate health decisions" (Ratzan & Parker, 2000, para.7).

Computer literacy is detailed in this chapter's section on accessing information on the Internet and in Chapter 5, "Devices as Adjunct to Being Healthy at Home." Security literacy is addressed primarily in both the chapters on personal health records and on devices. Here, an everyday security risk is presented to highlight steps on the path of health literacy. Phishing and infection from disabling agents can create chaos at the speed of a click.

Table 2.4 Media Fluency Landscape Definitions

Computer Literacy	Digital Literacy	Educational Technology	ICT Literacy	Information Literacy	Media Literacy	Technology Literacy	Internet Security
The ability to use a computer and its software to accomplish practical tasks.	Digital literacy is more than just the technical ability to operate digital devices properly; it comprises a variety of cognitive skills that are utilized in executing tasks in digital environments, such as surfing the Web, deciphering user interfaces, working with databases, and chatting in chat rooms.	Educational technology is a systemic approach to teaching and learning that promotes innovative teaching approaches to modernize and improve the school setting. Education technology combines technology equipment to support local, state, and national curriculum standard(s) and imbed 21st-century skills into curricular activities.	Information and communications technology (ICT) literacy is the ability to use technology to develop 21st-century content knowledge and skills, in support of 21st-century teaching and learning.	Information literacy is defined as the ability to know when there is a need for information, to be able to identify, locate, evaluate, and effectively use that information for the issue or problem at hand.	Media literacy is a 21st-century approach to education. It provides a framework to access, analyze, evaluate and create messages in a variety of forms—from print to video to the Internet. Media literacy builds an understanding of the role of media in society as well as essential skills of inquiry and self-expression necessary for citizens of a democracy.	Technology literacy is the ability to responsibly use appropriate technology to communicate, solve problems, and access, manage, integrate, evaluate, and create information to improve learning in all subject areas and to acquire lifelong knowledge and skills in the 21st century.	In the computer industry, refers to techniques for ensuring that data stored in a computer cannot be read or compromised by any individuals without authorization. Most security measures involve data encryption and passwords. Data encryption is the translation of data into a form that is unintelligible without a deciphering mechanism. A password is a secret word or phrase that gives a user access to a particular program or system.
National Forum on Information Literacy	*Eshet-Alkali & Amichai-Hamburger*	*State Educational Technology Directors Association*	*Partnership for 21st Century Skills*	*National Forum on Information Literacy*	*Center for Media Literacy*	*State Educational Technology Directors Association*	*Webopedia*

Source: Courtesy of State Educational Technology Directors Association (2007).

Table 2.5   Skills Framework for Digital Literacy

- Photovisual literacy: Reading instructions from pictures, icons, and symbols as "text"
- Reproduction literacy: Copy-and-paste culture of creativity
- Lateral literacy: Constructing knowledge from hypermedia-branching navigation
- Information literacy: "Trust nobody" critical thinking filter for quality and credibility
- Socioemotional literacy: Sharing and recognizing affective dimensions and avoiding traps

Source: Adapted from Eshet-Alkali & Amichai-Hamburger, 2004.

Consumers are increasingly at risk of *phishing* or viral attacks. Phishing occurs when fraudulent websites are set up with criminal intent. By mimicking a legitimate website, phishers often succeed at getting consumers to provide bank account numbers, home addresses, and other information that facilitates identity theft. Opening an unsolicited link may also be a way to become infected with malicious software. Understanding types of e-mail formats and the logic of the URLs may help consumers avoid these traps. HTML e-mail is basically a Web page that has been e-mailed. Just as any word can be a link to any other website using HTML, the same is true of HTML e-mail. Basically, it is *not necessarily what you see is what you get.* Terry Wolff, Director of Information Technology for the University of Southern California School of Social Work, provides some basic coaching on minimizing this risk (Table 2.6).

Health literacy will be discussed in detail later in this chapter.

Computer and Digital Literacy Variations with Age

For older adults, there are issues in becoming literate with respect to computer access to information online that goes beyond physical and cognitive considerations of aging (see Chapter 5). Computer literacy addresses the ability to engage with digital resources to access information, share information, and engage in interactive experiences. Computer literacy requires knowledge of the physical aspects of turning on the computer, negotiating websites, saving materials, and more. This topic is discussed in greater detail in this chapter's section on information online and in Chapter 5. Literacy skills specific to health information are presented later in this chapter.

Table 2.6 Everyday Internet Security Literacy: Phishing and Infectious Attachments

HTML E-mails

What you see:
- Nice fonts, graphics, etc.
- URL apparently critical to fixing bank account, charge card, e-mail account, etc.

What you don't see:
- The HTML e-mail is a Web page sent by e-mail with link
- Potentially malicious URL hiding behind the link
- Click takes you to fraudulent site for theft of your password, identity, account number, etc., as requested

Basically, it is *not necessarily what you see is what you get.*

Remedies

HTML e-mail:
- Do not click on embedded URLs, even from "known" sources
- Copy and paste the address sent to you into the browser to ensure a link to the actual Web page you are seeking, not hidden URL

Any e-mail with URL link (ALERT: look carefully at links from any e-mail):
- Subtle misspellings may be ignored by human brain
  - For example, http://www.wellfargo.com—missing the *s* in *Wells*
- User is taken to the fake Web page the user actually requested

Attachments:
- Ignore unexpected attachments
- Confirm unexpected attachment with known source
- Common alert: unexpected e-mail with attachment but no actual message
- Special alert: unexpected e-mail attachment with suscpicious generic message and known sender
  - e.g., "your eyes only"; "urgent attention required"

Source: T. Wolff, personal communication, July 17, 2009.

Computer Skills Training for Adults

One dilemma regarding compute literacy in older adults relates to the availability of training and support. Various models have been tried. Some adults learn at senior centers where peers, staff, or student volunteers may provide instruction, coaching, and support without the complication of family tutoring (Jordan-Marsh et al., 2006). Adults who depend on family members, old or young, for computer training may tap into complex dimensions of family relationships. This may create new stressors and exacerbate old ones.

Competition for computer use at home may be an issue as well. Individuals who are not literate might best be encouraged to explore options at community colleges, university extension programs, and community centers. Drawing on family members to supplement skills might be less complicated.

Age and Gender-Related Differences in Digital Information Performance

In a study of age differences in computer literacy performance, Eshet-Alkalai and Geri (2007) found that younger participants did better than older ones with photovisual and branching tasks. Unexpectedly, older adults did significantly better with reproduction and information literacy tasks. The latter is of particular concern for the younger generation as creativity and healthy skepticism are critical skills for the digital age, which will be increasingly dominant in their lives. Health professionals cannot expect that seemingly computer-competent younger adults have the requisite literacy skills in sorting out online health information. Interestingly enough, the researchers concluded that there is no clear body of evidence for gender differences.

HEALTH LITERACY AS THE FULCRUM FOR HEALTH TECHNOLOGY ENGAGEMENT

Health literacy is important because it has an impact on health outcomes, quality of care, and healthcare costs (Hargittai, 2002; IOM, 2009). These outcomes require specific abilities (Table 2.7). Consumers in the new, engaged,

---

Table 2.7   Core Health Literacy Skills

- Navigate the healthcare system, find providers, make appointments, and complete forms.
- Share personal and health information with providers and caregivers.
- Network to engage social support (Caring Bridge, e-mails).
- Engage in self-care and chronic disease management by documenting, monitoring, and learning.
- Participate in online social support and therapy applications.
- Use decision-support tools.
- Act on health-related news and announcements.

Source: Adapted from Hargittai, 2002.

active model of health care are expected to navigate the healthcare system on a geographic and payer level. They must find services within their ability to travel, work out eligibility for services, fill out forms, and monitor billing. Consumers will inform providers of their personal health status and lifestyle patterns, and outcomes of treatments attempted. Consumers are expected to engage in self-care and chronic disease management, adopt a healthy lifestyle, and act on the plethora of news and announcements related to health. Health literacy fact sheets that summarize key points are available from the Center for Health Care Strategies (Potter, 2005).

Health Literacy-Specific Skills

As eHealth is not yet widely known to either consumers or health professionals, it is important to appreciate the wide range of experiences that consumers encounter now and will be encountering soon. Table 2.8 presents a catalog of health-related experiences that are now or will be everyday experiences testing health literacy in the United States.

The National Assessment of Adult Literacy (NAAL) team (White, 2008) collected data in 2003 and documented that health literacy continued to be a major problem in the United States (see also Berkman et al., 2004; Institute of Medicine health literacy reports, 2004, 2009). All of these reports are readily available online (see reference list). The NAAL report provides an in-depth picture of the demands of health literacy in the usual consumer context where reading is required. The report did not address literacy related to listening, which is the most common information exchange in current health provider–consumer interactions. Readers interested in this nondigital dimension can search for literature on adherence and the patient–doctor, patient–provider visit. The NAAL report also did not address situations where the consumer or family member has developed a serious acute or chronic illness and is challenged by the literacy demands of his or her situation with special vocabulary and complex regimens with conflicting advice and research.

In the NAAL report, health literacy skills were assessed across three types of literacy: *document, prose, and quantitative.* These skills were examined in three health-task contexts: *clinical, prevention, and navigation.* Adults were sorted into four levels of performance: below basic, basic, intermediate, and proficient. These concepts are detailed in Figure 2.3. Each of these types is highly relevant to consumer health technology. Health-specific Internet interaction is still predominantly through text and visual material. Spoken material is increasingly available and will be essential to meeting the needs of the linguistically diverse population of the United States (see the section in this chapter on multilingual website issues in the United States).

Table 2.8   Everyday Experiences Testing Health Literacy for the United States[1]

- Articulating or recognizing personal health beliefs, resources, and habits
- Accessing and utilizing information from news announcements and decision aids
- Weighing risks and benefits in making decisions
- Incorporating US healthcare culture assumptions into personal decisions and interactions with providers (prevention, personal responsibility, proactivity, questioning, keeping track of medical history including reports, prescriptions, payment documentation, appointment system)
- Selecting from available healthcare options for compatibility with beliefs, language options, payment expectations, and travel demands
- Accessing local, affordable care across the continuum of primary, secondary, and tertiary promotion, prevention, treatment, and rehabilitation actions
- Distinguishing appropriate care sources and supports based on urgency: 911 emergency departments, urgent care, appointment centers, Internet applications, community-based classes, online groups
- Acting on the right to have an interpreter when provider and patient language differ
- Reading, interpreting, and acting on health-specific instructions and labels
- Using information about medical conditions, symptoms, treatment choices, and prognosis to make decisions
- Communicating questions and concerns to providers either face-to-face, on the telephone, or online
- Actively listening to provider responses and instructions, seeking clarification as needed
- Calculating dosages and adjusting regimen time intervals to personal schedule and events
- Completing forms such as intake, financial resources, and family history
- Seeking reasonable means of securing care (insurance, public benefits and agencies, clinical trials, payment plans, reduced fees)
- Read, interpret, and act on payment for care or eligibility instructions and forms
- Responding to a denial of claims orally or in writing
- *Disclosing information appropriately online to referral services, personal health records, online support groups, social networking sites, etc.*
- *Using personal health records to supply information, access reports, make appointments, secure prescriptions, records of vaccinations, return-to-work letters, monitor accuracy, and update appropriately*
- *Reading the healthcare environment: geography, roles, time cycles (shifts, rotations)*
- *Search and select from online information specific to personal, family, and community healthcare needs with attention to credibility and quality*
- *Using online aids to select from a range of healthcare payment plans and private, employer government options*

(continues)

[1]Italicized items are emerging in the new eHealth paradigm.

Table 2.8   Everyday Experiences Testing Health Literacy for the United States[1] (*continued*)

> - *Using rating systems of healthcare providers, hospitals, prescription plans, government, nonprofit groups, and other healthcare resources to make decisions about access*
> - *Selecting from, arranging installation, and interfacing with potential gadgets, sensors, and other digital resources to meet personal health needs*
> - *Collect and access data from gadgets, sensors, and other digital resources, appreciating trends and sentinel events and taking appropriate action: intervention, contacting healthcare provider or emergency services*

Source: Adapted from Glassman, 2008; Hargittai, 2002; Rosen, 2007; Singleton, 2003.

Figure 2.3   Overview of Literacy by Performance Level: NAAL Study

Level and Definition	Key Abilities Associated with This Level	Sample Health Literacy Tasks Typical of This Level
Below Basic indicates no more than the most simple and concrete literacy skills.	Adults at the ***Below Basic*** level range from being nonliterate in English to having the following abilities: • Locating easily identifiable information in short, commonplace **prose** texts • Locating easily identifiable information and following written instructions in simple **documents** (e.g., charts or forms) • Locating numbers and using them to perform simple **quantitative** operations (primarily addition) when the mathematical information is very concrete and familiar	• Searching a short, simple text to find out what a patient is allowed to drink before a medical test • Signing a form

Figure 2.3   Overview of Literacy by Performance Level: NAAL Study (*continued*)

Level and Definition	Key Abilities Associated with This Level	Sample Health Literacy Tasks Typical of This Level
Basic indicates skills necessary to perform simple and everyday literacy activities.	• Reading and understanding information in short, commonplace **prose** texts • Reading and understanding information in simple **documents** • Locating easily identifiable **quantitative** information and using it to solve simple, one-step problems when the arithmetic operation is specified or easily inferred	• Giving two reasons a person with no symptoms of a specific disease should be tested for the disease, based on information in a clearly written pamphlet • Entering names and birth dates in a health insurance application • Calculating what time to take a medication by combining two pieces of information
Intermediate indicates skills necessary to perform moderately challenging literacy activities.	• Reading and understanding moderately dense, less commonplace **prose** texts as well as summarizing, making simple inferences, determining cause and effect, and recognizing the author's purpose • Locating information in dense, complex **documents** and making simple inferences about the information • Locating less familiar **quantitative** information and using it to solve problems when the arithmetic operation is not specified or easily inferred	• Consulting reference materials to determine which foods contain a particular vitamin • Finding the age range during which children should receive a particular vaccine by using a chart that shows all the childhood vaccines and the ages when children should receive them • Determining a healthy weight range for a person of a specified height, based on a graph that relates height and weight to body mass index (BMI)

(*continues*)

Figure 2.3 Overview of Literacy by Performance Level: NAAL Study (*continued*)

Level and Definition	Key Abilities Associated with This Level	Sample Health Literacy Tasks Typical of This Level
Proficient indicates skills necessary to perform more complex and challenging literacy activities.	• Reading lengthy, complex, abstract **prose** texts as well as synthesizing information and making complex inferences • Integrating, synthesizing, and analyzing multiple pieces of information located in complex **documents** • Locating more abstract **quantitative** information and using it to solve multistep problems when the arithmetic operations are not easily inferred and the problems are more complex	• Comparing the power of attorney with a living will and determining the advantage of the power of attorney • Interpreting a table about blood pressure, age and physical activity • Computing the price per year of an insurance policy

Source: White, 2008. Used with permission.

Health Literacy Types: Prose, Document, Quantitative

The types of health literacy (photovisual, reproduction, visual, and branching literacies) were previously described in this chapter in terms of the task required (p. 59). *Prose literacy* is the knowledge and skills required for continuous texts (sentences organized in a paragraph). To be literate one must search, comprehend, and use information. Prose literacy tasks are performed in obtaining health information from brochures, instructional materials, and newspapers. Online, these skills are needed for reading blog, knol, and wiki postings, as well as website essays and reports and for searching for visual media.

Document literacy refers to the knowledge and skills required for searching, comprehending, and using formats where the text is not continuous (some examples are lists, rows, columns, matrices, graphs). Document literacy tasks include filling out health insurance forms, studying charts or graphs in health materials, searching a map to find a health service location, or finding the proper dose on a drug label. Online, users choose from a list of links to access other material, complete questionnaires, and update personal health records.

Quantitative literacy in the NAAL report refers to knowledge and skills needed to perform quantitative tasks using information and numbers embedded in printed materials. The relevant skills are identifying and performing computations, alone or in sequence. Quantitative tasks are performed when comparing health-care costs, performing on-the-spot calculations of the practical meaning of food labels, determining the timing of medications, or calculating how to adjust timing of medications or treatments when schedules change or unexpected events occur. Online, users may need to compare their medication dose to posted ranges. As personal health records become available, users will be looking at laboratory values with actual and usual ranges for contrast. White (2008) noted that quantitative tasks were the most challenging because they usually required prose, document, and computational skills.

Health Literacy Tasks: Clinical, Preventive, Navigational

The NAAL report (White, 2008) described three major health literacy tasks. *Clinical tasks* are those activities specific to the patient–provider interaction around screening for and treatment of illnesses. This includes understanding instructions for medication doses and treatment procedures and preparing for screening procedures. *Preventive tasks* are more independent and focus on self-care and self-management to maintain and improve health and prevent illness. These are tasks that require understanding guidelines for preventive health services and establishing habits to build a healthy lifestyle. The third task was labeled *navigation* of the healthcare system, which White described as covering rights and responsibilities specific to eligibility for assistance, finding the location of services, and "later interpreting" the bill (White, 2008, p. 7). In the future, assessment of navigation skills could include finding and interacting with health-specific resources on the Internet.

All of these tasks are affected by website design. The design of a healthcare website is a critical factor in supporting consumers across literacy levels. One of the most comprehensive guides for constructing health information technology applications is available at the Agency for Healthcare Research and Quality (AHRQ) website and is titled "Accessible Health Information Technology (IT) for Populations with Limited Literacy: A Guide for Developers and Purchasers of Health IT" (Eichner & Dullabh, 2007). AHRQ is tracking the number of hits and downloads from this page, but there is no current information on who is using the guide and what their experience is (Brach, 2009). Dissemination of this guide and evaluation of its effectiveness and implementation would significantly enhance the experience of consumers with limited health literacy.

Rule of Three for Online Information

Consumers going online for information and support face a particular challenge if they or their significant others are struggling with chronic conditions.

There is an emerging consensus (Isham, 2009) that people can juggle only three concepts at a time. Similarly, a standard of website design that is gaining popularity is the 3-clicks rule (Brach, 2009). Beyond three links, the assumption is that the searcher will discontinue the search and leave the website. It is not clear whether these limitations will persist as individuals gain skill in manipulating their searches, saving them, and creating new personally relevant composite searches from preexisting material.

Health Literacy Tasks of the Future: Navigating Electronic Records and Games

As the nation moves to electronic health records and provides the personal health record component, new "navigation" skills will be required. Also, at the time of the NAAL report, few instances of health-related digital games were available, so gaming was not presented as a context (Brown, 2009). However, as noted in Hawn (2009), digital games with a wide range of peripherals and sensors are showing promise in promoting health and recovery from trauma. Playing a digital game calls on document and quantitative literacy, minimally on prose literacy.

However, there is a whole separate literacy of gaming that is not obvious to the uninitiated. The required literacies for gaming include knowing how to get started, understanding of achievement through levels, knowing when to collect prizes or pass them by, how to link with friends who are also playing, and accessing games that are free versus one-time purchase or a continuous subscription. Health-specific literacies of gaming are also related to safety behaviors—both preventive of physical damage by using equipment improperly and preventive of physical damage from overdoing. Appreciating the difference between the game core play and embedded minigames can make play more pleasant. As the "game-care revolution" (Brown, 2009) plays out, users will need to learn how to report game play to health professionals—such as length of play, outcomes, and choice of games. Chapter 6 of this book discusses health games.

Technology as a Resource for Improving Health Literacy and Health Outcomes

Pignone, DeWalt, Sheridan, Berkman, and Lohr (2005) did an extensive review of the literature on interventions designed to improve health literacy. They looked at over 3000 studies held from 1980 to 2003. Only 20 met the criteria of rigorous research. Whether the outcome was health knowledge, health behaviors, proxy measures, prevalence, or severity of disease, the results were too mixed for practice recommendations. Paasche-Orlow, Schillinger, Greene, and Wagner (2006) suggest that technology will advance the ability to tailor interventions to specific needs, skills, and preferences of the consumer. They referred, in particular, to nascent health dialog systems as an emerging resource in overcoming literacy limitations.

Health Dialog Systems for Health Information and Behavior Change

The expectation that consumers will take more responsibility for their health comes at a time when providers have less time for coaching and counseling. Bickmore and Giorgino (2006) find that there has been progress in automating the delivery of *static media* (printed materials, Web pages) for health outcomes. However, in their review, they noted that when delivery is static, tailoring to an individual's needs is *asynchronous* if the provider is not close at hand. Consumers may want information to be rephrased if it is not clear, they want to ask questions, and pace the flow of information.

Bickmore and Giorgino (2006) note that gaining information necessary for sound diagnosis and relevant treatment plans is difficult for providers in the current healthcare system. Patients have an equally difficult time in making sense of what they are to do about what they are told. Bickmore and Giorgino comment on the constraints put on patients by the time pressure of a healthcare appointment. Such appointments are routinely less than 15 minutes. Patients become reluctant to ask questions or take time to process information and personalize it. Bickmore and Giordino note another, less often discussed drawback of the live interaction: *fidelity* (p. 557). As they note, providers do not always follow clinical practice guidelines, thus creating variation that might be undesirable to the agency. Providers also can get distracted by unexpected issues that arise in the visit and may not get to all the critical points. Bickmore and Giordino also remind us that personal convenience and financial and scheduling issues limit consumer access to all the resources they might prefer.

Bickmore and Giorgino (2006) argue that simulations or health dialog systems "may even be better than interacting with a human provider" (p. 556). Simulations and health dialog systems are interaction innovations consumers sometimes label as "talking to the robot." This is a system where, instead of a person interviewing the patient, an intelligent query and response computer interaction is set up. Bickmore and Giorgino are at the forefront of designing friendly, true-to-life voice tones and phrases—removing the robot element. A well-designed dialog system technology can overcome time pressure and translation issues. Other advantages they cite are novel interaction formats where consumers engage in role playing with scripted "peer" characters. These systems can be totally telephone-based and require only basic touchtone phone technology and skills once the agency produces the program.

Dialog systems are ideal, Bickmore and Giordino (2006) assert, for moving from the paternalistic norms of professional–client interactions. In the new eHealth model, "health professional and client work together on an equal footing to come up with a treatment plan that fits into the client's life" (p. 559). Natural language *argumentation* systems with social, emotional, and relational dimensions are emerging that build an anthropomorphic relationship between the consumer/patient and the computerized dialog system. These systems will move forward in providing true interactive *counseling* that is finely tailored to "personal characteristics, the current situation, and all that has been communicated before" (p. 465). Achievement of this match will take eHealth well beyond providing health education to promoting lifestyle health behavior change and chronic disease management. These applications advance from building literacy to conducting telehealth without real-time engagement of a health professional. Asynchronous, data store, and forward technology allows convenient, time-of-urgency telehealth access for the consumer and builds a database for systematic analysis by the health professional and researchers. Telehealth or telecare and its complexity is covered in the first and final chapters.

VISUAL LITERACY

The Significance of Visual Literacy

In contemporary health care, consumers and health professionals alike are confronted with a wide array of visual stimuli in digital format. These can come as instructional materials, video clips, Web searches, online applications of learning and behavior change, financial systems, appointment systems, and more (Table 2.9).

One can encounter these visuals at any time in the continua of interaction with the healthcare system, when trying to navigate online information, social networking, completing eligibility forms, interpreting instructions for health-related devices, monitoring remote progress, and in any engagements with virtual worlds.

Visuals are increasingly important to surviving and thriving in a digital world where social capital and health capital are conveyed by images as much as by words. Information literacy is no longer possible without strong visual literacy skills. Visuals document, validate, communicate, inform, engage, expose, politicize, and provoke the viewer (Metros, 2008b).

Visuals are thrust upon the users of the Internet and digital devices for the purpose of marketing, instructing, and influencing decisions health consumers will make. Visual literacy is important to critical analysis of materials presented by others to advance their agendas. Images may be juxtaposed, edited, and manipulated to achieve a desired message. Although drug companies may come to mind as using visuals to sell their products, consumer groups with a point of view use the same tactics, especially regarding such controversial subjects as abortion or vaccination.

Table 2.9   Variations in Visual Depictions of Data, Information, and Knowledge

Type	Description
Chart/graph	Representation of tabular numeric data and/or functions that may show growth or change over time
Table	Matrix for organizing large quantities of numerical data
Flowchart	Hierarchical branching structure that indicates steps in a process or procedure or decision points in diagnosing a problem
Diagram	Visual representation of concepts, ideas, constructions, relations, statistical data, anatomy, etc.
Mind or concept map	Nonlinear diagram depicting relationships between ideas and concepts
Storyboard	Graphic organizing device that depicts a sequence of illustrations or images for the purpose of planning and envisioning a motion graphic or interactive media sequence
Schematic	Technical drawing illustrating parts of an object and their relationship to each other
Blueprint	Technical drawing documenting an architectural or an engineering design or more generic detailed plan
Map	Simplified depiction of a space that highlights relationships between components

(continues)

Table 2.9   Variations in Visual Depictions of Data, Information, and Knowledge (*continued*)

Type	Description
Symbol	Object, character, figure, sound, or color used to represent an abstract idea or concept
Icon	Image, picture, symbol, or mark that signifies or represents an object or concept
Signage/label	Graphic displaying way-finding or identifying information
Photograph/video	Actual object or scene captured and recorded through the lens of a camera or other imaging device
Drawing/painting	Two-dimensional, artistic representation created using artist tools such as pencil, ink, crayon, paint, charcoal, pastel, and/or digital software
Illustration	A visualization such as a drawing, painting, or photograph created to elucidate or embellish something described in text
Cartoon/caricature	Illustration that humorously or satirically depicts a current event or exaggerates a likeness
Simulation	Computerized, sometimes animated, representation or modeling of characteristics, actions, or events for the purpose of running alternative scenarios and/or testing and observing behavior
Immersive environment	Artificial, interactive, computer-created scene or "world" often used in video and online games in which users feel like they are part of the simulated "universe"

Source: Adapted from Metros, 2008b.

A new development in the era of eHealth is the ability, and expectation, for ordinary consumers and health professionals to create visuals. Health professionals increasingly must develop their own visual literacy in order to act in concert with consumers, and to take leadership in providing true peer review of teaching materials, websites, games, and other digital media. Consumers will be motivated to create images to tell the story of their health and illness journey. The impetus for this use of visuals will come from social networking site experiences and engagement in personal health records (see the section in Chapter 2 on personal health records).

Levels of Visual Literacy

Metros (2008a) proposed levels of visual literacy. The first is *observer*; many people fit in this category.[1] This would describe individuals who are surrounded by visuals, may enjoy them overtly or engage mostly at a subliminal level. These individuals do not deliberately create visuals other than perhaps documenting faces, events, and places in snapshots. Judgments are primarily aesthetic and practical: "Do I have a record?" "Is this a good picture of…?" Sharing images is limited to posting by mail or to an Internet site.

The next level of visual literacy would be *stimulated*. At this level, the individual is aware of living in a visually saturated world, interacts with visuals every day, is an amateur producer and manipulator, imitates rather than innovates, and lacks knowledge to judge visuals produced by self or others. The stimulated individual is at risk of visual overload. The third level is *literate*. At this level, the individual understands design vocabulary and concepts; is an informed viewer, decoder, and consumer; is an effective communicator who can encode and produce original works or unique composites of preexisting works; and is an informed critic of visual information. The components of critiques are discussed in a subsequent section of this chapter. Literate individuals have strategies for resolving visual overload.

The fourth level, *fluent*, occurs when the individual is a knowledgeable and highly skilled innovator, designer, composer, and producer. At the level of fluency, the individual is able to prevent as well as diagnose the risk of visual overload. Metros (2008a) notes that part of building skill and advancing in literacy levels is recognizing one's preferred style of learning (auditory, kinesthetic, visual, or textual). Fluent individuals are skilled in recognizing and supporting individuals whose preferred style of learning is predominantly visual. In addition to the skills specific to each level and recognition of preferred learning styles, health professionals will need new vocabularies. The vocabulary and concepts components of construction and analysis of visuals proposed by Metros (2008a) include elements, attributes, and relationships, in addition to the message itself. The details of each component are listed in Table 2.10. See also the section in this chapter on creating visually skillful materials. A detailed tutorial is beyond the

---

[1]First level added by M. Jordan-Marsh on conferring with S. Metros (personal communication, August 1, 2009).

Table 2.10   Components of Visuals: Construction and Analysis

Elements	Attributes
• Point	• Color/tone
• Line	• Texture
• Form	• Volume
	• Size
Relationships	Function
• Structure	• Document
• Balance	• Validate
• Contrast	• Communicate
• Position	• Inform
• Motion	• Engage
	• Expose
	• Politicize
	• Provoke

Source: Metros, 2008a. Courtesy of Susan E. Metros.

scope of this book. Readers are referred to a video of Metros describing her approach: http://unescochair.blogs.uoc.edu/23032009/susan-metros-visual-literacy-conference-video.

Critical Analysis of Visuals for Health Technology Consumers

Design concepts include font selection, navigation, layout, hierarchy of information, and attention to the components of construction and analysis of visual images. For health technology consumers, in-depth knowledge of design-specific components of imagery is not required (i.e., elements, attributes, and relationships of imagery details). Rather, the savvy consumer will appreciate that these components can be arranged to manipulate their response to visual images. For example, color and tone can be changed to signal displeasure or emphasize negative aspects of an image. Portraying a person in muddy colors with words overlaid can suggest criminal tendencies without saying a word. A frequently presented example can be found by searching "magazine covers OJ Simpson." One blog (http://www.museumofhoaxes.com/hoax/photo_database/image/darkened_mug_shot) describes the manipulation and gives the link to the *Time* magazine apology. Positioning can also be used to make a point. A common strategy for inflating results is to switch the angle of presentation. For example, examine before-and-after pictures that use full frontal photos of the undesirable state (fatness, acne, etc.) and then use a profile to show the positive results of a product. The profile view is more limiting and can exaggerate the message that minimal improvements are major changes.

Understanding and recognizing the intended *function* of the designed image is very important for consumer visual literacy. Analyzing the goal of the image designer can be very informative in making a decision about how to respond after viewing a visual presentation. A visual may be presented simply to document or provide evidence of something. In a new personal weight-management program, some individuals may take photos of themselves to document their baseline. Serial photos may be used to validate that progress is being made. In some programs, the photos may be shared with health professionals to inform the provider that the client is engaged in weight management. The photo series may be shared to communicate progress and to engage the provider in coaching or reinforcement.

If individuals are doing weight management together, one may use a photo at a party to expose an unhealthy behavior in an attempt to provoke their partner to do better. Some public health advocates are using photos of overweight children to politicize the discussion of the seriousness of the obesity epidemic. The level of literacy needed for analysis of visuals requires being informed about potential functions and biases surrounding a health issue or health behaviors. The literate consumer decodes the presentation of the image to analyze the function and the corresponding message. Recognizing one's response to an image designed by another is a requirement for being literate.

Creating Visually Skillful Instructional Materials

Images for instructional materials include diagrams, graphs, tables, figures, photographs, videos, symbolic pictorials, and graphics that range from abstract to complex in detail, color, and motion. Advances in digital media mean that health professionals have the ability to instantly insert photos or symbolic images from stock collections. This gives rise to the expectation that anyone can create instructional materials spontaneously. However, reviews of the literature on pictorial aids suggest that creating instructions is a complex process (Houts, n.d.; Katz, Kripalani, & Weiss, 2006; Metros, 2008a). Consumers in the eHealth paradigm will be expected to view a wide range of images, rate their credibility and quality, to build skills and form attitudes and use them in decisions about health actions.

Visuals as Behavioral versus Conceptual Triggers

Increasingly, patient education materials are shifting from having a traditionally heavy focus on concepts and knowledge to a focus on behavior. The emphasis is on providing what the consumer *needs to do* rather than what the user *needs to know* (Seligman et al., 2007). As awareness of the limitations of literacy independent of language grows simultaneously with new digital options for manipulating images, visual aids receive more attention. In constructing visuals for behavior change, designers are encouraged to revisit the table on critical analysis of visuals (Table 2.10). This analysis will also be helpful in coaching patients and consumers on "reading" visuals.

Adherence and Image or Text Blends

The extant literature (Houts, n.d.; Katz et al., 2006; Seligman et al., 2007) clearly validates the incorporation of pictorials or photographs with instructions on health actions. Providing images incorporated with appropriate text has been repeatedly shown to increase retention of information and adherence to proposed regimens. Interestingly, the use of photographs has not necessarily created an advantage over pictorials that are symbolic and suggestive rather than photographic.

Culture and Imagery

Culture plays a large role in determining effectiveness (Houts, n.d.). A photograph makes clear the match or discrepancy between the individual portrayed and the gender, age, dress, body image, and ethnicity or race of the learner. The consumer may rate the information as lacking relevance. The author did a trial of a pain management scale using photographs to indicate levels of pain (Jordan-Marsh et al., 2004). Although the nurse could offer a Caucasian, Asian, or African American version, little girls sometimes refused to "tell me which picture shows how much hurt you have now" as they were presented with only little boy pictures. The girls said, I "only see boys."

In addition, photographs of health professionals with learner consumers can create similar incongruities (Houts, n.d.). In the past, the typical healthcare professional was a white male. Health education materials increasingly are including more diverse people as professionals and patients. However, given the broad range of human beings, more attention should be paid to tailoring materials to the audience. Houts recommends including representatives of the target audience when creating materials. When healthcare groups can use technology to incorporate images congruent with the patient–provider population, there may be powerful advantages.

Seligman et al. (2007), in their report of engaging consumers in design and production of materials, learned that low-literacy learners disliked pictorials

Figure 2.4   Using the Patient's Voice to Offer Concrete Behavior-Change Suggestions

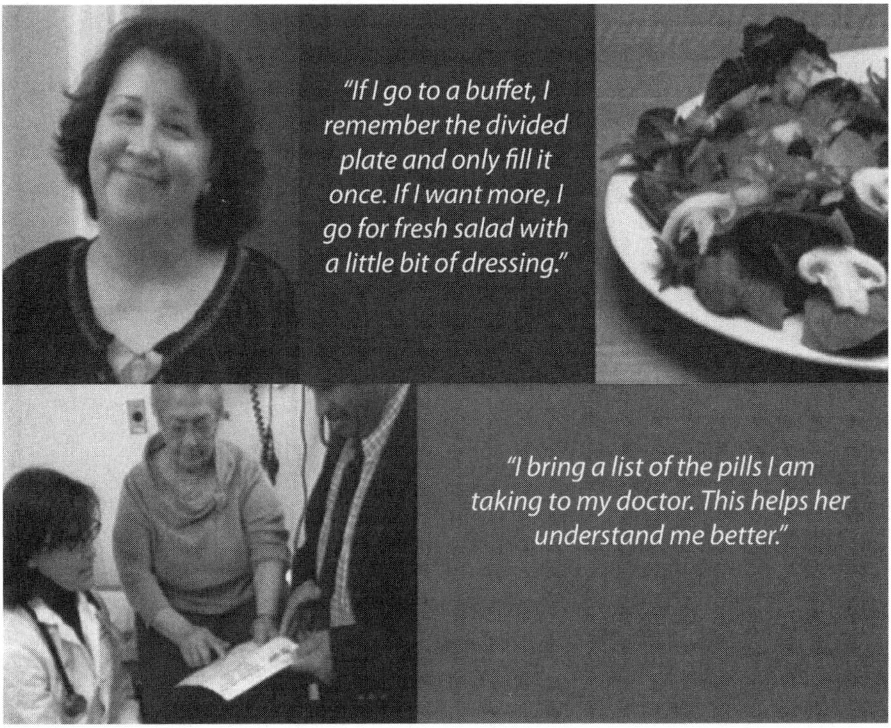

"If I go to a buffet, I remember the divided plate and only fill it once. If I want more, I go for fresh salad with a little bit of dressing."

"I bring a list of the pills I am taking to my doctor. This helps her understand me better."

Source: Seligman et al., 2007, p. S77. Used with permission.

and preferred photos. For adults, a mix of genders, body sizes, and ethnicities might be very effective (Figure 2.4). Advances in technology are such that for a small cost, developers of health education materials might supply a template and a range of photos to insert given the target audience. No reports of this kind of tailoring were found, however. When materials-rich programs fail to obtain expected results, a study of the match of images to target participants might be enlightening.

Clear, simple text to accompany the pictures is essential (Houts, n.d.; Katz et al., 2006; Seligman et al., 2007). The slide presentation assembled by Houts (n.d.) illustrates these issues (see http://healthliteracy.worlded.org/visuals_in_ health.pdf). A graphic example is given in Figure 2.5.

In fact, Houts (n.d.) suggests that we shift from the common assumption of fifth-grade literacy to an expectation of second-grade literacy. He proposes a "caption" approach to combinations of text and pictorials. He provides a link to captions approved by second-grade teachers (http://www.frycomm.com/ags/eldercare/caregiving_handout_MSWord.pdf).

Designers may want to consider the wide range of visual charts that can convey an idea. Lengler and Eppler have provided an interactive display as a periodic table of visualization methods that is available at http://www.visual-literacy.org/periodic_table/periodic_table.html#. The table arranges methods by their purpose using labels such as a Venn diagram. Running a cursor over the specific method evokes a visual example of the method.

HEALTH NUMERACY

Definition of Health Numeracy

Health numeracy is the "Productive use of quantitative health information, i.e., the effective use of quantitative information to guide health behavior and make health decisions" (Ancker & Kaufman, 2007, p. 713). The consumer, in this model, is required to obtain, process, and apply information to accomplish core tasks in managing health care. Ancker and Kaufman propose four components to health numeracy: *basic quantitative skills, ability to use information artifacts* (e.g., navigating documents), *ability to communicate orally, and information design*. As personal health records become a standard part of health management, the ability to digitally record personal health values obtained at

---

Figure 2.5   Clear Labels May Allow Images to Communicate Important Concepts Without Having to Read Additional Text

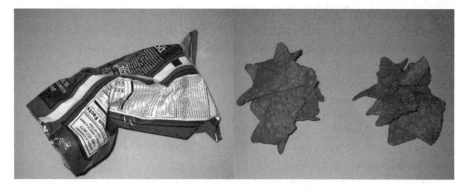

Source: Adapted from Seligman et al., 2007.

home and to communicate such quantitative information by e-mail or other applications such as Facebook will increase in importance.

For the health professional who has completed a college education, it will be difficult to appreciate the extent to which these skills present a challenge for others, especially older adults. As we shift to greater consumer empowerment and responsibility, new skills are required. A number of the increasingly common self-health management tasks have large quantitative components that may intimidate many consumers. A list is offered in Table 2.11.

We have long expected consumers to collect data about their body temperature, although it is important to note that the task is sufficiently complex that multiple devices have evolved to simplify the process. This includes disposable devices that provide a digital readout. Increasingly, measures of blood pressure are done at home. As body computing advances, there will be many devices that collect numbers that contribute to decisions about health behaviors, including medication choices. The Nike link to a device embedded in a shoe that counts steps, miles, and minutes is one example of new applications that challenge health numeracy (see http://www.apple.com/ipod/nike). Pedometers and accelerometers are becoming more common in promoting physical activity for any age.

Table 2.11   Health Numeracy Skill Challenge Examples

- Appointment slips: Interpreting, balancing multiple providers
- Online appointment scheduling
- Medication schedules: Routine and adaptations for missed dose
- Diluting concentrations: Medicated shampoos, infant and adult formulas
- Procedure and treatment regimens
- Nutrition information: Reading labels
- Food value ratios: Balancing fat, fiber, calories
- Weight management
- Behavior counts: Recording, reviewing
- Health game scores
- Laboratory values: Consumer-initiated action, contact provider
- Vital sign measures
- Bone density reports: Improvement in face of negative values
- Risks and benefits of therapies
- Billing reports: Accuracy, fraud watch
- Insurance plan choices, including Medicare drug plan
- Data entry for consumer-collected data: Personal health records, EHR

(continues)

Table 2.11   Health Numeracy Skill Challenge Examples (*continued*)

- Accelerometer or pedometer data
- Daily vitamin requirements: Food and supplement balance
- Risk ratio and prevalence data for decisions
- Interpretation of trend data: Positive and negative slopes, significance of spikes

Significance of Health Numeracy

Inadequate numeracy can be linked to poor health outcomes (Rothman, Montori, Cherrington, & Pignone, 2008). In fact, Rothman and colleagues note that people with adequate literacy for printed text may be unable to work with numbers. "Numeracy may be a unique explanatory factor for adverse outcomes beyond the explanations provided by overall literacy" (p. 585). As they summarize, many of the tasks of self-management for chronic illness require numeracy skills

> such as reading food labels, refilling prescriptions, measuring medications, interpreting blood sugars or other clinical data, and understanding health risks…. These tasks often require patients to deduce which mathematical skills to use and then to use these in a multistep fashion. (p. 585)

Before patients can compute, estimate, or interpret data, they must acquire it, often from documents, scales, or other information artifacts. Three interrelated skills (representational fluency, document literacy, and graphical literacy) have been described as necessary for using information artifacts in health care (Ancker & Kaufman, 2007). This means that consumers will have to interpret what certain configurations of numbers represent, make sense of them in documents discussing ideal physiological parameters (e.g., blood pressure), and use graphical displays to note progress or comparison to similar patients. Consumers will be able to, and be expected to, upload information collected by these devices. It will be important to read uploaded entries for accuracy, use graphs of progress that are generated by accompanying software, compare personal data to guidelines based on age and gender, and set reasonable goals. All these tasks require numeracy and digital literacy skills.

Whether patients successfully use their everyday life numeracy skills to advantage in managing their health depends on both the consumer/patient and the provider. Ancker and Kaufman (2007) describe four factors that contribute to patients' success (see Table 2.12). These include basic quantitative skills, ability to use "information artifacts" such as graphs and device readings, oral communication skills to communicate clearly, and, by implication, access to good design.

Table 2.12   Factors Contributing to a Patient's Ability to Use Quantitative Information for Health

	Factor	Definition	Examples
Patient factors	Patients' quantitative skills	Basic computational skills (such as addition, multiplication, and use of simple formulas), estimation, and statistical literacy	Computing calorie content; comparing computation to determine whether it is correct; understanding concept of randomization in a clinical trial
	Patients' ability to use information artifacts	Ability to navigate documents, interpret graphs, and translate between different representations of the same information	Obtaining nutrient information from a nutrition label; comparing personal health data as displayed on different meters or devices
	Patients' oral communication skills	Ability to speak clearly about quantities and understand spoken information	Reporting a previous medication regimen accurately to a new physician
	Information design for patients	Arrangement of information media and symbols to support comprehension and cognition	Designing a patient interface for an electronic health record that provides graphics to illustrate numerical information
Provider factors	Providers' oral communication skills	Ability to communicate quantitative concepts clearly to the patient	Explaining a new medication regimen to a patient in an understandable fashion
	Providers' quantitative skills	Basic computational skills, estimation, and statistical literacy	Converting between units of measure; understanding the positive predictive power of a diagnostic test
	Providers' ability to use information artifacts	Ability to navigate documents, interpret graphs, translate between representations of the same information	Interpreting a graph of patient lab values over time; applying the numerical output of a decision support system to an individual case
	Information design for providers	Ability of a system or document to support the provider's cognition	Designing a provider interface that provides automated conversions between units of measure

Source: Ancker & Kaufman, 2007, p. 713. Used with permission.

Definitions of the factors and how they apply in health situations to patients and to providers are detailed in the table. Research on the effectiveness of new personal health records calling on quantitative skills requires attention to these variables and not simply to outcomes. Failure to achieve desired outcomes of new information enabled by personal health records may be a failure related to these potential mediators as much as any limitation of the new record system interface or structure.

The Numeracy Challenge of Interpreting Risk

One major task consumers face is related to assessing risk in terms of a treatment choice. Making a truly informed choice requires statistical literacy (Ancker & Kaufman, 2007). Risk is related to complex concepts, they note, such as chance and uncertainty, sampling variability, margins of error, and randomization in clinical trials. These concepts are even difficult for some physicians to comprehend. New ways of conveying risk will be possible as both consumers and health professionals gain visual literacy. The Internet already provides interactive approaches to understanding risk.

Numeracy Assessment by Task

Although tools are available for assessing the "readability" level of documents (some word-processing programs offer it as a feature), there are no similar tools that characterize quantitative demands. Similarly, instruments are available to assess aspects of numeracy in patients, but no assessments have been developed to evaluate providers' ability to create materials containing information about numbers that their patients can understand. Rothman et al. (2008) provide a detailed table of numeracy assessment tools without endorsing any one as meaningful. Some are quite limited, as in assessing only the ability to read a nutrition label. As with health literacy in general, Rothman and colleagues raise the question of the potential harm of embarrassing clients by revealing their inadequacies.

Potential of Technology to Minimize Numeracy Demands

Rothman and colleagues (2008) list interventions to minimize poor numeracy skills:

> Potential interventions could include color-coded measuring devices that replace measurement-related numeracy, picture- or table-based materials that replace medication instructions, simplification of current labels to ease interpretation,

and computerized interventions that convert mathematical problems or instructions into goal-oriented text, pictures, or verbal instruction. (p. 593)

Internet applications will make these changes readily accessible if they are conceptualized with digital literacy skills in mind.

Paasche-Orlow and Wolfe (2008) have made a strong case against screening selected patients for their level of literacy. They point out that available tools seem to test general reading ability rather than health literacy. They argue that available tests do not take into account that consumers with a specific health issue may have developed adequate levels of literacy for that condition. This competence would not be addressed with current tools. Paasche-Orlow and Wolfe indicated that such screening, if targeted, has the potential to embarrass patients to the point of anxiety that interferes with critical learning and collaboration.

Mancuso (2009) reviews available screening tools and is equally dismissive of their value. She notes that the two best-known tools, ReALM and S-TOFHLA were designed for use in internal medicine contexts and are not relevant to pediatrics. She also suggests a purpose-specific measure with attention to language and culture. The eHeals scale (Norman & Skinner, 2006) is cited as an example. This tool is available free at http://www.jmir.org/2006/4/e27. The eHeals scale is reported to have high reliability and internal consistency, is translated into multiple languages, and in use in 10 countries. Although the tool has been cited by others, reports of use for adults have not surfaced as of 2009 other than by Norman (2009).

Paasche-Orlow et al. (2006) make a strong case for offering assistance with literacy on a "universal precautions" philosophy. This would mean assuming that all consumers need assistance and allowing them to demonstrate skills to the contrary. The author once had a family physician who was fond of saying, "I know you are a nurse and probably teach this, but, I have a rule that everybody gets...." He would then offer a variety of assistive resources (pamphlets, tutorial, demonstrations). This universal precaution approach is particularly valuable when patients are receiving difficult news. Anxiety may overwhelm usual coping skills, including numeracy. The alternative is potential embarrassment and subsequent reluctance to engage with health professionals.

Sample Task with Numeracy Challenges: AskBlue Website

Numeracy challenges abound in the healthcare environment. As indicated earlier, dealing with insurance plans, choosing a plan, and ensuring claims are processed accurately is a task of health literacy. Numeracy challenges (and digital literacy challenges) are illustrated in an interactive application from Blue

Shield and Blue Cross. If a consumer read a news story about the new Blue Shield/Blue Cross service called AskBlue and searched for it on the Internet but did not notice that there was no space between the words "Ask" and "Blue," then the consumer was taken to an irrelevant website. If the user scrolled to the proper link on the search page, he or she would find http://www.bcbs.com/innovations/askblue. Clicking on that link brought the user to a suspiciously named link: http://ic.jellyvision-conversation.com. This actually is the page for sorting out costs of possible insurance plans. But the challenges don't end there.

The next difficulty arises in trying to enter the birth date of the potential insured in the application form. Failure to use the correct digital format of two digits for every month (09 for September) and four digits for the year (2001) simply results in a message that the birth date is invalid. Users are not directed to an example of a correct entry or coached on potential problems. This frustration occurs long before the actual comparison of health plans. Clearly, this is a failure in user-centered design. Over time, as more consumers check out the site, given the structure of search engines, the link to a college humor website and YouTube videos may be displaced in the rank ordering. The challenges of website designs were discussed earlier with a link to relevant resources.

HEALTH TECHNOLOGY LITERACY: LANGUAGE AS A BARRIER

For American immigrants, finding health information in another language can be very difficult. With respect to health, *linguistic literacy* becomes important as families struggle to support the sharp increase in older adults who have new health challenges. Illness, new diagnoses, and new expectations in this age of self-care create anxieties. Anxious people can be more comfortable if information is available in their preferred or first language. There are a variety of ways that first-language health information is available. For example, MedlinePlus offers information in over 40 languages. SPIRAL is a website that makes Asian language health information accessible: http://www.library.tufts.edu/hhsl/spiral/index.html.

However, the first linguistic literacy challenge is appreciating where the information is available. Savvy health professionals who speak only English might search *health information Chinese* and get to these resources. A specific topic search of *diabetes Chinese language* will get searchers to SPIRAL and other resources. The same phrase using *Korean* retrieves a variety of resources, and SPIRAL is one of the lower listed resources.

Multilingual Website Issues in the United States

For the health professional, or family member who did not learn the older adult's language, there are multiple challenges. On MedlinePlus, the English language user has no information or cues as to the comparability of materials in other languages. The next challenge is that the user must select the language searching. The complication of this sequencing is that the health professional is not able to look up a health topic, see what is available, skim for relevance, and then click a language. On MedlinePlus, if you are on the topic page and use the search bar to insert *Chinese*, for example, the results list is not relevant.

On SPIRAL, if one searches by topic, the English language reader can see links to available materials in multiple languages, and English is always one choice. The description of criteria for selection of materials to post states that an "English language version is available for comparison." This gives the health professional or caregiver some confidence. Another advantage of the SPIRAL website is the links to other Web resources for translated materials.

The 24 Languages Project could be a very useful resource in that there are sound recordings for many of the entries (http://library.med.utah.edu/24languages). For each language page, there is a note that an English version is available. The non-English entries have sound and some have videos. The English entries seem to be only PDF files. However, there is no search function. You simply click on a language and surf to see what topics have been posted. This website also provides links to other URLs with language flexibility.

Sustaining a website with up-to-date links is very difficult in that the content and sponsorship are dynamic. Sites may be well designed, but not up-to-date. For some health problems, this may not be an issue. However, for many topics, there are changes in thinking as new technology allows new questions and finds more rigorous solutions. The WHERE project at University of Southern California is an example of a burst of intense activity and then virtual abandonment. A review of the website, available at http://sowkweb.usc.edu/projects/where/publication.htm, reveals the site has not been updated since 2005. Language choice is limited to English and Chinese. A lack of funding for this kind of resource limits willingness of individuals to sustain websites. Although readers may be directed to use Babelfish in some instances, it is very unsatisfactory. There is apparently no medical dictionary, so key medical diagnoses are not translated. Sentence construction is very awkward, and the whimsy of some translations distracts from the content.

Challenges of International Health Websites

Another alternative is that users can go directly to health information sites in other countries. This option may provide excellent direction and comfort to the user. However, there are several dilemmas. One issue is that in the United States, we assist clients in finding credible information by suggesting that they take note of the domain. Domains with the extension dot-com (.com) exist primarily to sell a product or service. Domains with .org or .gov are less likely to be selling a product or service. In Asia, this domain distinction is not universal, and health organizations may use either dot-com or dot-org or dot-gov.

A second complication is that the information on the website may reference drugs and treatments and protocols not available in the United States. For most international health websites, English translation is not available. The health professional or family member who is not literate in the language of that website will not be able to assist in evaluating the credibility of the site or in making sense of the recommendations. See the discussion in Chapter 3 of the Health on the Net Foundation, which sets standards for credible health information. The Health on the Net icon can provide some confidence in the quality of the website. However, dialogue among professionals and non-English-speaking people in the care situation will be difficult. Although some states have passed laws requiring a healthcare agency to provide interpreters, the opportunities for misunderstandings are almost infinite.

INFOMEDIATION

Moderating access to information is a strategy of digital inclusion. Infomediaries can be websites that are moderated by external reviewers, collaborative content experiences without expert review, or information stores. Infomediaries have historically been librarians, but increasingly they may be consumers or health professionals. Infomediaries have become more important to consumers of health information and advice as the content of the Web has expanded to include seemingly limitless resources of unknown provenance.

History of Information Mediation

Librarians have been critical information brokers or mediators in a taxonomy-driven search world of journal subscriptions and geography-bound book collections. A long-standing information-mediated service is when a librarian conducts a search as a salaried employee for university-affiliated scholars, schools, and public libraries. In the past, commercial groups that wanted confidence in the state of knowledge and science before undertaking a new enterprise would hire an in-house librarian or pay a freelance librarian on a fee-for-service basis. The need for these assisted searches was grounded in the arcane search-term taxonomy in place at the time. In addition, key health resources were restricted to subscribers, individuals, libraries, and corporate entities. Today, we are all "subscribers" to the wide range of information on the Web in a zero-geography search world—one independent of phone or physical access to a library collection or librarian.

As a result, consumers are more likely to conduct their impromptu searches across multiple databases on their own. In most cases, this is sufficient for broad health topic searches. Most consumers can successfully search the Web using tags or bookmarks that have emerged based on user attempts to frame their questions and to rediscover satisfactory answers/Web pages. User-generated tags are especially helpful for returning to material that might not have seemed specific enough on first try but later haunts the searcher who wishes to return. User-generated tags will be discussed later in the chapter as part of information literacy.

The Deep Web as Unexplored Resource

In some instances, consumers with health issues are frustrated by an inability to find the information they need and assume exists somewhere. This is the "iceberg" that is the *deep Web*. As early as 2001, Bergman observed that search engines were probably accessing only 1 of the 3000 pages available on a topic (Figure 2.6).

The usual search engines crawl across the surface of the Web accessing only documents that are static and have multiple links or were submitted by individuals. What the user receives in a search is a list ranked by "popularity" or links to links. For those who are frustrated with their inability to retrieve needed information, there is the deep Web. In addition to the material retrieved through search engines such as Google, Bing, and Yahoo, there are topic-specific databases and resources with content that may not be discovered by usual search strategies. These resources are part of the deep Web (Bergman, 2001). A directed query is often required for accessing the deep or highly focused and dynamic documents that get compiled daily on the Web. These queries can be accomplished through topic- or discipline-focused databases. Complete Planet (available at http://www.completeplanet.com) is one free resource designed for navigating the deep Web to find these databases. It presents a broad topic list and then links you to relevant sites that might not be found by the popular search engines.

Deep Web for Health

For health, deep Web content is available through the PubMed database and other information portals. The National Library of Medicine's online archive,

Figure 2.6   Comparison of Search Engine and Deep Web Directed Query Results

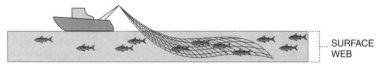

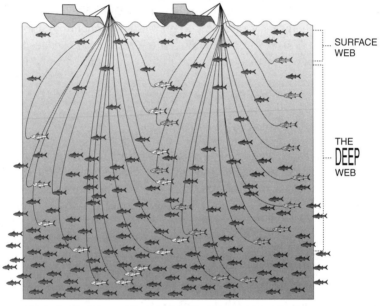

Source: Reproduced courtesy of Michael K. Bergman and BrightPlanet.

PubMed, has abstracts of journal articles free to the public. Full-text articles are available 1 year after publication in a journal. This is a change in federal public health access policy (see Consolidated Appropriations Act, 2008 [H.R. 2764]). Websites and information portals increase access. MedLinePlus, for example, will link users to documents produced for that website, to other websites with very narrowly focused information, and in some cases to publications.

Academics and many health professionals have access to subscription-only direct-query databases online. Librarians at those institutions and in public libraries may assist with direct-query requests for the public. Health professionals who do not find the resources they need should always contact a librarian for assistance. In some institutions, the library policy encourages those conducting a search on behalf of patient care, for research, or teaching, to contact the librarian before embarking on all but the most casual search. The librarian-guided search can be extremely productive in a brief time—both for finding references and arranging access to full-text resources. Coaching on searching for health resources using direct queries of databases is beyond this text. Readers are referred to their librarian and to the PubMed search tutorial at http://www.nlm.nih. gov/bsd/disted/pubmedtutorial. A similar resource is the Ovid Medline search tutorial available through the George Washington University Medical Center Himmelfarb Library at http://www.gwumc.edu/library/tutorials/ovidmed.

Consumer-Driven Health Information Searches

Many consumers conduct searches for health-related resources without librarian guidance. In some cases, this is because their access to the library during service hours is limited, they do not have access to a skilled health information librarian, or equally likely, because of personal preference. In some cases, language is a barrier between the consumer and the available librarian contacts. See discussion of language issues in this chapter's section, "Health Technology Literacy: Language as a Barrier."

Posing Questions and Rediscovering Answers: Folksonomies and Tag Clouds

A common dilemma for older adults going online is their limited skill in asking pertinent questions (Kerr & Kerr, 2003, as cited in Godfrey & Johnson, 2009). A major skill requirement for accessing the Internet is not only asking the right question but being able to engage in what Trant (2009, p. 2) labels "personal rediscovery"—getting back to pages users have encountered in the past. Developing a functional question and finding that answer again in the future requires the ability to guess at the best term that will lead the user to the most relevant data. Students and scholars in the past relied heavily on librarians to guide them in posing questions and retrieving answers using discipline-specific taxonomies. A taxonomy is a structure that arranges knowledge terms in a hierarchical manner of increasing detail, and it is specific to a database of literature for both paper-bound and online materials.

The evolution of the Internet in the Web 1.0 era was such that labels, or tags for information, were developed by people with very specialized backgrounds.

Often, the same technoculture groups that inserted "fatal error" and "illegal operation" as signals of problems with software applications are the group determining online category labels and other Internet conventions. Alternatively, there were subject matter experts who were as likely to use highly technical vocabularies or cultural idioms that led to confusion in a highly diverse world. Some health professionals avoid technical vocabulary to the point of dysfunctional communication. Zeng and Tse (2006) give an example where instead of saying to the patient "You have pulmonary congestion," a phrase such as "water in the lungs," was used. This led a patient to take creative steps to get rid of the water (Zeng & Tse, 2006)! The patient (the daughter of a plumber) proceeded to "empty the pipes" of her lungs by inducing vomiting and urinating frequently in bed. She worked to remove the water overload!

In Web 2.0, more user-generated content and labeling is possible than in Web 1.0. A major example of consumer engagement is the evolution of tag clouds (see Figure 2.7). These clusters of tags help users make connections with relevant material that otherwise might not be apparent. This cluster of discontinuous text is useful in conducting searches as well as retracing steps.

Tagging, or allowing user-generated key words, may be a core strategy for building Internet information literacy for consumers of health technology. When these tags are shared (social tagging), users are led to new content. Trant (2009) proposes that a folksonomy results in a sense of ownership of content and develops social cohesion. *Folksonomy* is defined as a "collective vocabulary (with a focus on knowledge organization)" that is a valuable tool for navigating in the

---

Figure 2.7   Example of a Tag Cloud: Searched by "Health Nurse"

Alternative Health Care alternative health care medicine attractive Healthy body Bachelor in Nursing best career in nursing best weight loss products care of health Causes of Hypertension diabetes medication Diet for a maturing education of nursing school exercise first aid to safe the life fitness Fitness Lifestyle Good health good looking healthy body Health Advices Health Care Health body Healthy Diet Healthy Lifestyle Healthy Tips Healthy Tips for Bad Breath home nursing course hospital guides Hypertension medical dictionary natural medicines normal values of blood pressure nursing Nursing Health Care Nursing Health Care Training nursing jobs Nursing School Nutrition nutritional supplements online health advices online health Hospital guides Public Health Care Public Health Nurse Public Health Nursing Training of First Aid to Safe Life Weight Loss What is Hypertension

Source: NursingLife.net. http://www.nursinglife.net/tag/public-health-nurse. Used with permission.

"environment of abundance" that is the Internet (Trant, 2009, p. 4). Encouraging social tagging can be a key strategy in building a community of support or the digital circles of support under construction by Godfrey and Johnson (2009).

A challenge in building support groups is creating trust and shared experiences. Online groups are further challenged by the absence of face-to-face contact and the social gathering experiences of coffee, social chitchat, walking out together, and so on (Godfrey & Johnson, 2009). A folksonomy (shared vocabulary) takes advantage of consumers' compulsion to share (Trant, 2009). A common experience then is created by the expectation that a tag does not have to be forced into a hierarchy or taxonomy based on consensus. The group needs only to label similar material with the same tag when they can agree. Over time, some people change their vocabulary. However, others can retain their preferred tags for their idiosyncratic use. The quick turnaround and responses from the group provide incentives to collaborate (Udell, 2005, as cited in Trant, 2009). Examples provided include tagging in a photo-sharing group and Internet information group. Flickr allows you to specify other users as contacts, friends, or family and see views of just their material. Delicious allows you to "subscribe" to other users' lists. Table 2.13 provides an overview of some examples of ways consumers can tag material they have found for personal rediscovery.

Infomediary: Sponsored Sites and Government

Free stand-alone websites that are constructed to provide comprehensive health information can be private or government based. WebMd and MedlinePlus are two examples. Another type of sponsored website is one that is tethered to a particular organization, such as the Kaiser Permanente Thrive site or the Mayo Clinic and Cleveland Clinic. Some parts of tethered websites may be restricted to customers or clients of the healthcare agency. These websites per se will not be discussed in depth here (see Chapter 3).

Recently, the US Department of Health and Human Services (DHHS) launched a new and timely public private initiative for community-based health care performance improvement (DHHS, 2010). The apparent philosophy is that by making interactive data sets available for free that stakeholders at multiple levels will participate in pressure to improve health care performance. The website promises that the data is new and not previously available and will include material at the "national, state, regional, and potentially county level…on prevalence of disease, quality, cost and utilization…[and] information on evidence based programs and policies that have successfully improved community performance" (DHHS, para. 5). Although not explicitly labeled, the approach is quintessentially

Table 2.13   Websites for Organizing and Sharing Internet Discoveries

Rediscovering Internet information is a key part of sustained literacy. The Web services listed here assist users to track their finds for the future and share them in the present. The labeling is through a folksonomy or social tagging mechanism.

Delicious—Formerly referred to as "de.li.cious," this is a social bookmarking website in which users tag, share, save, and manage a variety of Web pages from one central location. This website uses community social networking to allow users to discover new resources and manage their own bookmarks from any computer.

http://www.delicious.com

CiteULike is a free service that allows users to organize, save, and share scholarly papers over the Internet. Scholarly work of interest to you may be added to a personal CiteULike library with one click. The entire citation will be transferred and can be used on any computer with access to the Internet. It is also possible to share libraries among users, which helps others discover new relevant papers.

http://www.citeulike.org

Technorati was the first blog search engine founded and is currently collecting, organizing, and distributing online conversation globally. This website appeals to both bloggers and advertisers who are able to communicate through blogs and have the opportunity to gain revenue and visibility.

http://www.technoratimedia.com

Flickr is a secure online photo management and sharing website available free to the public. Through this website users are able to upload and retrieve photos and videos through the Web, mobile devices, home computers, and many other technological methods. In addition to sharing, users are able to organize their own photos and videos with the help of their friends and family.

http://www.flickr.com

ecological (see Figure 2.8). This development has profound implications for literacy demands for healthcare professionals and consumers. The Community Data Initiative (CDI) from DHHS will directly facilitate the empowerment predicted by the socioecological framework for health literacy (see Figure 2.1). DHHS has anticipated the transitions precipitated by the recently enacted healthcare reform. The CDI promises to provide data so that leaders in the community and health professionals can collaborate to distill core information to discern and predict patterns (knowledge) so that available capital can be assessed and wise decisions can be made. Those consumers and health experts who wish to have influence will be challenged to appreciate the capital made available in this initiative and to develop the skills to move beyond data.

Figure 2.8   The Ecology of the DHHS Community Data Set Initiative

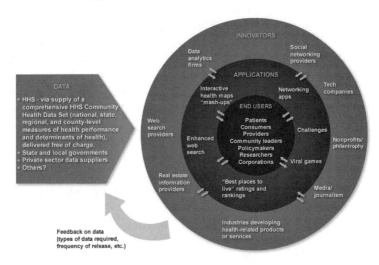

Source: DHHS, 2010.

As indicated on the website links, familiarity with downloads, interactive data sets, widgets, and RSS feeds will be expected. The website also provides a list of illustrative examples of applications, each of which imply the full range of literacy skills described in this chapter and related subsequent chapters. The list from the "About" webpage (http://www.hhs.gov/open/datasets/about.html) includes:

- Interactive health maps on the Web that allow citizens to understand health performance in their area versus others with tremendous ease and clarity
- "Dashboards" that enable mayors and other civic leaders to track and publicize local health performance and issues
- Social networking applications that allow health improvement leaders to connect with each other, compare performance, share best practices, and challenge each other
- Competitions regarding how communities can innovate to improve health performance
- Viral online games that help educate people about community health
- Utilization of community health data to help improve the usefulness of results delivered by web search engines when people do health-related searches and further raise awareness of community health performance
- Integration of community health-related data into new venues, such as real estate websites, which could be highly effective disseminators of such information

Trust Signs for Health Information Websites

In this section, we are concerned with theory and research on how the sites attract and retain users. Song and Zahedi (2007) point out that users spend a great deal of time in the search process—probably due to inefficiencies in the user approach. Ease of use becomes very important and may be equated with lack of ability. In studies using the technology adoption model, ease of use has been one of the most important factors in building trust. Ease can be measured, they suggest, by the number of clicks made before linking to the desired information. Three clicks seems to be the threshold beyond which users will quit and begin another search. Another factor that creates difficulty for users is locked font sizes or styles that are difficult to read and are not adjustable to user preferences. The ability to adjust font size is particularly important for older adults (*Spry Foundation*, 2001). Confusing or difficult page navigation may discourage users also.

A notable study done with college students in two US universities suggests that trust signs are very important (Song & Zahedi, 2007). The signs on their list include statements about privacy and security that signal self-regulating policy, providing references for sources posted, ownership disclosure—such as an HMO or pharmaceutical company, third-party seals such as HON code, and customer communities that encourage feedback. In this study, students were directed to interact with WebMD and MedlinePlus and rate the sites on a variety of criteria. The results indicated that the reputation of the health infomediary was a factor in rating ability. Investing in simplifying information and helping users understand healthcare jargon were recommended.

The study findings validated the importance of reputation and the ability to personalize information in a custom format. The major recommendation emerging from the study was knowing the audience. Song and Zahedi (2007) noted that government agencies are designing health infomediary sites for members of the general public, who are predominantly novices at searching for health information on the Web. Simple explanations and minimal jargon are required. Failure to follow recommendations for building trust for naïve users may lead such users to seek other intermediary, proprietary, or fringe sites that are less reliable and not monitored. These sites can create health risks with unsubstantiated recommendations for products and treatments, and may generate a following for health policies that are detrimental to individuals and communities.

Infomediary as New Consumer Role: Seeking Peer Wisdom

The usefulness of information depends on its availability "at the right time—namely the point at which a decision about a course of action might be required" (Godfrey & Johnson, 2009, p. 635):

Information needs to be wide-ranging, unbounded by the interests of agencies and services; it must be personalized and tailored to facilitate option appraisal and make decisions; and it requires the engagement of [consumers] themselves in providing solutions tested through experience. (p. 637)

Godfrey and Johnson (2009) propose a model for building literacy that links information, advice, and advocacy. Information is data that is meaningful given a context that makes sense to the individual when considering a course of action. Advice is an opinion or recommendation shared between individuals that may affect the decision, and advocacy is "pleading the case" for an individual or collective group or a peer, volunteer, or professional (p. 635). Information, they note, for older adults is "perceived as a means to an end, namely to getting a service or resource or resolving a problem, and not intrinsically useful in itself" (p. 635). The implication, then, is that advocacy may be a tool to facilitating getting pertinent information, and advice is a means to moving adults to both sources of information and posing questions to ask.

A resource for bridging digital literacy limitations for health matters could be older adults who draw on their life skills to assist others—the Internet literate. Godfrey and Johnson (2009) propose structuring groups of older adults who foster Internet connectivity for information, advice, and advocacy in digital circles of support. An example of a digital circle of support can be found at Leeds information store, Leeds AgelinkPlus: http://www.olderpeopleleeds.info/view.aspx?id=15.

Circles of support have members range across the ecosystem of the individual. The habitat created by the digital circle reflects the nodes of support for the older adult Internet consumer: relative, friend, neighbor, social worker, health worker, community volunteer, or caregiver (Figure 2.9). Relationships in the circle are dynamic and diverse with a mix of collaboration, advice, and support bounded by the Internet as resource. Godfrey and Johnson (2009, p. 640) note that the roles include "teacher, helper, and evangelist." The dynamics of such circles are validated by a pre/post study of Web searching and social feedback (Lau & Coiera, 2008). In this study, to answer six health questions, undergraduates retrieved documents from PubMed, MedlinePlus, and HealthInsite. Feedback was provided on their answers by sharing postsearch answers of other searchers. Searchers who were not confident were more likely to change their answers after receiving feedback. Social feedback can be important, not only for those who are uncertain. Confident searchers may not be correct. Participation in a digital circle of support could act to increase accuracy in answering health questions.

In some instances, nodes in this ecosystem may disagree, share, or may be unaware of each other's role. Whose information is trusted and whose is discounted may vary with the context. In Figure 2.9, the interaction between the

Figure 2.9   Digital Circles of Support: Node Relationships

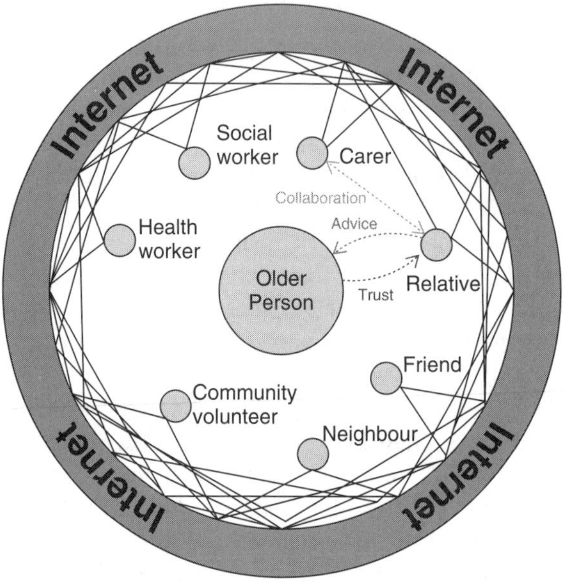

Source: Godfrey & Johnson, 2009. Used with permission from Elsevier.

relative and the older person is portrayed, but in fact, there will be complex networking across the circle (O. Johnson, personal communication, July 28, 2009). This intertwined and continually changing dynamic is difficult to portray in two dimensions. As indicated in Chapter 3, there are many bidirectional websites intended to provide information and support for the full range of consumers. What is unique about this model is the recognition that an intermediary can be critical when literacy is limited. New diagnoses, life events, or acute episodes of illness may create conditions that overwhelm usual coping strategies.

"Friending" and Confidentiality

As information stores linked to digital circles of support proliferate, issues of confidentiality arise. O. Johnson (personal communication, July 27, 2009) reflects that they are now exploring with the Leeds City Council the legal, ethical, and practical concerns about information sharing initiated by public-sector employees. In addition, as users become comfortable with their digital circle, they may forget to monitor privacy settings. As with other social networking sites, it is easy to link to friends of friends without appreciating the viral impact. Wikipedia (see Viral phenomenon, 2008) notes that a viral phenomenon occurs when exposure to an object leads to spreading copies or to another object becoming more like the original. There is an implication of rapid, uncontrolled response. Failure to review privacy settings may mean that a personal story or information may move across the globe as a user's friend list attaches it to every one of his or her friends, and so on. Just as health professionals caution people about not taking medications prescribed for others, or mixing medications indiscriminately, we need to warn consumers about privacy checks.

Life Events as Structure for Digital Circles of Support

Although Godfrey and Johnson (2009) have set up digital circles of support centered on older adults, the concept could easily be extended to other age groups. In fact, intergenerational linking has tremendous potential. For the digital circles of support there are three major contexts that trigger support opportunities: life course transitions, life events, and daily hassles. Older adults are particularly vulnerable to stressors related to changed relationships caused by death or disability and related to their own changes in abilities. However, children and their parents have the potential as well to be stressed by events in the lives of older family members. For some older adults, information, advice, and advocacy needs can escalate as their adult children and grandchildren experience life transitions, events, and daily hassles for which they ask or appear to need assistance from older adults in their lives.

User-Generated Content as Infomediary Resource

There are multiple ways that users can provide information and advice on the Internet. Some may be classified as community-driven knowledge sites (Kim & Han, 2009). These are collective social networking sites using a question-and-answer format. Yahoo!Answers is an example. Other user-generated content sites with relevance to health include Wikipedia, PatientsLikeMe, and knols. The risk inherent in health-related websites is the promotion of solutions that are unsafe and the aggregation of like-minded people who band together to perpetuate errors or pander to persistent fears (antivaccination groups, for example). The Yahoo!Answer site requires users to read a long string of answers, some of which are spam or deliberately posted as entertainment.

On the other hand, there are sites organized with built-in feedback loops. Wikipedia is one example where users post health information that is edited by other users—continuously. Authors are never owners of the content. Wikipedia editors note when a document is an "orphan"; lacking three or more links. The links are a way of triangulating information and advice that assists users in assessing credibility. In addition, citations are encouraged so that users can read original material for themselves. PatientsLikeMe is also a site with some moderation by experts and an overt expectation that users will review, reflect, and comment in an organized fashion.

Another resource that is emerging for dynamic development of content is the *knol*, which is available at http://knol.google.com/k. Google developed this resource to encourage experts and consumers to collaborate.

In the case of a knol, a draft of a document is posted and is open for collaboration for a defined period that is moderated by the author. Comments are reviewed for incorporation, and the knol is posted. There is a specific category for health. Although authors must sign in with their real name, some health knols post only a screen name and a declaration of credentials. Others post the name of the author and credentials. Knols are reviewed by users, and comments may be left even after collaboration is closed. One example is a knol posted by Ann Peters from the University of Southern California that received an award for most viewed and top quality (see Peters, 2009). Monsters and Critics Tech Features (2007) points out that authors may get a share of revenue for ads posted near the content. This potential conflict of interest is not declared. The potential of these resources has barely been explored.

Emergence of Referral Service Infomediaries: Searching for Wisdom

As the Internet and its potential becomes magnified, navigation becomes more complex. Tagging may not be sufficient. Experts who serve as intermediaries arise in an entrepreneurial environment such as that made possible by the Internet. Users are seeking wisdom from credible and reliable sources of influence to simplify their searches and their lives, in particular when a service is urgently needed. A mediator role for information sorting, screening, and tailoring becomes more attractive as complexity increases. Infomediaries seem to have been first conceptualized by Hagel and Rayport (1997) to describe ways that consumers could protect their privacy and yet learn about products of interest. Goldman (2005) summarized that in this model, the marketers would get access to prospective, relevant customers, and the infomediary would get a payment for their services. For consumers, key selling points he noted were saving time in searching and privacy. The costs of these services were hidden as commissions. However, Goldman reported that as of 2005, these commercial intermediaries had faded away and not become a significant market force with respect to consumer goods.

Information brokers have emerged who provide software and services for purchase. Bright Planet markets a companion product, Deep Query Manager, that harvests and organizes information across platforms on the Internet, going beyond Internet and intranet websites to search e-mail and internal documents. This product is for sale to anyone needing intense, state-of-the-art and state-of-the-science digitally available information. For most people, tools that are available without payment are more than adequate.

Costs of Health Referral Infomediaries: Dollars and Contact Exposures

Making health information readily available that is reliable and trustworthy is a major challenge for policy makers and healthcare professionals as well as for individuals and their families. A dilemma for those in the middle age and older adult category is their lifelong expectation that information is free when it is not gained face-to-face or is provided anonymously. Many adults do appreciate that if you meet with an expert in their office or engage consultants or assistants to carry out specific tasks on your behalf, someone must pay.

Fee for service, financial retainers for expert advice, and sales commissions are common arrangements with those with the ability to pay. Others who have experience being in the low-income segment of the population are well aware that they must be screened and deemed eligible for services for which the government or a charitable group will pay. However, with the Internet, many individuals and groups take advantage of the online resources with limited awareness of how these resources are supported. The role of advertisements or commissions is unknown or ignored. Exceptions occur when consumers become annoyed by advertisements that slow website loading or that are overtly tailored to information gathered by cookies. HTTP cookies are described on Wikipedia (see HTTP cookie, 2009) as bits of text generated by the Web browser to aid in tracking user behaviors, authenticating users, remembering preferences, and maintaining electronic shopping carts.

Google introduced a fee-for-service answer website that was mediated by experts in searching. Users registered, offered a bounty for answers, and the search was done by experts. The service was considered experimental and had multiple issues (see Google Answers, 2009). Google retired the service as a failed experiment.

Independent of cookies that collect personal information in the background, consumers increasingly provide personal information as the "cost" of accessing "free" websites. This is the registration process. Unless one reads very carefully, client information may be sold or shared freely with others. This can start a cascade of contact exposures. These contacts may result in marketers using the phone numbers or e-mail addresses supplied on registration. If these phone numbers and e-mail addresses are your business contacts, you might be overwhelmed at work. Alternatively, you may receive phone calls at home that disrupt your routines.

Free Referral Sites: Hidden Costs

Internet-based "free referral" services are an example of creating unanticipated infomediary costs. In this case, the marketing feature is matching available services to potential consumers. The implicit promise is experts have vetted or reviewed the products or services and are skilled in sorting and prioritizing them for specific consumer preferences. These free services have multiple pitfalls. Elder care provides an excellent example. As the population of older adults explodes there are multiple challenges to traditional arrangements. Today, many families are geographically separated, younger families live in housing unsuited to sharing generational space, and the women who used to care for older adults are fully employed outside the home. These conditions mean supervision at home or supervised senior housing is eagerly sought. Consumers need to be cautious and exert skepticism as they access referral sites.

Free Referral Sites: Elder Care Search Example

Patricia Grace, a senior living consultant who has authored multiple websites, recently warned about the hidden consequences of registering for "free referrals" (Grace, 2009). The referral website, she notes, is a way to generate leads for elder care providers to contact potential customers. The provider pays a fee and the website owner gets a commission. This information is not usually disclosed to the consumer. In some cases, Grace notes, that financial information clients supply is used to steer them to the care provider that pays the highest commission. Client information may not be given to providers that pay smaller fees. Consumers, she reports, can be surprised and overwhelmed by a cascade of phone calls from persistent recruiters.

In the blog comments that follow Grace's (2009) piece, users are advised to appreciate the difference between broker services and care coordinator services. The broker usually breaks the connection once you supply the information and may not even track any complaints. Blog commenters claim that a fee-for-service care coordinator works with consumers until their needs are met. The assertion is that fee-for-service arrangements have quality assurance built in.

Finding reputable referral services and care coordinators is beyond the scope of this book. However, it is not a major stretch to realize that consumers will be turning to the Internet to get referrals for care coordinators—leading to the same problems. Alternate free resources include the Medicare website for comparing nursing homes based on responses to Medicare questionnaires and data collected by nonprofit groups such as California Advocates for Nursing Home Reform.

However, as Godfrey and Johnson noted, government sources can be perceived as "too official, complex, cautious, and general to have much meaning" (Godfrey et al., 2004, as cited in Godfrey & Johnson, 2009, p. 639). Consumer advocacy sites have their own problems tied to sponsor relationships. For example, the California Advocates for Nursing Home Reform has been criticized for overt bridging to lawyers who take on cases of elder abuse or elder care malpractice on contingency. An alternative view is offered by an attorney who notes that the lawyers pay a fee to the nonprofit site, which allows it to exist. The nursing home screening is an independent function. Without the referral fee for those independent situations where consumers wish to consult an attorney, the service would not exist. New norms and funding arrangements are needed.

Strategies for Retaining Control of Referral Contact Exposures

Teaching clients (and professionals) to review the About Us and Contact Us features is key. Watching for check boxes that are automatically filled usually means you are opting in to a choice that is best for the website owner. For example, a well-known collaborative software program is set up so that when you add a new member to your group, it "automatically" grants them access to all projects and messages. The user must uncheck the choice. Similarly, Facebook in 2007 had a default where your online purchases were revealed to your friends unless you deliberately opted out (Wheaton, 2007). Some airlines have a similar screen that comes up when you are checking in online that automatically signs you up for costly options. Becoming literate in website interactions includes strategies to make the outcome manageable (Table 2.14).

In addition, some clients may need to be coached on the value of using answer machines and voicemail services to screen calls. Good hygiene or Internet security practices can minimize risks of interactions with malicious digital technology.

CHALLENGE AND PROMISE OF HEALTH LITERACY

The empowerment of consumers is expected to save money and rescue the beleaguered healthcare system—and improve health. A case has been made that literacy skills are a form of capital essential to realizing these lofty goals.

Table 2.14   Everyday Experience of Web Registrations: Digital Footprints

- Check privacy policy: What promises are made?
- Be alert to "default" choices: Will information automatically go to Facebook, etc.?
- Consider intent of website: "Referral" means sharing your information.
- Choose personal and work phone numbers and e-mail addresses that will be the least intrusive.
- Set up a task-specific e-mail address to control flow of messages.
- Never provide Social Security or bank account numbers online.
- Consider opening a credit card just for Internet purchases.
- Create an "information only" password dissimilar to bank, insurance, health records, etc.
- Create a record of your passwords that is not stored under "passwords" on any medium and is not on devices easy to lose (flash drives, cell phones, etc.)
- Do not follow links supplied in unsolicited e-mails, even when apparently from trusted sources.
- Conduct your own search for sites seeking personal information rather than following unsolicited links to minimize phishing consequences.

Literacy skills will vary with the consumers' acceptance of the new priority for learning, documenting, and communicating about their health and their environment—social and physical. There seems to be agreement that literacy skills can be taught but that the requirements and expectations will be continually in flux (Norman, 2009; Wien-Peckham, n.d.). A particular challenge is the lack of rigorous research with comparable variables (Pignone et al., 2005). In the review by Pignone and colleagues, very few interventions actually changed health literacy. Additionally, as more consumers buy in to the new empowerment model, vocabulary and literacy skills will become more of an issue. The dilemma of whether to assess certain clients for health literacy or employ a "universal precautions" model (Paasche-Orlow & Wolf, 2008) will become more urgent. Focusing on the socioecological aspects of literacy (see Figure 2.1) related to health will be a powerful framework for engaging all of the stakeholders in making the most of the Internet and related digital devices.

In this chapter, it is clear that there are many views of what literacies are required and what skills and abilities are inferred. Many different labels are being promoted. Advances in research and practice will be limited until consensus can be obtained on core attributes, vocabulary, and approaches to assessment and evaluation. At present, the only consensus seems to be that literacy is a requirement for empowering individuals and communities to develop both health and social capital.

REFERENCES

Ackerman, K. (2009, January 29). *Consumers tap online tools to better manage their health.* Retrieved August 12, 2009, from http://www.ihealthbeat.org/Features/2008/Consumers-Tap-Online-Tools-To-Better-Manage-Their-Health.aspx

American Nurses Association. (2008). *Nursing informatics: Scope and standards of practice.* Silver Spring, MD: American Nurses Association.

Ancker, J. S., & Kaufman, D. (2007). Rethinking health numeracy: A multidisciplinary literature review. *Journal of the American Medical Informatics Association, 14*(6), 713–721. Retrieved July 8, 2009, from http://www.jamia.org.libproxy.usc.edu/cgi/content/abstract/14/6/713

Armstrong, S., & Warlick, D. (2004, September 15). The new literacy. *Tech and Learning.* Retrieved October 16, 2009, from http://www.techlearning.com/article/2806

Barak, A., Boniel-Nissim, M., & Suler, J. (2008). Fostering empowerment in online support groups. *Computers in Human Behavior, 24,* 1867–1883.

Bergman, M. (2001). The deep web: Surfacing hidden value. *Journal of Electronic Publishing, 7*(1), doi: http://dx.doi.org/10.3998/3336451.0007.104. Retrieved August 8, 2009, from http://www.techlearning.com/article/2806

Berkman, N. D., Dewalt, D. A., Pignone, M. P., Sheridan, S. L., Lohr, K. N., Lux, L., et al. (2004). Literacy and health outcomes. *Evidence Report: Technology Assessment (Summary), 87,* 1–8. Retrieved August 12, 2009, from http://www.ncbi.nlm.nih.gov/books/bv.fcgi?rid=hstat1a.chapter.32213

Bickmore, T., & Giorgino, T. (2006). Health dialog systems for patients and consumers. *Journal of Biomedical Informatics, 39*(5), 556–571. doi: 10.1016/j.jbi.2005.12.004.

Brach, C. (2009). A guide for developing and purchasing successful health information technology. *Health literacy, eHealth, and communication: Putting the consumer first: Workshop summary* (pp. 73–77). Washington, DC: National Academies Press. Retrieved August 11, 2009, from http://books.nap.edu/openbook.php?record_id=12474&page=73

Brown, J. (2009). *Game-care revolution: A health care game changer?* Center for Connected Health. Retrieved June 22, 2009, from http://www.connected-health.org/about-us/get-connected-discussion/discussion/game-care-revolution-a-healthcare-game-changer.aspx

Coleman, K., Austin, B. T., Brach, C., & Wagner, E. H. (2009). Evidence on the chronic care model in the new millennium. *Health Affairs, 28*(1), 75–85. doi:10.1377/hlthaff.28.1.75.

Consolidated Appropriations Act, 2008 (H.R. 2764). (2007). Retrieved October 16, 2009, from http://thomas.loc.gov/cgi-bin/bdquery/z?d110:H.R.02764:

Department of Health and Human Services (DHHS). (2010, June 1). About the initiative [Community health data sets]. Retrieved June 4, 2010, from http://www.hhs.gov/open/datasets/about.html

Eichner, J., & Dullabh, P. (2007). Accessible health information (IT) technology for populations with limited literacy: A guide for developers and purchasers of health IT. (Prepared by the National Opinion Research Center for the National Research Center for Health IT.) AHRQ publication No. 08-0010-EF. Rockville, MD: Agency for Healthcare Research and Quality. Retrieved September 23, 2009, from http://healthit.ahrq.gov/portal/server.pt/gateway/PTARGS_0_803031_0_0_18/LiteracyGuide.pdf

Eshet, Y. (2002). Digital literacy: A new terminology framework and its application to the design of meaningful technology-based learning environments. *Proceedings of World Conference on Educational Multimedia, Hypermedia and Telecommunications 2002,* 493–498. Retrieved March 22, 2010, from http://www.editlib.org/p/10316

Eshet-Alkali, Y., & Amichai-Hamburger, Y. (2004). Experiments in digital literacy. *CyberPsychology & Behavior, 7*(4), 421–429. doi:10.1089/cpb.2004.7.421.

Eshet-Alkalai, Y., & Geri, N. (2007). Does the medium affect the message? The influence of text representation format on critical thinking. *Human Systems Management, 26*(4), 269–279.

Eysenbach, G., & Kummervold, P. E. (2005). "Is cybermedicine killing you?"—The story of a Cochrane disaster. [Comment]. *Journal of Medical Internet Research, 7*(2), e21. Retrieved November 7, 2007, from http://www.ncbi.nlm.nih.gov/pubmed/15998612

Federal Interagency Forum on Aging-Related Statistics. (2008). *Older Americans 2008: Key indicators of well being.* Washington DC: U.S. Government Printing Office. Retrieved March 22, 2010, from http://www.agingstats.gov/agingstatsdotnet/Main_Site/Data/2008_Documents/OA_2008.pdf

Fox, S., & Jones, S. (2009). *The social life of health information.* Washington, DC: Pew Internet and American Life Project. Retrieved August 23, 2009, from http://www.pewinternet.org/Reports/2009/8-The-Social-Life-of-Health-Information.aspx

Godfrey, M., & Johnson, O. (2009). Digital circles of support: Meeting the information needs of older people. *Computers in Human Behavior, 25*(3), 633–642. doi: 10.1016/j.chb.2008.08.016.

Goldman, E. (2005). *Infomediaries: Where are they? Technology and marketing blog.* Retrieved July 30, 2009, from http://blog.ericgoldman.org/archives/2005/03/infomedieswh.htm

Google Answers. (2009, September 24). In *Wikipedia, The Free Encyclopedia.* Retrieved October 16, 2009, from http://en.wikipedia.org/w/index.php?title=Google_Answers&oldid=316000983

Grace, P. (2009). *The truth about free eldercare Internet referral placement services.* Retrieved July 30, 2009, from http://www.examiner.com/x-13909-Senior-Care-Examiner~y2009m7d14-The-truth-about-free-eldercare-internet-referral-placement-services

Hagel, J., & Rayport, J. F. (1997). The coming battle for consumer information. *Harvard Business Review, 75*(1), 53–55, 58, 60–65.

Hargittai, E. (2002). Second-level digital divide: Differences in people's online skills. *First Monday, 7*(4), 1–20. Retrieved July 8, 2009, from http://firstmonday.org/htbin/cgiwrap/bin/ojs/index.php/fm/article/view/942/864

Harris, L., & Friedman, C. P. (2009). Health literacy, health information technology, and Healthy People 2020. *Health literacy, eHealth, and communication: Putting the consumer first: Workshop summary* (pp. 78–80). Washington, DC: National Academies Press. Retrieved August 11, 2009, from http://books.nap.edu/openbook.php?record_id=12474&page=73

Harris Poll. (2009). *Internet provides public with health care information that they value and trust and which often stimulates discussion with their doctors.* Retrieved August 12, 2009, from http://harrisinteractive.com/harris_poll/pubs/Harris_Poll_2009_07_28.pdf

Hawn, C. (2009). Games for health: The latest tool in the medical care arsenal. *Health Affairs, 28*(5), w842–w848. doi:10.1377/hlthaff.28.5.w842.

Horrigan, J. (2007). *A typology of information and communication technology users.* Washington DC: Pew Internet and American Life Project. Retrieved August 11, 2009, from http://pewinternet.org/Reports/2007/A-Typology-of-Information-and-Communication-Technology-Users.aspx?r=1

Horrigan, J. (2009). *Home broadband adoption 2009.* Washington DC: Pew Internet and American Life Project. Retrieved August 11, 2009, from http://www.pewinternet.org/Reports/2009/10-Home-Broadband-Adoption-2009.aspx

Houts, P. (n.d.). *Using pictures to improve health communication.* Unpublished manuscript. Retrieved July 30, 2009, from http://healthliteracy.worlded.org/visuals_in_health.pdf

HTTP cookie. (2009, October 14). In *Wikipedia, The Free Encyclopedia.* Retrieved October 16, 2009, from http://en.wikipedia.org/w/index.php?title=HTTP_cookie&oldid=319888107

Improving Chronic Illness Care. (n.d.). Retrieved October 16, 2009, from http://www.improvingchroniccare.org

Institute of Medicine. (2004). *Health literacy: A prescription to end confusion.* Washington DC: National Academies Press.

Institute of Medicine. (2009). *Health literacy, eHealth, and communication: Putting the consumer first: Workshop summary.* Washington, DC: National Academies Press. Retrieved August 5, 2009, from http://www.iom.edu/CMS/3793/31487/64643.aspx

Ioannidis, J. P. A. (2005). Contradicted and initially stronger effects in highly cited clinical research. *JAMA: The Journal of the American Medical Association, 294*(2), 218–228. doi:10.1001/jama.294.2.218.

Isham, G. (2009). Discussion. In Institute of Medicine (IOM), *Health literacy, eHealth, and communication: Putting the consumer first: Workshop summary* (pp. 77–78). Washington DC: National Academies Press.

Jordan-Marsh, M. (2008). Health habitat aspects of software as a service (SAAS/WEB2.0) reinforcing diabetic self-confidence: The PHRddBRASIL case. *DESAFIO International Symposium: Diabetes, Health Education and Guided Physical Activities,* 39–42.

Jordan-Marsh, M., Hubbard, J., Watson, R., Deon Hall, R., Miller, P., & Mohan, O. (2004). The social ecology of changing pain management: Do I have to cry? *Journal of Pediatric Nursing, 19*(3), 193–203.

Jordan-Marsh, M., McLaughlin, M., Chi, I., Brown, C., Moran, M., Jung, Y., et al. (2006). *St. Barnabas Cyber Café evaluation report 2004–2005.* Los Angeles: University of Southern California, School of Social Work, Annenberg School of Communication, Davis School of Gerontology. Unpublished manuscript.

Katz, M. G., Kripalani, S., & Weiss, B. D. (2006). Use of pictorial aids in medication instructions: A review of the literature. *American Journal of Health-System Pharmacy, 63,* 2391–2397.

Kim, B., & Han, I. (2009). The role of trust belief and its antecedents in a community-driven knowledge environment. *Journal of the American Society for Information Science and Technology, 60*(5), 1012–1026. Retrieved August 5, 2009, from http://proquest.umi.com.libproxy.usc.edu/pqdweb?did=1682801341&Fmt=7&clientId=5239&RQT=309&VName=PQD

Lau, A. Y., & Coiera, E. W. (2008). Impact of web searching and social feedback on consumer decision making: A prospective online experiment. *Journal of Medical Internet Research, 10*(1), e2.

Mancuso, J. M. (2009). Assessment and measurement of health literacy: An integrative review of the literature. *Nursing & Health Sciences, 11*(1), 77–89.

Metros, S. E. (2008a). *Visual literacy in the age of the big picture. Fighting the digital divide through education.* The Open University of Catalonia's UNESCO chair in E-learning Fifth International Seminar, Barcelona, Spain [Videotape]. Retrieved March 22, 2010, from http://unescochair.blogs.uoc.edu/23032009/susan-metros-visual-literacy-conference-video

Metros, S. E. (2008b). The educator's role in preparing visually literate learners. *Theory into Practice (TIP), 47*(2), 102–109.

Monsters & Critics Tech Features. (2007, December 14). Google unveils anti-Wikipedia project "knol." Message posted to http://www.monstersandcritics.com/tech/features/article_1381136.php/Google_unveils_anti-Wikipedia_project_Knol

Nelson, R. (2002). Major theories supporting health care informatics. In S. P. Englebart & R. Nelson (Eds.), *Health care informatics: An interdisciplinary approach* (pp. 3–27). St. Louis, MO: Mosby.

Nelson, R., & Joos, I. (1989, Fall). On language in nursing: From data to wisdom. *PLN Vision,* p. 6.

Norman, C. D. (2009). Skills essential for eHealth. *Health literacy, eHealth, and communication: Putting the consumer first: Workshop summary* (pp. 10–15). Washington, DC: National Academies Press. Retrieved August 11, 2009, from http://www.jmir.org/2006/2/e9

Norman, C. D., & Skinner, H. A. (2006). eHEALS: The eHealth literacy scale. *Journal of Medical Internet Research, 8*(4), e27.

Paasche-Orlow, M. K., Schillinger, D., Greene, S. M., & Wagner, E. H. (2006). How health care systems can begin to address the challenge of limited literacy. *Journal of General Internal Medicine, 21*(8), 884–887.

Paasche-Orlow, M. K., & Wolf, M. S. (2008). Evidence does not support clinical screening of literacy. *Journal of General Internal Medicine, 23*(1), 100–102.

Peters, A. (2009, June 6). Type 2 diabetes: Managing your numbers to achieve greater health. [Internet]. Version 83. Knol. Retrieved October 16, 2009, from http://knol.google.com/k/anne-peters-md-facp-cde/type-2-diabetes/NWhjxSXZ/lg_ybA

Pew Internet & American Life Project. (n.d.). What kind of tech user are you? Retrieved October 16, 2009, from http://pewinternet.org/Participate/What-Kind-of-Tech-User-Are-You.aspx

Pignone, M., DeWalt, D. A., Sheridan, S., Berkman, N., & Lohr, K. N. (2005). Interventions to improve health outcomes for patients with low literacy: A systematic review. *Journal of General Internal Medicine, 20*(2), 185–192.

Potter, L. (2005). *Health literacy fact sheets.* Retrieved October 16, 2009, from http://www.chcs.org/publications3960/publications_show.htm?doc_id=291711

Ratzan, S., & Parker, R. (2000). Introduction. In C. Selden, M. Zorn, S. Ratzan, & R. Parker (Eds.), *National Library of Medicine current bibliographies in medicine: Health literacy.* NLM Pub. No. CBM 2000-1. Bethesda, MD: National Institutes of Health, U.S. Department of Health and Human Services.

Resnick, P. (2001). Beyond bowling together: SocioTechnical capital in human–computer interaction in the new millennium. In J. M. Carroll (Ed.), *Human–computer interaction in the new millennium* (pp. 647–672). Boston: Addison-Wesley. Retrieved March 22, 2010, from http://www.si.umich.edu/presnick/papers/stk/ResnickSTK.pdf

Rothman, R. L., Montori, V. M., Cherrington, A., & Pignone, M. P. (2008). Perspective: The role of numeracy in health care. *Journal of Health Communication, 13*(6), 583–595.

Seligman, H. K., Wallace, A. S., DeWalt, D. A., Schillinger, D., Arnold, C. L., Shilliday, B. B., et al. (2007). Facilitating behavior change with low-literacy patient education materials. *American Journal of Health Behavior, 31*(Suppl. 1), S69–S78.

Shih, F., & Kagal, L. (2009). Policy-aware pipes: Support accountability in mashup service of linked data. Paper presented at the 3rd International SMR2 2009 Workshop on Service Matchmaking and Resource Retrieval in the Semantic Web. Retrieved June 4, 2010, from http://dig.csail.mit.edu/2009/Papers/ISWC/policy-aware-pipe/paper.pdf

Song, J., & Zahedi, F. (2007). Trust in health infomediaries. *Decision Support Systems, 43*(2), 390–407.

Spry Foundation: Evaluating health information on the world wide web. (2001). Retrieved June, 1, 2006, from http://www.spry.org

State Educational Technology Directors Association. (2007). Definitions: ICT media fluency landscape. *Leadership Summit Toolkit 2007.* Retrieved August 23, 2009, from http://www.setda.org/c/document_library/get_file?folderId=213&name=Matrix_Defiinitions_FINAL-1.pdf

Tatsioni, A., Bonitsis, N. G., & Ioannidis, J. P. A. (2007). Persistence of contradicted claims in the literature. *JAMA: The Journal of the American Medical Association, 298*(21), 2517–2526. doi:10.1001/jama.298.21.2517.

Trant, J. (2009). Studying social tagging and folksonomy: A review and framework. *Journal of Digital Information, 10*(1), 1–42. Retrieved August 5, 2009, from http://dlist.sir.arizona.edu/2595/01/trant-studyingFolksonomy.pdf

van Bronswijk, J. E. M. H. Bouma, H., Fozard, J. L., Kearns, W. D., Davison, G. C., & Tuan, P-C. (2009). Defining gerontechnology for R&D purposes. *Gerontechnology, 8*(1), 3–10.

Viral phenomenon. (2008, December 21). In *Wikipedia, The Free Encyclopedia*. Retrieved October 16, 2009, from http://en.wikipedia.org/w/index.php?title=Viral_phenomenon&oldid=259406532

Wagner, E. H. (1998). Chronic disease management: What will it take to improve care for chronic illness? *Effective Clinical Practice, 1*(1), 2–4.

Wheaton, S. (2007, November 29). Facebook bows to privacy protest. *New York Times*, Retrieved August 5, 2009, from http://thecaucus.blogs.nytimes.com/2007/11/29/facebook-bows-to-privacy-protest

White, S. (2008). *Assessing the nation's health literacy. Key concepts and finding of the National Assessment of Adult Literacy (NAAL)* (No. OP423908). American Medical Association Foundation. Retrieved August 5, 2009, from http://www.ama-assn.org/ama/pub/about-ama/ama-foundation/our-programs/public-health/health-literacy-program/assessing-nations-health.shtml

Wien-Peckham, J. (n.d.). *Redefining literacy*. Retrieved August 12, 2009, from http://users.accesscomm.ca/smilingbuddha/jwp_on_redefiningliteracy_essay_1.htm

World Health Organization. (2010). *Track 2: Health literacy and health behavior*. Retrieved June 4, 2010, from http://www.who.int/healthpromotion/conferences/7gchp/track2/en

Zeng, Q. T., & Tse, T. (2006). Exploring and developing consumer health vocabularies. *Journal of the American Medical Informatics Association, 13*(1), 24–29.

CHAPTER 3

Health Information Seeking Behavior on the Web

Maryalice Jordan-Marsh and Shuya Pan

DIGITAL INCLUSION OR DIGITAL DIVIDE

The widespread diffusion of the Internet has transformed the ways people are accessing health information. The Internet cannot only provide swift access to large quantities of health information, but also to communication channels (e.g., e-mail, instant messaging, discussion boards, social networking sites) through which people can exchange health information and social support with others in similar situations and with similar concerns.

According to recent data collected by the Pew Internet and American Life Project (2009), 74% of the adult population in the United States has used the Internet. Looking for health information was one of the most popular online activities described in the report. Approximately 80% of all Internet users in the United States have sought health information online (Fox, 2006). Data shows that those who are most likely to seek health information online are women, younger than 65, college graduates, those with more online experience, and those with broadband access at home (Fox & Jones, 2009). Meanwhile, another Pew report (Fox, 2007) indicates that a slightly higher number of Internet users (86%) living with disability or chronic illness have looked online for health information. Older adults, ages 65 and over, were found to be least likely to search online for health information compared to other age groups; only 6% of online health seekers are ages 65 and older, compared to 23% among ages 18–29; 45% among 30–49; and 23% among 50–64 (Fox, 2006).

Substantial research efforts have been made to explore people's online health information search behaviors. Major topic areas include:

- Consumer motives and needs (Shuyler & Knight, 2003; Tang & Lee, 2006)
- Theories to explain people's health information seeking behaviors (Johnson & Meischke, 1993; Afifi & Weiner, 2004)

- Barriers and challenges in using the Internet for health information, especially the quality concerns of online health information and the development of evaluative tools to filter unreliable information (Anderson, 2004; Breckons, Jones, Morris, & Richardson, 2008; Jimison et al., 2008)
- Consumer search and evaluation strategies (Josefsson, 2006; Sillence, Briggs, Harris, & Fishwick, 2007)
- The effect of online health information search behaviors on health status and patient–provider relationships (Czaja, Manfredi, & Price, 2003; Jimison et al., 2008)

People who use the Internet less than average, such as older adults, are more likely to become disenfranchised and disadvantaged. The dramatic technological advancement in contemporary society might accelerate the marginalization of less technology-literate groups and prevent them from fully benefiting from the digital age.

Focus of This Chapter

This chapter summarizes and discusses the findings about these critical issues. It also pays specific attention to older adults and minorities and examines the potential impact of the Internet on their health behaviors. A socioecological view of health and the Internet assists consumers and health professionals to ensure that digital inclusion is a global strategy rather than deepening the digital divide. Hargittai (2002) and others note that we have moved to the phase where discussions of equity in access must be balanced with attention to skills when given access. Sociotechnical capital, the ability to engage with digital resources (Resnick, 2002) as a means to interact with personal and professional support, is a new goal for consumers of health technology and the healthcare system. In this chapter, the potential for accessing information that can become knowledge consumers can use in making decisions is discussed. Approaches for understanding Internet behaviors and strategies for building sociotechnical capital based on accumulating wisdom are presented.

THE SOCIOECOLOGY OF HEALTH TECHNOLOGY: A FRAMEWORK FOR EMPOWERMENT

Consumer-Centric Health in an Information Age

The paradigm of consumer and provider relationships is shifting (Institute of Medicine, 2009). Consumers are taking on more responsibility and correspondingly becoming more empowered as participants. This is what *patient-centered* health care means. A socioecological focus can guide both consumers and health professionals in taking into account the environmental context in which health is sustained or challenged. Obtaining information and learning how to use it is a core skill of empowerment. Understanding online information behaviors and resources is important to maximizing digital inclusion and is the focus of this chapter.

Consumers in the age of telehealth may be hooking up to sensors that generate *data* on their health status. Some want to go online to understand why this *data* is connected to treatments that are started or stopped. Some consumers surf the Internet seeking more *information* on what they can expect after a diagnosis. In some cases, they simply want to absorb what they were told by their healthcare provider—they want to become more *knowledgeable* about their clinical situation and options. The Internet supplements or complements consumers' ability to cope with or solve problems or take advantage of opportunities by accessing personal, social, and professional *wisdom*.

The Socioecological Conceptual Framework

As displayed in Figure 3.1, health professionals and consumer advocates promote empowerment by acting as though "everything is connected" and appreciating the potential of a digital world where *zero geography* (location does not matter) is the context for interacting (Hames, 2007).

Figure 3.1   The Socioecology of Health Literacy: The Empowerment Cycle

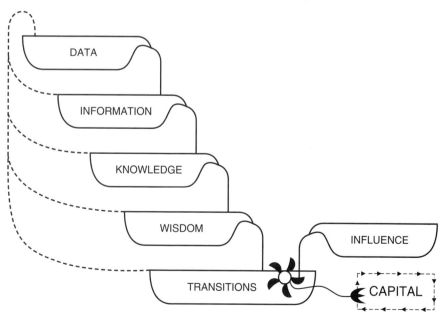

Illustration: Jin DePaul.

The socioecological framework builds from the Nelson Data-to-Wisdom Continuum (Nelson, 2002). She added *wisdom* to the categories developed by Blum in 1986 (as cited in Nelson). For this book, an ecological perspective of connection is proposed to reflect the process flow. New research and experience suggests that in order to assess and undertake interventions, the patient (and family) and healthcare professionals can increase success if they take into account the environmental resources of *capital* and *influence* (social dynamics) for any *transitions*. The explanations of the flow of data, information, and knowledge that accumulates in wisdom, as portrayed in Figure 3.1, are based on those presented by Nelson and expanded by Staggers and Nelson (2009).

Data are uninterpreted bits (age, time of day, number of people signed on to a website, a single vital sign). *Information* results when data bits are processed and put in context. Trends in data that signal normalcy or unusual patterns are information that may require action. *Knowledge* emerges as patterns are recognized and relationships drawn. Knowledge is perspective, often built around a conceptual framework or theory. Experienced patients and health professionals can put these trends in context, using a framework from experience, research, and theory. Knowledge is how we make sense of information in considering a decision at the point of a transition. Knowledge for practice (or behavior) takes into account information on *influences* in the environment and available capital. *Wisdom*, in a socioecological framework, is the use of knowledge to take advantage of opportunities, to create peace of mind, or to cope with or solve problems—to move through a transition. *Transitions* occur when a change is triggered, or fails to happen. For example, a much-wished-for pregnancy does not occur, a mammography alert is resolved without a diagnosis of cancer. Transitions prompt people to reconsider their attitudes and behaviors, they respond to data, seek information, accumulate knowledge and, hopefully, act wisely. A consumer's ability to take action is enhanced (or limited) by available *capital*. The direction of actions is shaped by *influences* in the environment.

Expanding on Nelson's (2002) notes, wisdom for health requires combining values, experience, and knowledge (human capital) that encompasses empirical evidence (*data*), ethical principles, aesthetic appreciation, and awareness of self. As consumers interpret and connect these patterns using personal, community, and Internet resources, they gain *knowledge* that will assist them to feel reassured about their health situation, develop new attitudes and behaviors, and prepare for making decisions. Building on personal *wisdom*, or connecting with others who are sources of *influence* (in the real or virtual world), empowered consumers to come to decisions that work for them.

Wisdom creates *influence* or a push to act or stabilize. In this process, consumers are influenced by charismatic individuals, groups, and media, including websites and digital games and applications. *Charisma* is the power and energy that motivates behaviors and attitudes. It is the magic of interaction that is personal and can be generated by manipulating visual and aesthetic elements in the presentation of information—the power of advertising.

Consumers' access to and ability to use wisdom is directly and indirectly influenced by the capital available to them. *Capital* is the environmental context of values and resources on which individuals, groups, and communities draw to survive. These values and resources range from economic to psychological/emotional, health, human, and social capital. Capital comes in several forms and consists of values, support, skills, and tangible items including human capital (education and attitudes), economic capital (financial), social capital (values and support available from friends, family, health professionals, etc.), and sociotechnical capital. Sociotechnical capital is critical to participating in the emerging eHealth initiatives. This involves skill in using digital resources for social networking including data reporting, gathering information, and building knowledge and wisdom (Resnick, 2002).

Across the globe there are great inequities that affect the relevance of digital resources to building and sustaining a healthy life with technology. These inequities must be taken into account and are noted in the discussions of telehealth (see Chapter 7), but they will not be detailed in this book.

The Health Habitat as Context for the Conceptual Framework

People are using the Internet in multiple ways to meet their different health needs. They use the Internet for gathering health information, managing their health records, booking a doctor's appointment, accessing other healthcare services, using interactive tools to help make healthcare decisions, and more importantly, finding people with similar health situations and building a wider social support system with each other than could be built without the Internet. These interactions broaden the *health habitat* and increase resources available to consumers of health technology. As described in Chapter 1, the health habitat is the ecological construct that describes the range of environments and resources (capital) in which individuals and families carry out their lives and struggle or thrive. The outcome of struggles or opportunities can be greatly enhanced by digital resources and a recognition that everything is connected (Hames, 2007). This ecological framework promotes appreciation of how data can be collected, aggregated, and viewed online so that patterns of information emerge (refer to Figure 3.1).

Theoretical Models for Understanding Online Health Search Behaviors

A number of theories have been developed to explain the process of health information-seeking behaviors. Johnson and Meischke (1993) proposed a comprehensive model of information-seeking that integrates the factors from three theoretical perspectives: the health belief model, uses and gratifications research, and a model of media exposure and appraisal. The comprehensive model of information seeking postulates that four health-related factors (demographics, direct experience, salience, and beliefs) determine people's perceptions of the characteristics and usefulness of information, which in turn influences health information-seeking actions.

Another theory, the Theory of Motivated Information Management proposed by Afifi and Weiner (2004), integrates the key factors that influence the information-acquisition process, such as uncertainty, experience with an illness, and expectations about the outcomes associated with acquiring information. More specifically, the theory states that the information-seeking process starts with a gap between desired and actual uncertainty about certain issues. Such a gap will lead to uncertainty-related anxiety, which can motivate people to assess the usefulness of various information management strategies by evaluating their outcome and efficacy. In the end, individuals choose what they consider to be the best strategy based on their judgment of physiological, cognitive, social, and behavioral concerns.

Two other theoretical frameworks, the uses and gratifications theory (Rubin, 1994) and the selective exposure theory (Atkin, 1985), both from communication perspectives, are also applied in the realm of health information processing. These two theories articulate that individuals select media to use based on their needs and interpret media messages that are consistent with their existing attitudes and beliefs. For example, Dutta-Bergman (2004) used selective exposure theory and demonstrated that those who were highly engaged in health-related issues were more likely to seek out health-specialized media content than the individuals who were not involved in issues of health. As indicated in these theories, research has demonstrated that such variables as one's perception of uncertainty (Brashers, 2001), the degree to which a health threat is salient (Johnson & Meischke, 1993), health information needs (Dutta-Bergman, 2004), or the perceived outcomes associated with acquiring health information (Afifi & Weiner, 2006) play a central role in health information-seeking behaviors.

Several theorists also attempt to categorize online health information search activities and patterns. Josefsson (2006) used Wilson's (1997) general model of information behavior and identified four types of information-seeking behaviors online: passive attention, passive search, active search, and ongoing search. Passive attention involves information acquisition without intentional seeking. Passive search occurs when an individual comes across limited and random sets of health information that happen to be relevant to his or her health condition, through interpersonal or physician recommendations or while reading or searching for other information. Active search occurs when the individual actively seeks out health information relevant to his or her health condition, whether through search engines or medical sites. Active searches often yield a large and almost unlimited amount of information and bring about opportunities to interact with fellow patients for social support through forums such as discussion groups, self-help groups, and e-mail lists. In an ongoing search, individuals have settled on favorite sites for relevant health information and continually go back in order to further refine and develop their knowledge. The information found is then processed and used.

Niederdeppe et al. (2007) also identify two types of health information-seeking behaviors: information seeking and scanning. Information seeking is defined as an active and purposeful information-seeking behavior, while information scanning is defined as the exposure to health information less purposively. Their study suggests that health information scanning more frequently happens among information seekers than health information seeking. Xie (2009) investigated the online and offline health information behavior of older adults and developed a conceptual framework of health information wants. The framework identifies four types of health information needs that influence healthcare decisions and the relationship with the healthcare provider. Information needs range from basic to complementary. Individuals who are type 1 (basic) depend highly on professionals in making direct healthcare decisions, and individuals who are type 4 (provider) are highly involved in health information gathering and tend to make their own decisions about providers, diagnosis, and treatment. Meanwhile, type 2 (advanced) wants as detailed health information as is possible to obtain, and type 3 (complementary) are interested in information about alternative treatments. The Internet can be used to provide medical information in simpler language (type 2) or help patients search for nontraditional or complementary remedies (type 3). The sources for nontraditional remedies specific to cancer, it turns out, are most likely to have errors on the website (Bernstam, Shelton, Walji, & Meric-Bernstam, 2005). Given the nature of alternative or complementary medicine, it is likely that errors are commonly found in websites that discuss nontraditional health care for other conditions. In 2008, BBC Health removed the complementary health section of their website due to difficulties in sustaining quality (Williams, 2008). A registry has been proposed as a strategy for setting standards. Health professionals will want to specifically initiate coaching on information seeking for clients who express interest in complementary or alternative medicine. It is important to clarify that legitimate news stations may report sensationalized health stories because they are of public interest and not necessarily because the event or therapy is legitimate. Adverse reactions to established treatments or vaccinations can go "viral"—spread around the globe to highly diverse audiences, especially if a dramatic video is posted. All health information searchers on any topic would benefit from triangulation—finding information on a specific topic from three different sources. For example, coaches on information seeking might recommend following up blog statements or videos with searches of PubMed, university medical center affiliated, government, or professional association websites.

Personal Traits as Variable in Information Seeking

Efforts also have been made to identify the personal traits related to the desire to seek health information. Dutta-Bergman's (2004) research indicates that those who use the Internet as a primary source for health information are more health conscious, more concerned about their health, and more likely to engage in healthy behaviors than those who did not use the Internet as a primary information source.

In addition, a review of the literature by Mills and Sullivan (1999) identified a number of disease-related factors that may predict information needs and activities. These include time since diagnosis, type of cancer, type of treatment, and stage of disease. For example, Luker et al. (1996) suggest that the time since diagnosis may influence the type of information needed and where and how intensely the information is sought. Flynn, Smith, and Freese (2006) found that those with diagnosed conditions or illnesses were more likely to have ever sought health information online.

Internet self-efficacy is another important variable in examining online health information-seeking behavior. Self-efficacy is a key component in social cognitive theory (Bandura, 1986). Bandura (1997, 2004) notes that self-efficacy does not concern the skills one actually possesses, but how one perceives his or her abilities in doing something. Self-efficacy is critical to determine how much effort and persistence one is willing to put forth, as people with low self-efficacy may feel their efforts will just end in failure, whereas people with high self-efficacy believe they can overcome obstacles and attain their goals (Bandura, 1997, 2004). Self-efficacy is also domain specific, varying across different circumstances and tasks.

Internet self-efficacy is one's perception of his or her ability to use the Internet, which in this context, is the ability to acquire health information online (Eastin & LaRose, 2000). Hong (2006) found that individuals who had a high degree of Internet self-efficacy were more successful at locating high-quality health websites than those lacking efficacy. Rains (2008) found that the effect of Web experience on the perceived success of an online health information search was mediated by Internet self-efficacy. Similarly, self-efficacy about computers (and lower anxiety about aging) was a better predictor of enrollment in a cybercafé than previous experience with computers (Jung et al., 2010). This is especially relevant as access was simple: the cybercafé was in the room visible to participants in a daily meal program for seniors (Jung et al., 2010). Therefore, simply offering individuals access to the Internet cannot guarantee they will have a positive and effective experience in acquiring useful health information online. It is important for practitioners to know that improving a sense of efficacy is critical in overcoming the barriers to online health search. To improve self-efficacy for online health searches, it is important that training is conducted in a relaxed and supportive environment so that trainees do not feel rushed or frustrated. In short, to understand online health information search behaviors, it is necessary to take into account personal characteristics, information needs, psychological variables, demographic variables, and role-related and interpersonal factors, as well as environmental characteristics and source characteristics.

Online Tools to Aid Decision Making

The Internet has also become an important means for helping people make healthcare decisions (Fox & Rainie, 2002). Decision-making aids are intervention tools that help patients make specific and deliberate choices for treatment (or other care) in the way that they prefer by providing information on the options and outcomes relevant to their health status (O'Connor et al., 2009). Decision aids range from simple paper-and-pencil tools to complex multimedia computer programs (O'Connor et al., 2009).

Online guides and tool kits have also been developed that help patients with decision making (Murray, Burns, See, Lai, & Nazareth, 2005). For example, the Ottawa Hospital Research Institute (OHRI) has a website devoted to Patient Decision Aids (http://decisionaid.ohri.ca). The OHRI website provides an inventory of decision aids, a tutorial, a kit for developing decision aids, and a link to the Cochrane Decision Aid Registry for managing resources. This website offers both a general decision-making aid that can be used when making any health-related (or other life) decision, as well as an extensive selection of decisions aids designed for specific medical conditions. These decisions aids present facts about the medical condition, compare the benefits and risks of options, provide questions to capture your feelings about the options, and then ask questions about how to decide what to do next. In O'Connor et al.'s review (2009), a quality decision-making aid must:

1. "Provide evidence-based information about a health condition, the options, associated benefits, and risks.
2. Help patients to recognize the value-sensitive nature of the decision and clarify, either implicitly or explicitly, the value they place on the benefits and risks. Strategies that may be included in the decision aid are describing the options in enough detail that clients can imagine what it is like to

experience the physical, emotional, and social effects; and guiding clients to consider which benefits and risks are most important to them.

3. Provide structured guidance in both decision making and communicating their values with others involved in the decision (e.g., clinician, family, friends)." (p. 3)

In a variety of studies, decision-making aids have improved user knowledge, led to more realistic expectations, reduced decisional conflict relating to feeling informed, and increased active participation in decision making (Green et al., 2004; Murray et al., 2005; O'Connor et al., 2009). However, Murray et al. (2005) also called for more research to determine the best type and best way to deliver decision aids, and to examine how these decision-aid tools may have effects for different groups of people. There is very little information on cultural variations or gender differences in responses on decision-aid tools.

Barriers and Challenges in Information Seeking

As the Internet plays an increasing role in delivering health information and health care, those people with limited Internet access and skills will be highly disadvantaged. As shown in Table 3.1, people who are over 65 years old, from rural areas, have less education, and have lower incomes are less likely to go online. Meanwhile, the data also shows that the racial and gender differences in access to the Internet have diminished, and most remaining differences can be explained by other basic factors such as age, income, and education (Pew Internet & American Life Project, 2009).

Table 3.1   Demographics of Internet Users

	Use the Internet (%)
Total adults	74
Men	74
Women	74
Race/ethnicity	
White, non-Hispanic	76
Black, non-Hispanic	70
Hispanic (English- and Spanish-speaking)	64

Table 3.1   **Demographics of Internet Users (*continued*)**

	Use the Internet (%)
Age	
18–29	93
30–49	81
50–64	70
65+	38
Household income	
Less than $30,000/yr	60
$30,000–$49,999	76
$50,000–$74,999	83
$75,000+	94
Educational attainment	
Less than high school	39
High school	63
Some college	87
College+	94
Community type	
Urban	74
Suburban	77
Rural	70

Source: Pew Internet & American Life Project, 2009. Used with permission.

Jimison et al. (2008) reviewed the research on the barriers to the use of interactive health information technology by the elderly, those with chronic conditions or disabilities, and the underserved. In this very extensive review of studies of interactive consumer health information technology (IT), the authors concluded that "several types of consumer health IT were usable and effective in multiple settings and with all of our populations of interest (p. v). The reviewers emphasized that a feedback loop was the most consistent variable in achieving desired outcomes. This meant a cycle of monitoring data on patient status, interpreting the data in the context of information about the individual, adjusting care plans combining the professional's expertise and knowledge of the patient, and sharing wisdom with the patient.

Jimison et al. (2008) reported that the most common factor influencing the successful use of interactive technology was that the consumers perceived a benefit from using the technology. In sum, they listed the following barriers we should pay attention to when promoting new health information technologies, including Web-based ones:

- Lack of perceived benefit
- Technology intervention did not fit their lifestyle
- Lack of trust in the system
- Technological malfunctions
- Technology is too cumbersome
- Confusion with the technology and content
- Specific barriers with interactive reminding technologies
- Clinician use of patient-retrieved information
- Cost
- Age, disabilities, and other physical limitations

The existing digital divide presents a great barrier to accessing and using online health information and health services, especially for older adults and those with lower socioeconomic status. Joint efforts from public, private, and nongovernmental sectors are needed to bridge this "technology gap" so that all people can have equal access to online health information.

In addition, DiMaggio, Hargittai, Neuman, and Robinson (2001) suggest that the digital divide cannot be simply understood as an access issue. There is a "second-level digital divide," which refers to the lack of skills to accomplish a set of technological tasks. As discussed in detail in Chapter 2, a wide range of literacies is required to thrive in the digital age. This indicates that, besides the solution to access issues, it is equally important to deliver effective trainings and technical support to those in need of help in acquiring online health information. This need is especially strong for groups such as seniors who may experience difficulties using computers and the Internet. A focus on digital inclusion has been proposed as reflective of new potentials—with costs dropping, broadband availability in more neighborhoods, and more community resources for coaching and support. Generalizing from concerns about stigma attached to literacy screenings, a universal precautions approach is proposed to establishing access issues.

SOCIAL NETWORKING AS A MAGNET FOR INTERNET ENGAGEMENT

Currently, thousands of online health-related peer-to-peer support groups are available on the Internet in the form of mailing lists, chat rooms, and discussion forums (Demiris, 2006). Members in these online support groups share common problems, assist each other toward mutual goals, and support each other through good and bad times (Preece, 2001). Numerous studies have demonstrated that the participation in these online support groups can lead to increased knowledge of one's health condition and improved psychological well-being and health status, such as decreased stress, depression, and anxiety, and increased disclosure, self-esteem, and coping skills (Carlbring et al., 2005; Gustafson et al., 1999; Lieberman et al., 2003; Meier, Lyons, Frydman, Forlenza, & Rimer, 2007; Rodgers & Chen, 2005; Tate, Jackvony, & Wing, 2003).

These online groups are an important means of moving bits and reams of data that consumers now can collect and pool to share information. As groups interact, new knowledge emerges for individuals, group members, and the professionals monitoring these sites. Many consumers turn to their social networks for wisdom so they can make good choices or feel reassured about choices made or offered to them. Online groups have the potential of becoming a powerful influence on health behaviors and decisions. To date, there is scant evidence of such change, but online support groups have been very effective in empowering participants to take a more active role in their health care (Barak, Boniel-Nissim, & Suler, 2008). It is not clear to what extent information mediation (see Digital Circles of Support in Chapter 2) would increase the effectiveness of the groups.

Social Networking Sites for Health Purposes

It has been widely claimed that the next generation of the Internet will be centered around the development of Web 2.0 technologies, which emphasizes the potential of the Internet in facilitating more effective and productive communication and collaboration among social members (Eysenbach, 2008; Sarasohn-Kahn, 2008). Social networking technologies are central to the Web 2.0 applications, and have been used for health-related purposes. The use of social networking features is expected to foster more intimate relationships, thus enhancing the exchange of information and social support. Rau, Gao, and Ding (2008) found that people on social networking sites are connected in a person-to-person manner while traditional online communities (e.g., online forums) are more likely to center around a specific topic. Mayfield (2005) concluded that traditional online communities are usually top-down, topic-driven, and centralized, whereas social networking sites are usually bottom-up, people-focused, and decentralized.

The features of social networking technologies are believed to be able to greatly empower patients by providing a powerful tool for social collaboration and connection. Technology provides a means to reshape the picture of medical research and patient–provider dynamics. For example, members in PatientsLikeMe (2010) can use specific visualization tools to chart their medical histories and share their personal experiences about their current treatments, symptoms, and outcomes with one another (Arnst, 2008). Like normal social networking sites, members in PatientsLikeMe have their own profile pages with photos, real names, and other personal information. Fox (2009) notes that such peer-to-peer advice and support has a powerful influence on patients' health-related behaviors. According to a survey of HIV community members on PatientsLikeMe, two thirds of respondents reported that they were more knowledgeable about a treatment because of advice from other users at PatientsLikeMe, and 70% of respondents said that participating in PatientsLikeMe had increased their attention to the results of tests ordered by the doctor treating their HIV (Fox, 2009).

Currently, most support sites such as PatientsLikeMe (2010) take a hybrid form that combines different communication technologies, including discussion forums, information resources, and social networking features. Users of PatientsLikeMe can review and discuss their common health concerns and strategies for managing their illness or condition by participating in the discussion forums, using private messaging, and making comments posted on each other's profile pages (Frost & Massagli, 2008). In general, members of these sites can post and read messages about specific health conditions; can find information resources and learn about illnesses, treatments, and medication options; and can also have more personal interactions with other users by using social networking components. PatientsLikeMe and related sites can make important contributions to accumulating knowledge about drugs and treatments and disease progression on an everyday basis. The website recently was awarded a prize as having contributed to knowledge of post-marketing drug data (Journal of Medical Internet Research [JMIR], 2009).

The combination of these features in one online community greatly benefit the members and gratifies their various needs for health information and social support. There are many interactive websites created for people who are seeking health information. These websites have been developed to cover general health information and many medical conditions (Table 3.2), as well as websites that are dedicated to specific health issues, such as breast cancer or diabetes

(Table 3.3). Barak, et al. (2008) found that benefits of participating in online support groups can be feelings of empowerment, well-being, a sense of control, self-confidence, feelings of independence, and social interactions. However, users should be aware of potential risks, such as developing dependence and distancing from in-person contacts, but most reported empowerment and improvement in their well-being.

Table 3.2   Health Information Websites for General Health Purposes

- Tursera (www.tursera.com)
- Health Chapter (www.healthchapter.com)
- Wellescent (www.wellescent.com)
- Hope Cube (www.hopecube.com)
- Inspire (www.inspire.com)
- Daily Strength (www.dailystrengh.org)
- Tools To Life (www.toolstolife.com)
- Live Strong (www.livestrong.org)
- Revolution Health (www.revolutionhealth.com)
- Medicare Interactive Counselor (www.medicareinteractive.org)
- Caring.com (www.caring.com)
- Medline Plus (www.medlineplus.gov)
- National Business Group on Health (www.businessgrouphealth.org)
- Health Finder (www.healthfinder.gov)

Table 3.3   Health Information Websites for Specific Health Issues

- My Cancer Place (www.mycancerplace.com), Live Strong (www.livestrong.org), and No Surrender (www.no-surrender.org) for cancer
- My Crazy Sexy Life (www.crazysexylife.com) for breast cancer
- Planet Cancer (www.planetcancer.org) for young adults with cancer
- Prostate Cancer InfoLink (www.prostatecancerinfolink.ning.com) for prostate cancer
- Psych Central (www.psychcentral.com) for mental health
- Sober Circle (www.sobercircle.com) for alcoholism
- Diabetic Connect (www.diabeticconnect.com), TuDiabetes (www.tudiabetes.com), and SugarStats (www.sugarstats.com) for diabetics
- Daily Plate (www.thedailyplate.com) for dieting and eating
- BrainTalk (http://brain.hastypastry.net/forums) for neurological disorders
- Caring (www.caring.com) for elder care
- PatientsLikeMe (www.patientslikeme.org) features multiple conditions

Advancing Normative Health Behaviors with New Social Media Tools

Health professionals and consumers are becoming more aware of the social dimension of health behaviors and outcomes. Sharing information with each other using new social media may be a way of attracting the holdouts and motivating those who are reluctant to get engaged.

Social media tools are key in the repertoire of health professionals and consumer health advocates. These tools are the Internet-age basics: "to reinforce and personalize messages, reach new audiences, and build a communication infrastructure based on open information exchange" (Centers for Disease Control and Prevention [CDC], 2009, para. 1). These tools are a powerful means of sharing information, promoting shared decision making, and setting the expectation that the wisdom of the social network might be a key influence on health-related behaviors and beliefs.

Research with adolescents makes clear that beliefs about how others are behaving is key in setting norms for one's own behavior (Rice, Stein, & Milburn, 2008). How this operates for adults is less clear. Researchers and practitioners may have focused so narrowly on peer influences as a key feature of adolescence that such norm-checking studies may simply not have been carried out for adults. As we bring social aspects back to the ecological perspective on health, adults across the life span may be more influenced than previously appreciated. Healthcare providers and consumer health advocates will enrich their outreach efforts by providing their content using social media tools. New, desirable norms are promoted through media selected by the consumer and may become more widely adopted as they are perceived as group wisdom.

As health resources go more mobile, it is important for purveyors of resources to have a variety of access points. There is a dynamic tension between "push" and "pull" technology. In a pull mode, the consumer must keep track of how to find his or her preferred sources and remember to check them periodically. These "go-to" references include websites, blogs, and podcasts. Thus, the user pulls the content and decides each time whether to store the information, link to related resources, e-mail to self or others, post on a personal website, add to favorite blogs, or ignore it. For many people, a "push" approach is preferred. In this case, the consumer sets up an automatic link, and the content appears through e-mail, podcasts, emergency text messages, RSS feeds, or widgets. Often, the consumer can indicate a preference for a digest format, so that material is not constantly appearing. A week is a common interval to choose to have information condensed.

The Centers for Disease Control and Prevention (CDC) website provides an excellent overview of common social media networking tools with examples from their applications. The explanation of social media tools is available at http://www.cdc.gov/SocialMedia, with links to such resources as an inventory of current social media tools. In that section, CDC provides links that show examples and provide instruction for using the CDC versions of each tool (Table 3.4).

Table 3.4   Social Media Formats with CDC-Linked Examples

Blogs

Read a CDC blog on a topic ranging from occupational health to HIV prevention and control.
http://www.cdc.gov/SocialMedia/Tools/Blogs.html

Bloginars

CDC hosts bloginars on important and timely topics as a tool to reach out to bloggers and provide information about outbreaks or public health events.
http://www.cdc.gov/SocialMedia/Tools/Bloginars.html

Buttons and Badges

CDC uses buttons and badges, or graphic elements with links to websites to share health messages.
http://www.cdc.gov/SocialMedia/Tools/ButtonsBadges.html

CDC-INFO

As CDC's National Contact Center, CDC-INFO provides a single source of accurate, timely, consistent health and safety information 24 hours a day, 7 days a week. CDC-INFO plays an important role in our integrated eHealth communications efforts.
http://www.cdc.gov/SocialMedia/Tools/CDC-INFO.html

Content Syndication

Partners can use CDC's content syndication technology to display fresh Web content on the partners' Web pages.
http://www.cdc.gov/SocialMedia/Tools/ContentSyndication.html

eCards

Send an electronic greeting card, or eCard, to encourage healthy living, promote safe activities, or celebrate a health-and-safety-related event.
http://www.cdc.gov/SocialMedia/Tools/eCards.html

eGames

Play an interactive, electronic game for fun and creative ways to learn about health and safety information.
http://www.cdc.gov/SocialMedia/Tools/eGames.html

E-mail Updates

Get e-mail updates when CDC refreshes the content on CDC.gov Web pages.
http://www.cdc.gov/SocialMedia/Tools/emailUpdates.html

(continues)

Table 3.4   Social Media Formats with CDC-Linked Examples (*continued*)

Image Sharing

Share public health images provided on one of CDC's photo-sharing spaces.
http://www.cdc.gov/SocialMedia/Tools/ImageSharing.html

Micro-blogs

Follow one of CDC's status updates on Twitter.
http://www.cdc.gov/SocialMedia/Tools/MicroBlogs.html

Mobile

Stay informed on the go with health and safety information designed for your mobile device.
http://www.cdc.gov/SocialMedia/Tools/Mobile.html

Online Video

Watch one of CDC's online videos to engage with CDC content in a fun, visual, and interactive way.
http://www.cdc.gov/SocialMedia/Tools/OnlineVideo.html

Podcasts

CDC produces podcasts to provide health information in a portable format.
http://www.cdc.gov/SocialMedia/Tools/Podcasts.html

RSS

Stay updated by subscribing to one of many RSS, or Really Simple Syndication, feeds.
http://www.cdc.gov/SocialMedia/Tools/RSS.html

Social Networking Sites

Connect with CDC on one of their social networking profiles. You can find CDC's information on Facebook, MySpace, or Daily Strength.
http://www.cdc.gov/SocialMedia/Tools/SocialNetworking.html

Virtual Worlds

Learn more about CDC's involvement in the virtual worlds of Second Life and Whyville.
http://www.cdc.gov/SocialMedia/Tools/VirtualWorlds.html

Widgets

Add a CDC widget to your Web page, social networking profile, or blog, and stay informed with up-to-date, credible health and safety content.
http://www.cdc.gov/SocialMedia/Tools/Widgets.html

Source: CDC, 2009.

Two rather new approaches are described here. RSS feeds are defined by CNN as a Really Simple Syndication (CNN, 2010). This *feed* or *push* tool is for sharing and distributing Web content, such as news headlines. It is much like a subscription: the user signs up, agrees to a set of conditions posted by the syndicator, and an icon appears on the user's desktop when new information has arrived. A widget is an online application built on one website that can be automatically directed to another website. Widgets are particularly suited to groups of people who enjoy interfacing through their mobile phones.

Widgets as Decision Aids

The Centers for Disease Control and Prevention offers a new resource for decisions about healthcare issues—the CDC widgets. The CDC already uses e-mail updates, podcasts, emergency text messages, and RSS feeds to provide current health information and decision guides. The new widgets display featured content directly on a personal Web page or cell phone application page. The widget is designed for easy embedding in blogs, home pages, and social networking sites. Once the consumer determines the topics of continuing interest, installing the widget reduces searching and browsing time and facilitates sharing more easily than an RSS feed. CDC widgets are available at http://www.cdc.gov/Widgets. The widget posting extends the reach of CDC exponentially as friends on the social network site encounter the resource. In addition, making the link public encourages the easy dissemination of accurate, CDC-vetted prevention and disease control information throughout the Web, as Wikipedia-like information is often unreliable (E. Rice, personal communication, September 2, 2009).

Twitter as Microblogs

Twitter is an example of user-generated content, a form of social media that can be highly relevant in health care (Hawn, 2009; Terry, 2009). Terry defines twitter as "an Internet-based way to stay in touch, waste time, and kill productivity" (p. 507). He cites Kvedar as defining Twitter as "mass communication" and goes on to provide updates on how Twitter might be useful to healthcare consumers and providers.

The Twitter website provides a variety of support resources (www.twitter.com). Terry (2009) provides an excellent comparison of text messaging (160 characters) sent by cell phone to specific recipients with Twittering (140 characters and tiny URLs) to anyone else following a specific Twitter account. Tiny URLs compress the usual multicharacter URL to meet Twitter limitations and promote linking to relevant websites. Sign up is required. Subscribers can "follow" anyone they want continuously—on the Twitter home page or by requesting messages be "pushed" to or from a mobile device. *Tweet* is the name given to the message, and users may be continuously tweeting, alone or with others, in a variety of settings.

Consumer Health Applications

In health care, Terry (2009) reports that providers can simultaneously communicate with team members—handy for cancelled appointments. Baumann's list of nurse-generated healthcare uses for Twitter are highlighted on his blog post (see www.philbaumann.com). Trialx, which is a clinical trials finder tailored to specific consumer profiles, uses Twitter to increase information sharing about clinical trials open to enrollment. CDC countered "unreliable, ridiculous gossip" about H1N1 with CDC Twitter feeds (Terry, 2009, p. 509). CDC offers CDC-eHealth, which drives traffic to other social content available at CDC: a feed related to generic flu information, an emergency feed for outbreaks of H1N1, product recalls, and other urgent health events.

Designing Training for Internet Engagement

Research has been conducted to examine the best way to deliver effective training. Rogers, Campbell, and Pak (2001) proposed a systems approach to address the factors to be taken account into while developing and evaluating computer training programs. In the systems approach to training, the characteristics of the person, the environment, and the technology itself are considered through the following sequential stages: needs assessment, task/person analysis, selection and design of training programs, and evaluation.

Mayhorn, Stronge, McLaughlin, and Rogers (2004) applied this systems approach and reviewed a set of training programs for older adults. Mayhorn et al. provide recommendations for optimizing computer training for older adults (as shown in Table 3.5). The guidelines indicate that older users prefer written instructions, and that they want hands-on support from trainers throughout the class. It is recommended that instructions for the use of a computer and the Internet be provided in a written format, in plain language, so that individuals may refer to these instructions. Such instruction needs to be very simple, with every step included, and in a very easy-to-understand format. Table 3.5 depicts a number of general recommendations that can be used to optimize program design.

Table 3.5 Everyday Considerations for Computer Training for Older Adults

Class Arrangements

- Small class size
- Separation of students into levels based on skill, experience
- Adequate lighting
- Ergonomic furniture
- Café atmosphere
- Adequate tutor support
- Printer to capture accomplishments, reading at home

Design of Materials

- Minimize technical jargon
- Translate potentially alarming messages, such as "illegal operation" and other terms
- State purpose and objectives on materials
- Organize materials into brief units to avoid information overload
- Conduct task analyses for each computer task before instruction
- Use step-by-step format for instructions
- Provide hints for adapting to cognitive, visual, motor declines
- Create translated materials such that English and second language match placement for visual orientation of user and teacher

Spirit of Learning

- Instruction should proceed at a comfortable pace with built-in breaks
- Build in early successes and share personal learning challenges
- Use return demonstration approach: show, try, practice
- Keep learner in driver's seat: avoid "doing for"
- Make retrieval of learning materials easy to minimize embarrassment
- Encourage peer coaching model
- Consider starting point of interest to learner: printing photos, e-mailing, hometown news retrieval
- Consider cultural appeal of certificates of achievement

Sources: Jordan-Marsh et al., 2006; Mayhorn et al., 2004.

Cody, Dunn, Hoppin, and Wendt (1999) also proposed a "paced-format" method of training geared toward the different needs of adult learners. They found that some people left class because the tasks were too hard for them, while others left because they found the tasks were not as challenging as they had anticipated. It is important to tailor the instruction to the level of the individuals in the class. Jordan-Marsh et al. (2006) found that one-on-one instruction was very important for seniors. A combination of a paid coordinator for the cybercafé in a senior center, college student volunteers, and designated peer tutors was very effective. Seniors were willing to pay a small monthly fee for unlimited access during center hours. Many had Internet resources in their homes but desired supportive coaching and enjoyed the café atmosphere (computer stations surrounding a center of tables and chairs, a counter with coffee, tea, and pastries available), and the inexpensive printing in color was a big draw.

In addition, Anderson (2004) pointed out some other major barriers to the use of the Internet for health-related purposes, such as the potential threats to privacy, inaccuracy of information, problems in evaluating the quality of information and services obtained from the Internet, and physician disapproval. One of the most substantial challenges faced by consumers is locating high-quality information among a multitude of websites offering medical information and advice. This chapter specifically addresses this issue in the following section. Beyond the quality of health information available, consumers also face challenges understanding medical information written in complex or technical language (Berland et al., 2001) and identifying appropriate search terms for illnesses or conditions (Wolfe & Sharp, 2005).

MAKING USE OF THE INTERNET FOR HEALTH INFORMATION

Quality Concerns of Online Health Information

The Internet enables people to have timely and convenient access to a large amount of health information, so that they can be better informed about their health conditions and actively take part in the process of healthcare decisions. However, the potential downsides of online information access have not been fully studied. Unfortunately, a lot of what is available might be considered as data rather than information. Consumers can quickly get overwhelmed. There is a great variation in the quality of what is presented as health information online. Health information available on the Internet is not well regulated and might be inaccurate, confusing, and misleading to health seekers. The healthcare system has not instituted universal policies for reviewing information to see that it supplies the knowledge consumers need to make wise decisions. Influence may come from purveyors of expensive remedies or online subscriptions as easily as from valid experts, whether health professionals or consumer advocates.

The failure of health seekers to identify accurate health information might endanger their health. In addition, they may also be influenced by online advertising and marketing from medicine companies. Eysenbach, Powell, Kuss, and Sa (2002) conducted a meta-analysis of 79 studies that examined over 5900 health-related websites, reporting that consumers face "significant problems" locating accurate, complete, and quality health information websites (p. 2696).

Health seekers were also reported to have difficulty in understanding medical information written in complex or technical language (Berland et al., 2001). Anderson (2004) suggests that the use of the Internet for health-related purposes is also a potential threat to people's privacy. This is discussed in greater detail in Chapter 4.

Older adults are typically less experienced, skilled, and confident in generally using computer and Internet technologies. Consequently, older adults may have much greater challenges in finding needed and accurate online health information, and they are more vulnerable to the negative consequences of online health information searches. Various checklists and tools for consumers to assess the quality of health information on the Internet have been proposed, ranging from simple checklists to a portal that provides a scoring system to evaluate a site (Breckons et al., 2008). For example, the SPRY (Setting Priorities for Retirement Years) Foundation developed a specific guide to help older adults evaluate health information on the Web (SPRY Foundation, 2001). This guide contains a checklist of criteria that older adults can use to evaluate heath websites, including accuracy, authorship, copyright, contact information, site support, disclaimers and cautions, currency, intended audience, completeness of content, clarity of content, and privacy (Table 3.6). The full text of the guide is available online at http://www.spry.org/pdf/EvaluatingHealthInfo.pdf.

Some organizations also developed a scoring system for the evaluation of health-related websites. For instance, DISCERN developed an instrument to assess quality criteria for consumer health information (Charnock & Shepperd, 1997). Their instrument has 16 questions measured on a 5-point scale designed to judge quality and reliability of online health information.

Table 3.6   Checklist for Evaluating Online Health Information

1. Can you tell who **created the content**?	Yes ❑	No ❑
2. Are you given enough information to judge if the **author is reliable**?	Yes ❑	No ❑
3. Can you tell if the **content is current**?	Yes ❑	No ❑
4. Can you tell if the **content is accurate**?	Yes ❑	No ❑
5. Do you have confidence that your **privacy is protected**?	Yes ❑	No ❑
6. Is the content **copyrighted**?	Yes ❑	No ❑
7. Does the site provide complete **contact information**?	Yes ❑	No ❑
8. Is it clear who is **funding the site**?	Yes ❑	No ❑
9. Is there a clear **disclaimer posted**?	Yes ❑	No ❑
10. Does the site **provide references** for its content?	Yes ❑	No ❑
11. Is it clear who is the **intended audience**?	Yes ❑	No ❑

Source: Spry Foundation, 2001. Used with permission.

Some nongovernmental organizations (NGOs) have also taken action to ensure reliable health information on the Web. Health on the Net (HON) Foundation (www.healthonnet.org) is one such NGO that works to improve the quality of useful, reliable, and appropriate online health information. They developed the HONcode of conduct that sets standards and conditions for credible and ethical health information. Healthcare website developers or information providers can apply for HONcode certification and display the HONcode seal of approval and logo on their websites. HON also developed their own search engine and training tools for the public as an effort to guide people to trustworthy health information. Consumers can download the free HONcode toolbar, which installs a search engine they can use when browsing online health information. The HONcode toolbar checks the health website's certification status, and only displays those which have been accredited as trustworthy.

Introducing older adults to these guidelines and tools is believed to increase the likelihood that they find credible health information online. However, it does not seem that these guidelines are being widely used by the majority of older adults. Future research needs to explore the usability issues of these guidelines. Bernstam et al. (2005) suggested that any evaluation tool containing more than 10 criteria might be too long and time consuming for routine use. More effective and user-friendly guidelines and evaluation tools need to be identified and developed so that they can practically help older adults locate reliable, useful, and credible online health information. As noted in Chapter 2, the SPRY Foundation reported on the importance of the ease of attaining information online, highlighting the best practice of users only needing to click three times to get from a link to its destination (SPRY Foundation, 2001).

Another issue that needs further research is the efficacy of these evaluation tools. Bernstam et al. (2005) indicate that the majority of available instruments have not been systematically tested for their reliability or validity. Research on existing evaluation tools shows that there is poor agreement among users when ranking the quality of health websites (Bernstam et al., 2005; Breckons et al., 2008). Even researchers are likely to get poor agreement by using various criteria. Bernstam et al. (2005) examined the degree to which two raters could reliably assess 22 popularly cited quality criteria on a sample of 42 complementary and alternative medicine websites and found poor agreement on 8 out of 22. Future research is needed to identify the reasons for this, as well as more systematic evaluation of the efficacy of these guidelines.

Provost, Koompalum, Dong, and Martin (2006) proposed that one solution could be the standardization of evaluative tools. They developed their WebMedQual scale, which consists of 8 categories, 8 subcategories, 95 items, and 3 supplemental items to assess website quality. The criteria for evaluation include the following constructs: content, authority of source, design, accessibility and availability, links, user support, confidentiality and privacy, and e-commerce. Provost et al. claimed that their scale was the first step toward a standard easy-to-use tool. However, the feasibility of this proposal is not obvious.

Bernstam et al. (2005) argues that it may be useful to ask comprehensive questions about a site, but the usability of the instrument is also a factor. Breckons et al. (2008) questioned whether a 95-item scale, such as the WebMedQual scals, would be easy and fast enough for consumers to use when evaluating health websites. They propose that evaluation instruments should be easy to use, comprehensive, and current for maximum effectiveness (Breckons et al., 2008).

Consumers can go online for information to validate what they have been told by healthcare providers, to better understand what was quickly dispensed in a rushed visit, to make better decisions, and to engage social networks in understanding healthcare dilemmas and choices. And, as health care becomes less affordable and access more difficult, consumers are increasingly going online to self-diagnose or decide whether a visit to a healthcare professional is worth the effort and the cost.

The CDC has developed a variety of tools to provide consumers with reliable, scientific health information, such as blogs, podcasts, and online videos (refer to Table 3.4). Online health videos are gaining in popularity as an educational alternative to online health information in text format. Growing video libraries can be found at WebMD and MayoClinic.com, as well as websites devoted to specific conditions such as the American Cancer Society (www.cancer.org), Autism Speaks (www.autismspeaks.com), and Epilepsy.com (Painter, 2007). The Agency for Healthcare Research and Quality (AHRQ) (www.ahrq.gov) offers videos for consumers to help them ask the right questions at doctor visits so they can make better medical decisions and receive better care. Videos can be very helpful for those with limited text literacy, and the use of evocative images can assist with health literacy as well.

Other Concerns of Acquiring Online Health Information

There are some other concerns regarding reliance on the Internet for health information. As indicated by the theories discussed earlier, individuals may have different attitudes toward information provision and coping strategies. Some people want to know everything, whereas others truly believe that ignorance is bliss. Health information can be used to decrease uncertainty; however, it can produce converse effects that may create barriers for coping with health situations. Meanwhile, some level of uncertainty may sometimes promote hope and optimism. As Pinder (1990) points out, patients do vary in how much information they want, which is reflected in the efforts that patients make to obtain further information or to resist information that is offered to them. Pinder (1990) further notes that patients' information needs may also change during different stages of their illness.

Leydon et al. (2000) conducted in-depth interviews with 17 cancer patients, and the results showed that only 6 patients had made efforts to obtain as much information as possible, while the remaining 11 patients reported minimal efforts to obtain information in addition to that offered by hospital staff. Leydon et al.'s research showed that patients did not want information about everything all of the time, and patients selectively chose to know about different aspects of information at different times after their diagnosis. Patients who have different coping strategies for their illness may vary in their desire for information and their efforts to obtain it. Therefore, health information can be both positive and negative. The overwhelming amount of online health information may produce negative consequences for some people (Brashers, Goldsmith, & Hsieh, 2002). In short, health practitioners should attend to the variations in patients' desires for information and use different strategies to meet each patient's information needs.

Trends in Online Search Behaviors of Older Adults

Despite the good that Internet use might bring to older adults, they have not taken advantage of the full potential the Internet offers. A recent survey by the Pew Internet and American Life Project found that only 41% of people ages 65 and older use the Internet, compared to 72% ages 50–64, 82% ages 30–49, and 87% ages 18–29 (Fox & Jones, 2009). Meanwhile, the Pew project also reports that adults ages 65 and older are the least likely to search online for health information compared to other age groups (Fox & Jones, 2009). On the bright side, older adults are also a rapidly growing segment of the Internet-use population. According to a Pew report on Internet usage, the 70–75-year-old age group has the biggest increase in Internet use since 2005 (Jones & Fox, 2009). The Pew report on Internet usage also found that searching for health information is the third most popular online activity among seniors who are online, after e-mail and online nonhealth searches (Jones & Fox, 2009).

In an examination of the information needs of older adults in Singapore, Chong and Theng (2004) found that healthcare information was the second most popular topic of interest among the senior citizens in Singapore. Several studies suggest that the majority of online health information searchers in the older population are highly educated white females, with high socioeconomic status, and personal ownership and access to computers and the Internet (Campbell, 2004; Fox, 2006; Kaiser Family Foundation, 2005; Schwartz, Mosher, Wilson, Lipkus, & Collins, 2002). Over the next decade, as the more computer-literate young–olds, such as baby boomers, become the next generation of the older population, the number of older adults using the Internet is expected to increase dramatically (Alder, 2006; McDermott, 2001).

However, more research is needed on the patterns of online health information-seeking behaviors among older adults as compared to other age groups. A Pew report found that older adults were less likely than other age groups to go online for information about medical or health issues: only 27% of adults over 65 years of age, contrasted to 59% of those ages 50–64, 71% ages 30–49, and 72% ages 18–29 (Fox & Jones, 2009).

Hardt and Hollis-Sawyer (2007) surveyed adults ages 55 or older. They found that the Internet is not the leading source of health information for older consumers. In this study, male respondents did not mention the Internet as one of their top five sources for health information, whereas their female counterparts rated it as the fourth likely source to find health information. This finding is confirmed in recent research that demonstrated men were less likely than women to seek health information from the Internet (Tu & Hargraves, 2003). According to the Pew report, 57% of men surveyed had looked online for health information, versus 64% of women (Fox & Jones, 2009). Wicks (2004) interviewed older adults, and results indicated that they still strongly prefer in-person contact and print resources over electronic delivery for health information.

Most Frequently Searched Topics

The existing research also tells us some information about what kind of health information is searched for online. According to the Pew report about online health information-seeking behaviors, the top three searched topics by Internet users of all age groups were a specific disease or medical problem, a certain medical treatment or procedure, and exercise or fitness (Fox & Jones, 2009). Importantly, the Internet is a supplement to, rather than a replacement for, information from medical professionals: 86% of adults report asking a doctor or other health professional for information about medical issues, while 57% of adults search for health information online. Internet users ages 65 and older are much less likely than other age groups to search online for information about a specific disease or medical problem, certain medical treatments or procedures, and exercise and fitness.

One area of online search that has increased significantly over the years is searches about prescription and over-the-counter drugs (Fox & Jones, 2009). Forty-five percent of adults surveyed reported looking online for information about prescription or over-the-counter drugs, including a fair number of seniors: 41% of those 65 years or older, compared to 50% of 50–64-year-olds, 47% of 30–49-year-olds, and 38% of 18–29-year-olds.

Strategies for Online Health Searches

Several investigators have examined how people use the Internet to find health information. For example, Eysenbach and Köhler (2003) found that people who looked for online health information were likely to select the first few links that appear on search engines and tended not to look for information about site authors or disclaimers that sites might make. Sillence et al. (2007) proposed a stage model to explain how people select and filter online health information. They suggested that searchers normally made the decision to reject or accept a health website within the first few minutes, primarily on the basis of its design features. This is similar to the phenomenon described by Gladwell (2007) in his popular book *Blink*, in which he discusses how people tend to make unconscious judgments in the first few seconds when faced with a decision and how marketing manipulates these first impressions. Sillence et al. (2007) proposed that once searchers selected certain sites, they then evaluated the sites in more depth and mainly focused on the content rather than design factors. The final step Sillence et al. propose is when searchers develop a long-term trusting relationship with one or more particular sites.

More research is needed on the online health information search behaviors of older adults. Additionally, search strategies seem to be somewhat haphazard, so consumers need to be conscious of the way they are searching for and evaluating health information they find on the Internet. Generally, the literature supports the assumption that Internet searches for health information are growing in popularity among older adults. With the aging of baby boomers and increasing amounts of health care shifting to the home, the need for online health information will continue to increase.

Impact of Online Health Information

Information acquired online has been reported to lead individuals to feel more empowered in managing their own health, to improve their understanding of healthcare issues, increase their sense of control over their disease, influence their decision-making process, and change their approach to managing their health (Baker, Bundorf, Singer, & Wagner, 2003; Broom, 2005; Fox & Rainie, 2002; Hardey, 1999; Kivits, 2004; Sharf, 1997). Lau and Coiera (2008) found that searching across high-quality health information sources on the Web can improve consumers' accuracy in answering health questions. In another study, participants who used computers for health information reported making significantly more phone calls to their healthcare providers and decreased their need for doctor visits (Gustafson et al., 1999).

Helwig, Lovelle, Guse, and Gottlieb (1999) studied the effect of offering Internet access to consumers in an office waiting area. In this study, 94% of the patients found the Internet useful as a means of obtaining health information, 77% indicated they would change their behavior based on the information, 90% reported greater satisfaction with the office visit, and 92% stated they would use the system again. Oermann, Hamilton, and Shook (2003) assessed the value of using the Web to teach older consumers about their role in preventing medical errors. They developed a Web-based intervention that provided information for consumers about quality health care and their role in preventing medical errors. After being taught how to use the computer and Internet, seniors increased their knowledge about quality care and their own role in preventing medical errors, as well as learning how to locate highly rated websites.

Paradigm Shift to Truly Patient-Centered Care?

The process of searching online for health information is believed to have the power to challenge the historical hierarchical and physician-centered model in health care (Buckland & Gann, 1997). Hardey (1999) suggests that by breaking down the top-down model of health information giving, physicians may feel a loss of control over medical knowledge or deprofessionalization. Light (2001) argues that the Internet has the potential to lead to decentralized medical environments in which patients can participate in decision-making processes within health care. Recent developments in e-health validate this shifting paradigm (Institute of Medicine, 2009).

All these arguments seem to support the notion that the physician-centered model of health care is rapidly fading. However, the empirical evidence from the current research doesn't seem to support the argument that patient–provider dynamics have changed. For example, a Pew report (Fox & Jones, 2009) found that only 1 in 10 adults said that online health information had a "major" impact on their health care. A study conducted by Charles, Gafni, and Whelan (1997) showed little evidence of patient involvement in information exchange during prescription drug consultations. Sillence et al. (2007) suggested that physicians were still seen as the primary source of health information and advice despite the use of the Internet. In addition, research has shown a disconnection between information-seeking and decision-making preferences (Gaston & Mitchell, 2005; Hill & Laugharne, 2006; Robinson & Thomson, 2001), which means that although patients are very interested in having detailed health information, they tend to be much less interested in participating in decision making. Over time, consumers may be disappointed or unpleasantly surprised as the system shifts around them and is structured to require more responsibility on their part.

Changes in Patient–Provider Interactions

Research on how online health information access affects the quality of patient–provider communication shows mixed findings. Sillence et al. (2007)

reported that respondents perceived improved communication with physicians after online information access. However, it has been reported in earlier studies that health providers feel threatened by patients' information-seeking behavior and tend to react negatively to such behaviors in consultations (Anderson, Rainey, & Eysenbach, 2003; Henwood, Wyatt, Hart, & Smith, 2003). Broom's (2005) study also suggests that increased access to information and support online does not necessarily result in better provider–patient communication. He suggests that a patient attempting to engage actively in decision-making processes can sometimes result in hostility and irritation within a medical consultation. These findings indicate that physicians still tend to implicitly or explicitly discredit the ability and efforts of patients trying to become well informed via the Internet, which has presented a serious barrier to the establishment of a shared decision-making model in the healthcare system.

As indicated above, there has been much general discussion about the impact of the Internet on patient–provider relationships (Blumenthal, 2002; Gerber & Eiser, 2001; Wald, Dube, & Anthony, 2007). Yet, little is known about how older adults react to this ongoing transition of the decision-making model and corresponding shift to expectations of greater responsibility in health care. Unlike younger generations, many older adults learned to interact with their healthcare providers when the paternalistic model was dominant. This might make it even harder for them to take a more active and participatory role in health care. Meanwhile, age-related changes in cognition (Finucane, Mertz, Slovic, & Scholze-Schmidt, 2005) and emotional processing (Lockenhoff & Carstensen, 2007) have also been shown to make older adults' decision-making process differ from other age groups.

Research has widely confirmed that older people are less likely to get involved in both online health information-seeking and decision-making processes (Hill & Laugharne, 2006; Maibach, Weber, Massett, Hancock, & Price, 2006). According to the Kaiser Family Foundation (2005), among those seniors who were online health information seekers, only a third said that they had talked with a doctor or other provider about information they found online. Older Americans in the report also said that their doctors were not encouraging them to use the Internet for health information or to communicate with providers. Xie (2009) found that Internet use has not changed older adults' reliance on medical professionals for diagnostic and treatment decisions.

Campbell and Nolfi (2005) examined whether training in online health information seeking led to changes in older adults' perceptions of their interactions with healthcare providers. The study showed that although older adults were willing to use the Internet as a source for general health information, it did not translate into a willingness to take a more active role in their health care. They seemed to be more willing to stick to a physician-centered model of care when making decisions about their health.

Generational Differences

There is some evidence to support a generational difference in where people obtain health information. The Pew report (Fox & Jones, 2009) found that young adults were less likely than seniors to turn to doctors or other medical professionals when they needed health information: 79% of those ages 18–29 versus 89% of those ages 65 and up. In contrast, 72% of young adults said they looked online for health information, compared to 27% of adults 65 or older.

Although little evidence has thus far been presented to support the idea that the Internet has changed doctor–patient dynamics very much, both researchers and health practitioners confirm a trend toward fuller patient participation in health care with an increased number of more well-informed patients empowered by new technologies. McNutt (2004) suggests that the contemporary healthcare system should begin to encourage increased patient autonomy in making health decisions. For example, it has been recommended to include relevant knowledge in the medical school curricula about how to respond to more intelligent and empowered patients (Institute of Medicine, 2004). Some physicians have started to appreciate this transition and are adjusting to their changing roles in the healthcare system by giving more credit and encouragement to patients' health information-seeking behaviors and their participation in healthcare decisions. Hoch and Ferguson (2005), who are epilepsy specialists at highly respected medical centers in the United States, noted that they now are recommending or referring their patients to seek reliable health information and social support on the Internet.

Preparing Consumers for Increased Responsibility and Engagement

As patient–provider interactions are more likely to be shaped by a shared model of decision making, it has become critical to train older adults to become more independent consumers of health care. More research is needed to determine the factors that might facilitate or prevent older adults' participation in decision-making processes. Effective strategies must be identified in the future to make older adults not only more health literate but also more Internet and computer literate as an increasing volume of health information and services are now online (see Chapter 2). More importantly, actions should be taken to help older adults be more psychologically ready to actively participate in health care. To achieve this, Broom (2005) suggests that healthcare providers offer encouragement, guidance, and support to patients for health information seeking, either online or offline.

NEED FOR HEALTH INFORMATION AND SERVICES: OLDER ADULT ISSUES

Our society, with its rapid technological advancements, is also a society with dramatically rapid changes in demographics. According to the population data released by the US Census Bureau (2009), the number of persons ages 65 and older in the United States will increase 40% in the next 5 years and will double by 2050, rising from 39 million to 89 million. Meanwhile, the world's 65-and-older population is also projected to triple by 2050, from 516 million to 1.53 billion. The data also show that 100 countries are expected to have at least one-fifth of their total population ages 65 or older by 2050.

Research has shown that older adults tend to need health information and to use healthcare services at a far higher rate than younger adults (Oermann et al., 2003). Data from a survey conducted by DeFrances and Podgornik (2006) indicated a 24% increase in hospitalizations for patients 65 and older from 1970 to 2004. Because of these trends in increased numbers of hospitalized older adults and the subsequent economic and social consequences, there has been greatly increased pressure for healthcare agencies to provide sufficient health information, support, and services to the older population (Coleman, Austin, Brach, & Wagner, 2009; DeFrances & Podgornik, 2006; Levey, 2009; Scott et al., 2007). Furthermore, an increasing amount of health-related information, programs, and services has been placed on the Internet. It has become a common goal of public health advocates, government officials, and the medical community to use information and communication technologies as a promising way to meet these challenges.

Relieving Social Isolation of Aging

As individuals age, the loss of friends, parents, and other family members, in combination with functional impairment in mobility, vision, and hearing, leaves older adults at higher risk of social isolation. Numerous studies suggest that social and emotional isolation is associated with adverse health outcomes and diminished quality of life (Locher et al., 2005; Mullins, Sheppard, & Anderson, 1991; Thompson & Heller, 1990; Tomaka, Thompson, & Palacios, 2006). Computer- and Internet-based interactive technologies, such as discussion boards, chat rooms, instant messaging, and social networking tools, have a great potential to alleviate the social isolation and depression that are more common among older adults, especially those with disabilities and chronic conditions.

Innovations in Social Networking for Older Adults and Isolated Groups

Morris, Lundell, Dishongh, and Needham (2009) have piloted some spectacular tools for engaging older adults in social exchanges. These were discussed in some detail in Chapter 1 under telehealth. The Intel program coaches older adults, their families, and caregivers on the importance of social networking. A computer program that tracks social interchange activity is provided with a variety of displays. Early results have been very promising. It is not clear to what extent this resource will be part of the Intel/GE partnership called Health Guard.

Online Communities for Older Adults

One of the emerging Internet applications with the potential to relieve social isolation is senior-oriented online communities. One of most successful online communities for seniors is SeniorNet (www.seniornet.org), a nonprofit organization with the goal of providing education for, and access to, computer technology for older adults. SeniorNet consists of both an online community as well as computer learning centers where members can take classes. In China, a similar online community for older adults, OldKids (www.oldkids.com.cn), is also getting a good deal of attention from Chinese elders (Xie, 2005). Eons (www.eons.com) is a website similar to Facebook but designed specifically for baby boomers. On Eons, users can create a personal profile, stay in touch with family and friends who are on Eons, share pictures and videos, play games to stay mentally sharp, and join online groups according to their interests.

There are also emerging online communities that provide a platform for the caregivers of older adults to share resources, information, and support. These online communities differ by caregiver emphasis, data tools, and disease focus. For example, CAREgivinghelp (www.caregivinghelp.org) is an online community established by the Council for Jewish Elderly in Chicago, which provides information and support for caregivers regarding personal care, memory loss, handling difficult behaviors, relationship changes, and stress reduction (Chekal, 2007). Caring Bridge (www.caringbridge.org) allows users to create their own personalized websites that can be used to stay connected with family or friends during periods of illness and recovery. These online communities provide opportunities for older adults to extend their social networks and share social support, which has been shown to have potential benefits for the well-being of older adults (Wright, 2000).

Age-Related Changes Affecting Internet Experiences

Life span development researchers have identified biological changes in vision, audition, motor, and cognition accompanied with the aging process. People's visual acuity and accommodation, color perception, contrast and glare sensitivity, and adaption to darkness are affected as they become older. Such visual decrements make it harder for seniors to discriminate between certain colors, to perceive small elements on a computer display, or to locate relevant information on complex screens and low-contrast displays (Schieber, 2003). Age-related auditory declines also reduce older adults' sensitivity to high frequencies and the ability to distinguish among tones (Siewe, 2004). Motor abilities also decline over the years, and older adults experience decreased ability to manipulate very small controls and difficulty in coordination of movements (Rogers & Fisk, 2000; Scialfa, Ho, & Laberge, 2004). Cognitive abilities, such as memory, attention, spatial ability, discourse comprehension, and the speed with which information is processed also decline with the aging process (Craik & Salthouse, 2000; Greiner, Snowdon & Schmitt, 1996).

Research has demonstrated that these age-related changes in visual, auditory, motor, and cognitive abilities have become major barriers to older adults' learning and use of new information and communication technologies. For example, it has been reported that such age-related declines influence older adults' use of computer input devices such as the mouse and the keyboard (Czaja & Lee, 2007; Mead, Batsakes, Fisk, & Mykityshyn, 1999; Smith, Sharit, & Czaja, 1999; Walker, Philbin, & Fisk, 1997), and their efficiency in retrieving health information on the Internet (Echt, 2002; Mead, Lamson, & Rogers, 2002).

Guidelines for Designing Websites for Older Adults

Because of these physiological changes, efforts have been made to make online health information more accessible to older people and their caregivers. Various guidelines for interface and system designs have been developed that take into consideration older adults' age-related declines. For instance, a guideline developed by the National Institute on Aging and the National Library of Medicine (2002) introduces a checklist of design elements for websites intended to accommodate senior citizens, including 15 key usability factors such as minimal or no animation use to reduce screen clutter, simple language for text, definition of difficult words, use of plain typeface with 12- or 14-point font for body text, double-spaced body text with good contrast between text and background, and simple navigation from page to page.

Echt (2002) also proposed an extensive guideline of design principles for senior-friendly health websites, including aspects of layout, content organization, navigation, and graphics. A highly relevant website is found at www.usability.gov. The site provides an overview of basics: some templates, guidelines, an opportunity to blog, and a searchable site. For example, the tag *older adults* leads to newsletters that discuss the limitations older adults often have when searching or browsing on the Web—such as being easily diverted by unrelated content while searching for a topic or having a preference for bulleted lists.

Research suggests that senior citizens can benefit when websites make accommodations for the searching and browsing habits of older adults (Chaffin & Maddux, 2007; Clark, 2002). However, there is evidence that such guidelines haven't been well followed by many website designers. It has been noted that the majority of current websites are not accessible to older users (Echt 2002; Nielsen, 2002). A survey of award-winning software companies found that only 2 of the 19 companies were aware of usability and accessibility issues (Burgstahler, 2002). This means that there is still a strong need to reinforce the message about the benefits of developing senior-friendly applications and websites that are directly customized for the needs of the elderly population. The good news is that computer industry members such as Microsoft and IBM have started to focus on the older adult market and are designing senior-friendly Internet applications (SeniorNet, 2008).

In addition, it is important to keep in mind that most existing design guidelines have not been tested systematically and thoroughly (Echt, 2002; Mead et al., 2002). More research is needed to conduct a thorough examination of existing guidelines.

Cultural Differences

When we examine the behaviors related to health information seeking and healthcare use, it is important for us to take cultural factors into account. People with different cultural backgrounds may vary in health beliefs, health information needs, and the way health care is used. For example, Asian American older adults might have a higher interest in complementary and alternative types of health care, such as acupuncture, herbal medicine, t'ai chi exercise, and nutrition and diet. While treating this group, healthcare professionals and health information providers should consider their needs for traditional medicine and other forms of alternative medicine, rather than focusing only on conventional Western medicine.

Meanwhile, filial piety, which has been the core cultural concept in Chinese culture, may grant power to adult children and other family members in influencing Chinese elders' health information seeking and healthcare use patterns (Sung, 2001). The family has been the central social unit in Asian societies for thousands of years. Family members primarily rely on each other for their psychological, social, and physical needs. In the examination of the health seeking behaviors among Chinese elders in the United States, Pang, Jordan-Marsh, Silverstein, and Cody (2003) found that Chinese older adults were reluctant to seek help from health professionals. When encountering health problems, these Chinese elders first seek help and suggestions from family members and their personal networks, while doctors are the final resort in their pathway to healthcare seeking. They found that family members play a dominant role in providing health-related advice, information, decision making, and actual healing practice. One explanation for this is that these Chinese elders were not familiar with American health care and health insurance systems. In such a context, family members, especially adult children, are supposed to provide assistance in navigating through the complicated medical system, finding health information, and even making final medical decisions. These findings show that family members have a significant influence on the healthcare-seeking behaviors among Chinese elders in the United States. When promoting health-related behaviors among Asian elders and other groups close to their ethnic roots in the United States, it is important to make the best use of the influence of family members on these elders.

Similarly, professionals are urged to be cognizant of the wide diversity in family structure. American healthcare systems have been structured so that the family is defined in a narrow legalistic manner. Many ethnic groups and even some members of the majority use an expanded definition of family. Jordan-Marsh and Harden (2005) make a case for an inventory of social networks that includes what anthropologists call "fictive kin." Fictive kin are those individuals considered family even though there is no legal or blood tie. Validating and including socially expansive views of family is especially important for older adults who may be reluctant to seek help from family members (Jordan-Marsh & Harden). Such expanded views of the family are equally important for other groups, including emancipated minors and lesbian, gay, bisexual, and transgendered consumers whose preferred relationships are routinely ignored by standardized forms and interview protocols. A flexible electronic health record will assist health providers and consumers in bringing nontraditional relationships into the socioecological portrait.

Research has also indicated that older members of ethnic minority groups lag behind in their frequency of online health searches. According to the most recent

Pew report (Fox & Jones, 2009), more whites (65%) reported looking up information about health issues online as compared to African Americans (51%) or Hispanics (44%). In examining the different use patterns between Caucasian women and African American women of an online support group (CHESS) for women with breast cancer, McTavish, Pingree, Hawkins, and Gustafson (2003) found that the CHESS discussion group was used significantly less by African American women than Caucasian women. The study also indicated that the messages posted by African Americans more tightly focused on breast cancer issues, while the Caucasian women used the group far more broadly and were more likely to have conversations about day-to-day events. This study is only suggestive of cultural variation beyond language limitations.

Culture and language deserve careful attention. However, some experts are concerned that we have emphasized diversity at the expense of commonalities. "All campaigns and most experts in health communication act as if diversity matters. However, they do so with a remarkably thin evidence base" (Scrimshaw et al., 2002, p. 122, as cited in Institute of Medicine, 2002). It may be that how information is delivered is more subject to variations specific to diversity than the message itself. In their studies, the Pew Internet and American Life Project make the important assumption that there is more commonality than diversity in the way people respond to digital resource (Pew Internet & American Life Project, 2009). For example, men, women, e-patients of various levels of education, whites, African Americans, and Latinos are equally likely to post and make use of information provided by others on social networking sites.

In addition, the fact that most online health information is presented only in English imposes language barriers for non-English speakers, including older immigrants whose native language is not English. Research is needed to gain a deeper understanding of cultural differences in health-related beliefs and behaviors so that health information and health care can be more efficiently delivered to people with different cultural backgrounds.

Information Overload

All users of the Internet, whether patients, their advocates, or health professionals, are at risk of information overload. Applying the ecological framework of the interrelationship of capital and charisma to the progression from data to wisdom, which influences behavior and beliefs, the everyday experience of the consumer is well depicted in Figure 3.2.

There is a virtual explosion of applications to post data, locate information, exchange knowledge, and share wisdom related to health and health-related

Figure 3.2   The Everyday Experience of Engaging with Online Health Resources

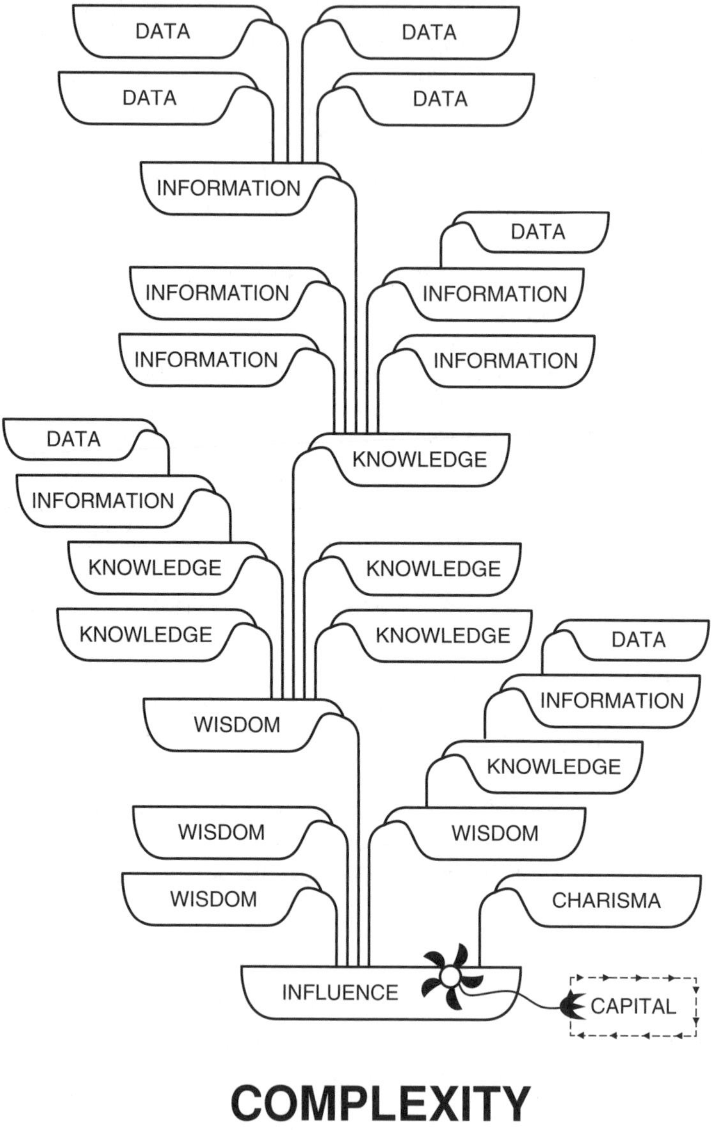

COMPLEXITY

Illustration: Jin DePaul.

behaviors and decisions. This creates a highly complex resource pool for consumers and health professionals. Navigating this eHealth scene calls for information mediation by advocates, peers, and health professionals. It is often difficult to sort out credible sites and even to analyze resources on known quality sites. The potential of information mediation as a strategy for coping with health literacy challenges and building both health and sociotechnical capital is described in Chapter 2. The goal should no longer be to simplify all health information to a basic level but to engage technology to filter available resources to the level desired by the searcher. Kerr, Murray, Stevenson, Gore, and Nazareth (2006) remind us that these needs may change as consumers and patients become both more knowledgeable and more empowered as they move along an illness or wellness journey.

SUMMARY

In conclusion, the Internet has become an important source for health information. Access to health information through the Internet has the potential to empower individuals by leading them to better manage their health needs, increase their ability to make more informed decisions, and improve their general quality of life. As Fox and Jones (2009) summarize, "Technology is not an end, but a means to accelerate the pace of discovery, widen social networks, and sharpen the questions someone might ask when they do get to talk to a health professional. Technology can help to enable the human connection in health care, and the Internet is turning up the information network's volume" (Overview, para. 2). It is unfortunate that around the globe, we cannot agree on a uniform review process such as Health on the Net to provide at least minimal credibility screening.

Health providers, advocates, and the entire health community need to reach out to health information consumers—lay and professional. The goal is to ensure that the information and tools consumers need are available, useable, and reliable, and that resources can be tailored to the personal preferences of all those who engage online on behalf of consumers. Abdicating this responsibility creates the risk that unstable sites like Wikipedia or commercially sponsored sites like WebMD are the "go-to" resources over noncommercial professional or governmental websites like Mayo Clinic and MedLinePlus. The danger is that consumer driven or commercially sponsored sites become very charismatic and agendas very subtle.

REFERENCES

Afifi, W. A., & Weiner, J. L. (2004). Toward a theory of motivated information management. *Communication Theory, 14*, 167–190.

Afifi, W. A., & Weiner, J. L. (2006). Seeking information about sexual health: Applying the theory of motivated information management. *Human Communication Research, 32*, 35–57.

Alder, R. A. (2006). *Older Americans, broadband and the future of the Net.* Retrieved January 2, 2009, from http://www.seniornet.org/research/SeniorNetNNPaper060606.pdf

Anderson, J. G. (2004). Consumers of e-health: Patterns of use and barriers. *Social Science Computer Review, 22*(2), 242–248.

Anderson, J., Rainey, M., & Eysenbach, G. (2003). The impact of cyber healthcare on the physician–patient relationship. *Journal of Medical Systems, 27*(1), 67–84.

Arnst, C. (2008) *Health 2.0: Patients as partners.* Retrieved April 2, 2009, from http://www.businessweek.com/magazine/content/08_50/b4112058194219.htm?chan=magazine+channel_in+depth

Atkin, C. (1985). Informational utility and selective exposure. In D. Zillman & J. Bryant (Eds.), *Selective exposure to communication* (pp. 63–91). Hillsdale, NJ: Erlbaum.

Baker, L. C., Bundorf, M. K., Singer, S., & Wagner, T. H. (2003). *Validity of the survey of health and the Internet, and Knowledge Network's panel and sampling.* Retrieved October 30, 2008, from http://www.knowledgenetworks.com/ganp/docs/Appendix%20Survey%20of%20Health%20and%20the%20Internet.pdf

Bandura, A. (1986). *Social foundations of thought and action: A social cognitive theory.* Englewood Cliffs, NJ: Prentice Hall.

Bandura, A. (1997). *Self-efficacy: The exercise of control.* New York: Freeman.

Bandura, A. (2004). Swimming against the mainstream: The early years from chilly tributary to transformative mainstream. *Behaviour Research and Therapy, 42*, 613–630.

Barak, A., Boniel-Nissim, M., & Suler, J. (2008). Fostering empowerment in online support groups. *Computers in Human Behavior, 24*(5), 1867–1883.

Berland, G. K., Elliott, M. N., Morales, L. S., Algazy, J. I., Kravitz, R. L., Broder, M. S., et al. (2001). Health information on the Internet: Accessibility, quality, and readability in English and Spanish. *Journal of the American Medical Association, 285*, 2612–2621.

Bernstam, E. V., Shelton, D. M., Walji, M., & Meric-Bernstam, F. (2005). Instruments to assess the quality of health information on the World Wide Web: What can our patients actually use? *International Journal of Medical Informatics, 74*(1), 13–19.

Blumenthal, D. (2002). Doctors in a wired world: Can professionalism survive connectivity? *Milbank Quarterly, 80*(3), 525–546.

Brashers, D. E. (2001). Communication and uncertainty management. *Journal of Communication, 51*, 477–497.

Brashers, D. E., Goldsmith, D. J., & Hsieh, E. (2002). Information seeking and avoiding in health contexts. *Human Communication Research, 28*, 258–271.

Breckons, M., Jones, R., Morris, J., & Richardson, J. (2008). What do evaluation instruments tell us about the quality of complementary medicine information on the Internet? *Journal of Medical Internet Research, 10*(1). Retrieved January 3, 2009, from http://www.jmir.org/2008/1/e3/HTML

Broom, A. (2005). Virtually healthy: The impact of Internet use on disease experience and the doctor–patient relationship. *Qualitative Health Research, 15*(3), 325–345.

Buckland, S. & Gann, B. (1997). *Disseminating treatment outcomes information to consumers: Evaluation of five pilot projects.* London: King's Fund Publishing.

Burgstahler, S. (2002). *Designing software that is accessible to individuals with disabilities.* Retrieved December 19, 2005, from http://www.washington.edu/doit/Brochures/Technology/design_software.html

Campbell, R. (2004). Older women and the Internet. *Journal of Women and Aging, 16*(1–2), 161–174.

Campbell, R. J., & Nolfi, D. A. (2005). Teaching elderly adults to use the Internet to access healthcare information: Before–after study. *Journal of Medical Internet Research, 7*(2). Retrieved December 12, 2005, from http://www.jmir.org/2005/2/e19

Carlbring, P., Nilsson-Ihrfelt, E., Waara, J., Kollenstam, C., Burhman, M., Kaldo, V., et al. (2005). Treatment of panic disorder: Live therapy vs. self-help via the Internet. *Behavior Research and Therapy, 43*, 1321–1333.

Centers for Disease Control and Prevention. (2009). *CDC social media tools.* Retrieved June 15, 2010, from http://www.cdc.gov/socialmedia/tools

Chaffin, A. J., & Maddux, C. D. (2007). Accessibility accommodations for older adults seeking e-health information. *Journal of Gerontological Nursing, 33*(3), 6–12.

Charles, C., Gafni, A., & Whelan, T. (1997). Shared decision-making in the medical encounter: What does it mean? *Social Science and Medicine, 44*, 681–692.

Charnock, D., & Sheppard, S. (1997). Retrieved August 24, 2009, from http://www.discern.org.uk/discern_instrument.php

Chekal, A. (2007). *Caregiver support Web sites grow: Online communities increase resources for older adult caregivers.* Retrieved July 12, 2009, from http://aginggrandparents.suite101.com/article.cfm/caregiver_support_websites_grow

Chong, S., & Theng, Y. (2004). A study of Web-based information needs of senior citizens in Singapore. In C. Stary & C. Stephanidis (Eds.), *Lecture notes in computer science: Vol. 3196/2004* (pp. 16–33). Heidelberg, Germany: Springer Berlin.

Clark, D. J. (2002). Older adults living through and with their computers. *Computers, Informatics, Nursing: CIN, 20*, 117–124.

Cody, M., Dunn, D., Hoppin, S., & Wendt, P. (1999). Silver surfers: Training and evaluating Internet use among older adult learners. *Communication Education, 48*(4), 269–286.

Coleman, K., Austin, B. T., Brach, C., & Wagner, E. H. (2009). Evidence on the chronic care model in the new millennium. *Health Affairs, 28*(1), 75–85.

CNN. (2010). *CNN RSS.* Retrieved July 2, 2010, from http://www.cnn.com/services/rss

Craik, F. I. M., & Salthouse, T. A. (2000). *The handbook of aging and cognition* (2nd ed.). Mahwah, NJ: Erlbaum.

Czaja, R., Manfredi, C., & Price, J. (2003). The determinants and consequences of information seeking among cancer patients. *Journal of Health Communication, 8*, 529–562.

Czaja, S. J., & Lee, C.C. (2007). The impact of aging on access to technology. *Universal Access in the Information Society, 5*(4), 341–349.

DeFrances, C. J., & Podgornik, M. N. (2006). *2004 National Hospital Discharge Survey.* Hyattsville, MD: National Center for Health Statistics. Retrieved May 5, 2006, from www.cdc.gov/nchs/data/ad/ad371.pdf

Demiris, G. (2006). The diffusion of virtual communities in health care: Concepts and challenges. *Patient Education and Counseling, 62*(2), 178–188.

DiMaggio, P., Hargittai, E., Neuman, W. R., & Robinson, J. P. (2001) Social implications of the Internet. *Annual Review of Sociology, 27*, 307–336.

Dutta-Bergman, M. J. (2004). Primary sources of health information: Comparisons in the domain of health attitudes, health cognitions, and health behaviors. *Health Communication, 16*(3), 273–288.

Eastin, M. A., & LaRose, R. L. (2000). Internet self-efficacy and the psychology of the digital divide. *Journal of Computer Mediated Communication, 6*(1). Retrieved July 15, 2004, from http://jcmc.indiana.edu/vol6/issue1/eastin.html

Echt, K. V. (2002). Designing Web-based health information for older adults: Visual considerations and design directives. In R. W. Morrell (Ed.), *Older adults, health information and the World Wide Web* (pp. 61–88). Mahwah, NJ: Erlbaum.

Eysenbach, G. (2008). Medicine 2.0: Social networking, collaboration, participation, apomediation and openness. *Journal of Medical and Internet Research, 10*(3), e22.

Eysenbach, G., & Köhler C. (2003). What is the prevalence of health-related searches on the World Wide Web? Qualitative and quantitative analysis of search engine queries on the Internet. *AMIA Annual Symposium Proceedings,* 225–229.

Eysenbach, G., Powell, J., Kuss, O., & Sa, E. (2002). Empirical studies assessing the quality of health information for consumers on the World Wide Web: A systematic review. *Journal of the American Medical Association, 287*(20), 2691–2700.

Finucane, M. L., Mertz, C. K., Slovic, P., & Scholze-Schmidt, E. S. (2005). Task complexity and older adults' decision-making competence. *Psychology and Aging, 20,* 71–84.

Flynn, K. E., Smith, M. A., & Freese, J. (2006). When do older adults turn to the Internet for health information? Findings from the Wisconsin Longitudinal Study. *Journal of General Internal Medicine, 21*(12), 1295–1301.

Fox, S. (2006). *Online health search.* Retrieved March 16, 2007, from http://www.pewinternet.org/pdfs/PIP_Online_Health_2006.pdf

Fox, S. (2007). *E-patients with a disability or chronic disease.* Retrieved October 20, 2008, from http://www.pewinternet.org/pdfs/EPatients_Chronic_Conditions_2007.pdf

Fox, S. (2009). *Uncle Sam and social media.* Retrieved August 25, 2009, from http://www.pewinternet.org/Commentary/2009/August/Uncle-Sam-on-Social-Media.aspx

Fox, S., & Jones, S. (2009). *The social life of health information.* Retrieved August 27, 2009, from http://www.pewinternet.org/Reports/2009/8-The-Social-Life-of-Health-Information.aspx

Fox, S., & Rainie, L. (2002). *Vital decisions: How Internet users decide what information to trust when they or their loved ones are sick.* Retrieved June 15, 2004, from http://www.pewinternet.org/PPF/r/59/report display.asp

Frost, J. H., & Massagli, M. P. (2008). Social uses of personal health information within Patients-LikeMe, an online patient community: What can happen when patients have access to one another's data. *JMIR: Journal of Medical and Internet Research, 10*(3), e15.

Gaston, C. M., & Mitchell, G. (2005). Information giving and decision-making in patients with advanced cancer: A systematic review. *Social Science and Medicine, 61,* 2252–2264.

Gerber, B. S., & Eiser, A. R. (2001). The patient–physician relationship in the Internet age: Future prospects and the research agenda. *Journal of Medical Internet Research, 3*(2), e15. Retrieved November 18, 2008, from http://www.jmir.org/2001/2/e15

Gladwell, M. (2007). *Blink: The power of thinking without thinking.* Boston: Back Bay Books.

Green, M., Peterson, S., Baker, M. W., Harper, G. R., Friedman, L. C., Rubenstein, W. S., et al. (2004). Effect of a computer-based decision aid on knowledge, perceptions, and intentions about genetic testing for breast cancer susceptibility: A randomized controlled trial. *Journal of the American Medical Association, 292,* 442–452.

Greiner, P. A., Snowdon, D. A., & Schmitt, F. A. (1996). The loss of independence in activities of daily living: The role of low normal cognitive function in elderly nuns. *American Journal of Public Health, 86*, 62–66.

Gustafson, D. H., Hawkins, R., Boberg, E., Pingree, S., Serlin, R. E., Graziano, F., et al. (1999). Impact of a patient-centered, computer-based, health information/support system. *American Journal of Preventative Medicine, 16*, 1–9.

Hames, R. D. (2007). *The five literacies of global leadership: What authentic leaders know and you need to find out*. San Francisco: Jossey-Bass.

Hardey, M. (1999). Doctor in the house: The Internet as a source of health knowledge and a challenge to expertise. *Sociology of Health and Illness, 21*(6), 820–835.

Hardt, J. H., & Hollis-Sawyer, L. (2007). Older adults seeking healthcare information on the Internet. *Educational Gerontology, 33*(7), 561–572.

Hargittai, E. (2002). Second-level digital divide: Differences in people's online skills. *First Monday, 7*(4), 1–20.

Hawn, C. (2009). Take two aspirin and tweet me in the morning: How Twitter, Facebook, and other social media are reshaping health care. *Health Affairs, 28*(2), 361–368.

Helwig, A. L., Lovelle, A., Guse, C. E., & Gottlieb, M. S. (1999). An office-based Internet patient education system: A pilot study. *Journal of Family Practice, 48*(2), 123–127.

Henwood, F., Wyatt, S., Hart, A., & Smith, J. (2003). Ignorance is bliss sometimes: Constraints on the emergence of the "informed patient" in the changing landscapes of health information. *Sociology of Health and Illness, 25*(6), 589–607.

Hill, S. A., & Laugharne, R. (2006). Decision making and information seeking preferences among psychiatric patients. *Journal of Mental Health, 15*(1), 75–84.

Hoch, D., & Ferguson, T. (2005). What I've learned from E-patients. *Public Library of Science Medicine, 2*(8), e206. Retrieved January 10, 2007, from http://medicine.plosjournals.org/perlserv/?request=get-document&doi=10.1371/journal.pmed.0020206

Hong, T. (2006). The Internet and tobacco cessation: The roles of Internet self-efficacy and search task on the information-seeking process. *Journal of Computer-Mediated Communication, 11*(2). Retrieved March 15, 2006, from http://jcmc.indiana.edu/vol11/issue2/hong.html

Institute of Medicine. (2002). *Speaking of health: Assessing health communication strategies for diverse populations*. Washington, DC: National Academies Press.

Institute of Medicine. (2004). *Improving medical education: Enhancing the behavioral and social science content of medical school curricula*. Washington, DC: National Academies Press.

Institute of Medicine. (2009). *Health literacy, eHealth, and communication: Putting the consumer first: Workshop summary*. Washington, DC: National Academies Press.

Jimison, H., Gorman, P., Woods, S., Nygren, P., Walker, M., Norris, S., et al. (2008). *Barriers and drivers of health information technology use for the elderly, chronically ill, and underserved* (Evidence Report/Technology Assessment No. 175, AHRQ Publication No. 09-E004). Rockville, MD: Agency for Healthcare Research and Quality.

Johnson, J. D., & Meischke, H. (1993). A comprehensive model of cancer-related information seeking applied to magazines. *Human Communication Research, 19*, 343–367.

Jones, S., & Fox, S. (2009). Generations online. *Pew Internet and American Life Project*. Retrieved on March 21, 2009, from http://www.pewinternet.org/pdfs/PIP_Generations_2009.pdf

Jordan-Marsh, M., & Harden, J. T. (2005). Fictive kin: Friends as family supporting older adults as they age. *Journal of Gerontological Nursing, 31*(2), 24–31.

Jordan-Marsh, M., McLaughlin, M., Chi, I., Brown, C., Moran, M., Jung, Y., et al. (2006). *St. Barnabas cyber café evaluation report 2004–2005.* Unpublished manuscript, University of Southern California, School of Social Work, Annenberg School of Communication, Davis School of Gerontology.

Josefsson, U. (2006). Patients' online information-seeking behavior. In M. Murero & R. E. Rice (Eds.), *The Internet and health care: Theory, research and practice* (pp. 127–147). Mahwah, NJ: Erlbaum.

Journal of Medical Internet Research. (2009, August 25). *Inaugural JMIR Medicine 2.0 award goes to PatientsLikeMe researchers.* Retrieved August 25, 2009, from http://www.jmir.org/announcement/view/27

Jung, Y., Peng, W., Moran, M., Jin, S., Jordan-Marsh, M., McLaughlin, M. L., et al. (2010). Low-income minority seniors' enrollment in a cyber café: Psychological barriers to crossing the digital divide. *Educational Gerontology, 36*(3), 193–212.

Kaiser Family Foundation. (2005). *E-Health and the elderly: How seniors use the Internet for health information.* Retrieved March 12, 2008, from http://www.kff.org/entmedia/upload/e-Health-and-the-Elderly-How-Seniors-Use-the-Internet-for-Health-Information-Key-Findings-From-a-National-Survey-of-Older-Americans-Survey-Report.pdf

Kerr, C., Murray, E., Stevenson, F., Gore, C., & Nazareth, I. (2006). Internet interventions for long-term conditions: Patient and caregiver quality criteria. *Journal of Medical Internet Research, 8*(3), e13.

Kivits, J. (2004). Researching the informed patient. *Information Communication & Society, 7*(4), 510–530.

Lau, A. Y., & Coiera, E. W. (2008). Impact of Web searching and social feedback on consumer decision making: A prospective online experiment. *Journal of Medical Internet Research, 10*(1). Retrieved January 2, 2009, from http://www.jmir.org/2008/1/e2/HTML

Levey, N. (2009, August 25). Getting cheaper, better healthcare at home? *Los Angeles Times.* Retrieved August 25, 2009, from http://www.latimes.com/news/nationworld/nation/healthcare/la-na-healthcare-housecalls25-2009aug25,0,1019530.story

Leydon, G., Boulton, M., Moynihan, C., Jones, A., Mossman, J., Boudioni, M., et al. (2000). Cancer patients' information needs and information seeking behaviour: In-depth interview study. *British Medical Journal, 320,* 909–913.

Lieberman, M. A., Golant, M., Giese-Davis, J., Winzelberg, A., Benjamin, H., Humphreys, K., et al. (2003). Electronic support groups for breast carcinoma: A clinical trial of effectiveness. *Cancer, 97,* 920–925.

Light, D. (2001). Managed competition, governmentality, and institutional response in the United Kingdom. *Social Science & Medicine, 52,* 1167–1181.

Locher, J. L., Ritchie, C. S., Roth, D. L., Baker, P. S., Bonder, E. V., & Allman, R. M. (2005). Social isolation, support, and capital and nutritional risk in an older sample: Ethnic and gender differences. *Social Science & Medicine, 60*(4), 747–761.

Lockenhoff, C. E., & Carstensen, L. L. (2007). Aging, emotion, and health-related decision strategies: Motivational manipulations can reduce age differences. *Psychology and Aging, 22*(1), 134–146.

Luker, K., Beaver, K., Leinster, S. J., Owens, R., & Glynn, B. (1996). Information needs and sources of information for women with breast cancer: A follow-up study. *Journal of Advanced Nursing, 23*(3), 4887–4895.

Maibach, E. W., Weber, D., Massett, H., Hancock, G. R., & Price, S. (2006). Understanding consumers' health information preferences: Development and validation of a brief screening instrument. *Journal of Health Communication, 11,* 717–736.

Mayfield, R. (2005). Social network dynamics and participatory politics. In J. Lebkowsky & M. Ratcliffe (Eds.), *Extreme democracy* (pp. 116–143). Lulu Press.

Mayhorn, C. B., Stronge, A. J., McLaughlin, A. J., & Rogers. W. A. (2004). Older adults, computer training, and the systems approach: A formula for success. *Educational Gerontology 30*(3), 185–203.

McDermott, A. (2001). *Report: More seniors see Web as fountain of youth*. Retrieved September 10, 2001, from http://www.cnn.com/2001/TECHInternet/06/04/web.seniors/index.html

McNutt, R. A. (2004). Shared medical decision making: Problems, process, progress. *Journal of the American Medical Association, 292*, 2516–2518.

McTavish, F. M., Pingree, S., Hawkins, R., & Gustafson, D. (2003). Cultural differences in use of an electronic discussion group. *Journal of Health Psychology, 8*, 105–117.

Mead, S. E., Batsakes, P., Fisk, A. D., & Mykityshyn, A. (1999). Application of cognitive theory to training and design solutions for age-related computer use. *International Journal of Behavioral Development, 23*, 553–573.

Mead, S. E., Lamson, N., & Rogers, W. A. (2002). Human factors guidelines for web site usability: Health-oriented web sites for older adults. In R. W. Morrell (Ed.), *Older adults, health information and the World Wide Web* (pp. 89–108). Mahwah, NJ: Erlbaum.

Meier, A., Lyons, E. J., Frydman, G., Forlenza, M., & Rimer, B. K. (2007). How cancer survivors provide support on cancer-related Internet mailing lists. *Journal of Medical Internet Research, 9*(2), e12.

Mills, M., & Sullivan, K. (1999). The importance of information giving for patients newly diagnosed with cancer: A review of the literature. *Journal of Clinical Nursing, 8*(6), 631–642.

Morris, M. E., Lundell, J., Dishongh, T., & Needham, B. (2009). Fostering social engagement and self efficacy in later life: Studies with ubiquitous computing. In P. Markopoulos, B. De Ruyter, & W. Mackay (Eds.), *Awareness systems: Advances in theory, methodology, and design* (pp. 335–349). London: Springer London.

Mullins, L. C., Sheppard, H. L., & Anderson, L. (1991). Loneliness and social isolation in Sweden: Differences in age, sex, labor force status, self-rated health, and income adequacy. *Journal of Applied Gerontology, 10*, 455–468.

Murray, E., Burns, J., See, T., Lai, R., & Nazareth, I. (2005). Interactive health communication applications for people with chronic disease. *Cochrane Database of Systematic Reviews, 4*, CD004274.

National Institute on Aging & National Library of Medicine. (2002). *Making your web site senior friendly: A checklist*. Retrieved December 19, 2005, from http://www.nlm.nih.gov/pubs/checklist.pdf

Nelson, R. (2002). Major theories supporting health care informatics. In S. P. Englebart & R. Nelson (Eds.), *Health care informatics: An interdisciplinary approach* (pp. 3–27). St. Louis, MO: Mosby.

Niederdeppe, J., Hornik, R. C., Kelly, B. J., Frosch, D. L., Romantan, A., Stevens, R. S., et al. (2007). Examining the dimensions of cancer-related information seeking and scanning behavior. *Health Communication, 22*(2), 153–167.

Nielsen, J. (2002). *Usability for senior citizens*. Retrieved February 1, 2008, from www.useit.com/alertbox/20020428.html

O'Connor, A. M., Bennett, C. L., Stacey, D., Barry, M., Col, N. F., et al. (2009). Decision aids for people facing health treatment or screening decisions. *Cochrane Database of Systematic Reviews, 3*, CD001431. Retrieved June 10, 2010, from http://decisionaid.ohri.ca/docs/develop/Cochrane_Review.pdf

Oermann, M. H., Hamilton, J., & Shook, M. L. (2003). Using the Web to improve seniors' awareness of their role in preventing medical errors. *Journal of Nursing Care Quality, 18*(2), 122–128.

Pang, E., Jordan-Marsh, M., Silverstein, M., & Cody, M. (2003). Health-seeking behaviors of elderly Chinese Americans: Shifts in expectations. *Gerontologist, 43*(6), 864–874.

PatientsLikeMe. (2010). Retrieved July 5, 2010, from http://www.patientslikeme.com

Pew Internet & American Life Project. (2009). *Demographics of Internet users.* Retrieved August 27, 2009, from http://www.pewinternet.org/Static-Pages/Trend-Data/Whos-Online.aspx

Pinder, R. (1990). *The management of chronic illness.* London: Macmillan.

Preece, J. (2001). Sociability and usability in online communities: Determining and measuring success. *Behavior & Information Technology, 20*(5), 347–356.

Provost, M., Koompalum, D., Dong, D., & Martin, B. C. (2006). The initial development of the WebMedQual scale: Domain assessment of the construct of quality of health web sites. *International Journal of Medical Informatics, 75*(1), 42–57.

Rains, S. A. (2008). Seeking health information in the information age: The role of Internet self efficacy. *Western Journal of Communication, 72*(1), 1–18.

Rau, P. L. P., Gao, Q., & Ding, Y. (2008). Relationship between the level of intimacy and lurking in online social network services. *Computers in Human Behavior, 24,* 2757–2770.

Resnick, P. (2002). Beyond bowling together: Sociotechnical capital in human–computer interaction in the new millennium. In J. M. Carroll (Ed.), *Human–Computer Interaction in the New Millennium* (pp. 647–672). Boston: Addison-Wesley.

Rice, E., Stein, J. A., & Milburn, N. (2008). Countervailing social network influences on problem behaviors among homeless youth. *Journal of Adolescence, 39*(5), 625–639.

Robinson, A., & Thomson, R. (2001). Variability in patient preferences for participating in medical decision making: Implications for the use of decision support tools. *Quality in Health Care, 10*(1), 134–138.

Rodgers, S., & Chen, Q. (2005). Internet community group participation: Psychosocial benefits for women with breast cancer. *Journal of Computer Mediated Communication, 10*(4), 1–42.

Rogers, W., & Fisk, A. (2000). Human factors, applied cognition, and aging. In F. I. M. Craik & T. A. Salthouse (Eds.), *The handbook of aging and cognition* (pp. 559–591). Mahwah, NJ: Erlbaum.

Rogers, W. A., Campbell, R. H., & Pak, R. (2001). A systems approach for training older adults to use technology. In N. Charness, D. C. Parks, & B. A. Sabel (Eds.), *Communication, technology, and aging: Opportunities and challenges for the future* (pp. 187–208). New York: Springer.

Rubin, A. M. (1994). Media uses and effects: A uses-and-gratifications perspective. In J. Bryant & D. Zillmann (Eds.), *Media effects: Advances in theory and research* (pp. 417–436). Hillsdale, NJ: Erlbaum.

Sarasohn-Kahn, J. (2008). *The wisdom of patients: Health care meets online social media.* Oakland, CA: California Health Care Foundation.

Schieber, F. (2003). Human factors and aging: Identifying and compensating for age-related deficits in sensory and cognitive function. In K. W. Schaie & N. Charness (Eds.), *Impact of technology on successful aging* (pp. 85–99). New York: Springer.

Schwartz, D. G., Mosher, E., Wilson, S., Lipkus, C., & Collins, R. (2002). Seniors connect: A partnership for training between health care and public libraries. *Medical Reference Services Quarterly, 21*(3), 1–19.

Scialfa, C., Ho, G., & Laberge, J. (2004). Perceptual aspects of gerotechnology. In S. Kwon & D. Burdick (Eds.), *Gerotechnology: Research and practice in technology and aging* (pp. 18–41). New York: Springer.

Scott, R. E., McCarthy, F. G., Jennett, P. A., Perverseff, T., Lorenzetti, D., Saeed, A., et al. (2007). Telehealth outcomes: A synthesis of the literature and recommendations for outcome indicators. *Journal of Telemedicine & Telecare, 13*(Suppl 2), 1–38.

SeniorNet. (2008). IBM reveals five innovations that will change our lives in the next five years. Retrieved November 5, 2009, from http://www.seniornet.org/jsnet/index.php?option= com_content&task=view&id=567&Itemid=2

Sharf, B. F. (1997). Communicating breast cancer on-line: Support and empowerment on the Internet. *Women & Health, 26*(1), 65–84.

Shuyler, K. S., & Knight, K. M. (2003). What are patients seeking when they turn to the Internet? Qualitative content analysis of questions asked by visitors to an orthopaedics Web site. *Journal of Medical Internet Research, 5*(4). Retrieved May 21, 2008, from http://www.jmir.org/2003/4/e24

Siewe, Y. J. (2004). *Understanding the effects of aging on the sensory system.* Oklahoma Cooperative Extension Service, Oklahoma State University. Retrieved March 23, 2007, from http://osuextra.okstate.edu/pdfs/T-2140web.pdf

Sillence, E., Briggs, P., Harris, P. H., & Fishwick, L. (2007). How do patients evaluate and make use of online health information? *Social Science & Medicine, 64*(9), 1853–1862.

Smith, M. W., Sharit, J., & Czaja, S. J. (1999). Aging, motor control, and the performance of computer mouse tasks. *Human Factors, 41,* 389–396.

SPRY Foundation. (2001). *Evaluating health information on the World Wide Web: A hands-on guide for older adults and caregivers.* Retrieved August 30, 2009, from http://www.spry.org/ pdf/EvaluatingHealthInfo.pdf

Staggers, N., & Nelson, R. (2009). Overview of nursing informatics. In D. McGonigle & K. Mastrian (Eds.), *Nursing informatics and the foundation of knowledge* (pp. 83–96). Sudbury, MA: Jones and Bartlett.

Sung, K. T. (2001). Elder respect: Exploration of ideals and forms in East Asia. *Journal of Aging Studies, 15*(1), 13–26.

Tang, E., & Lee, W. (2006). Singapore Internet users' health information search: Motivation, perception of information searches, and self-efficacy. In M. Murero & R. E. Rice (Eds.), *The Internet and health care: Theory, research and practice* (pp. 107–126). Mahwah, NJ: Erlbaum.

Tate, D. F., Jackvony, E. H., & Wing, R. R. (2003). Effects of Internet behavioral counseling on weight loss in adults at risk for type 2 diabetes: A randomized trial. *Journal of American Medicine, 289,* 1833–1836.

Terry, M. (2009). Twittering healthcare: Social media and medicine. *Telemedicine Journal & E-Health, 15*(6), 507–510.

Thompson, M. G., & Heller, K. (1990). Facets of support related to well-being: Quantitative social isolation and perceived family support in a sample of elderly women. *Psychology and Aging, 5,* 535–544.

Tomaka, J., Thompson, S., & Palacios, R. (2006). The relation of social isolation, loneliness, and social support to disease outcomes among the elderly. *Journal of Aging and Health, 18*(3), 359–384.

Tu, T., & Hargraves, J. L. (2003). *Seeking healthcare information: Most consumers still on the sidelines.* Retrieved May 12, 2009, from http://www.hschange.com/CONTENT/537/537.pdf

US Census Bureau. (2009). *The International Data Base.* Retrieved July 10, 2009, from http://www.census.gov/ipc/www/idb

Wald, H. S., Dube, C. E., & Anthony, D. C. (2007). Untangling the Web—The impact of Internet use on health care and the physician–patient relationship. *Patient Education and Counseling, 68,* 218–224.

Walker, N., Philbin, D. A., & Fisk, A. D. (1997). Age-related differences in movement control: Adjusting submovement structure to optimize performance. *Journal of Gerontology: Psychological Sciences, 52B,* 40–52.

Wicks, D. A. (2004). Older adults and their information-seeking. *Behavioral and Social Sciences Librarian, 22*(2), 1–26.

Williams, R. (2008). *Complementary medicine.* Retrieved November 9, 2009, from http://www.bbc.co.uk/blogs/bbcinternet/2008/02/complementary_health_site.html

Wilson, T. D. (1997). Information behavior: An interdisciplinary perspective. *Information Processing & Management, 33*(4), 551–572.

Wolfe, R. M., & Sharp, L. K. (2005). Vaccination or immunization? The impact of search terms on the Internet. *Journal of Health Communication, 10,* 537–551.

Wright, K. (2000). Perceptions of on-line support providers: An examination of perceived homophily, source credibility, communication and social support within on-line support groups. *Communication Quarterly, 48,* 44–59.

Xie, B. (2005). Getting older adults online: The experiences of SeniorNet (USA) and OldKids (China). In B. Jaeger (Ed.), *Young technologies in old hands—An international view on senior citizen's utilization of ICT* (pp. 175–204). Copenhagen, Denmark: DJOF Publishing.

Xie, B. (2009). Older adults' health information wants in the Internet age: Implications for patient–provider relationships. *Journal of Health Communication, 14,* 510–524.

CHAPTER 4

The Personal Health Record: Building Human Capital for Health

INTRODUCTION

In this new millennium, consumers are clearly expected to invest money, energy, and time in managing their health and health care. These investments have implications for consumers' quality of life. Consumers' ability to be successful at key transition points will be affected by the capital available to him or her. Four resources of immediate impact are human capital, economic capital, social capital, and sociotechnical capital. Economists describe human capital as characteristics that cannot be separated from the person—knowledge, skills, health, and values or attitudes. Building human capital is done through education and expenditures of money and time. Economic capital includes financial assets that span household income and the extent to which health expenses are covered by insurance or government plans. Social capital spans family, friends, and the professional experts available. When disposable income is limited, the design of accessible health care and sociotechnical skills to access digital resources become more important. (Sociotechnical skills refer to the interaction of people and technology—See Chapter 2, Literacy for an Age of eHealth). Information that is tailored to the individual and is available at the time and place the consumer desires is increasingly critical to eHealth. In this book, an empowerment cycle is promoted using a socioecological framework for health (see Figure 1.8 in Chapter 1). This cycle is fueled by *capital* available to the individual and is triggered by *transitions* where decisions are required. The cycle calls for making *wise* decisions at those trigger points. Decisions require access to *data* that can be transformed to *information* and linked to available *knowledge*. Wise decisions require awareness of and analysis of a range of factors (persons and media) that *influence* attitudes, and courses of action.

One of the most important human capital resources on the health and illness journey is information and related knowledge of optional courses of action. The consumer's ability to change his or her health-related attitudes and behaviors (aspects of human capital) toward recommended treatments is usually restricted, as most people can only see part of their overall health picture. Until recently, Americans have relied on their healthcare provider to be the custodian of information on their health status and needs. However, changes in the healthcare system itself, increases in costs attributed to chronic conditions (Robert Wood Johnson Foundation, 2009c), and changes specific to aging mean that dependence is no longer viable.

Healthcare records have traditionally been compiled and archived in a formal manner by health professionals and their affiliated agencies, institutions, or practice offices and payor sources to meet their own objectives. The choice of information to collect and store and the structure and vocabulary of archival healthcare records (charts) have long been the sole province of the health professionals and healthcare administrators. Electronic records are increasingly used for storing health data on individuals within their healthcare agency (Seidman & Eytan, 2008). This development has opened new horizons for sharing data among healthcare agencies and created a platform for consumers to become engaged in decisions and for research to be more meaningful.

Until meaningfully usable records are available, the ability of consumers to maximize their human capital with respect to their health is severely compromised. Consumers cannot bring to bear the best information and decision-making criteria as they lack basic data on their own situation. As some experienced consumers note, "Managed care means you manage your care." This consumer-centered chapter will make a case for the potential value of information coordination for health care. In addition, descriptions of personal health records and related issues are explored. eHealth will mean patients are empowered as partners in their care based on access to information and feedback (Sarasohn-Kahn, 2009).

GLOBAL AND NATIONAL INITIATIVES FOR ELECTRONIC RECORDS WITH PHRS

The World Health Organization (WHO) recommendations urging record access (RA) in a PHR form were summarized by Fisher, Fitton, and (2007). (A search by document title will lead to the draft document if the journal cited is not available to readers). In this document, congruence between the record and patient explanations is stressed. The WHO document makes clear that RA means that the patient and/or family can see or use the PHR information about his or her health. A wider range of potential benefits is promised.

There is a push for Web-based records in the United Kingdom with the National Health Service taking the lead with HealthSpace (Fisher, Fitton, Poirier, & Stables, 2007). HealthSpace is the free personal health record available to people living in England receiving care through the National Health Service (National Health Service, 2009).

The potential for health information coordination at a national level became a priority for the United States in 2004. President Bush set a deadline for linking electronic health records (EHRs) from public agencies to any healthcare agency hooked to the emerging Nationwide Information Network (U.S. Department of Health and Human Services [USDHHS], n.d.). Health records from the Department of Defense, Veterans Affairs, Medicare Beneficiaries, Federal Employee Health Benefit Administration, and the Indian Health Service are specifically to be included (USDHHS, n.d.). Applications from third-party entrepreneurs would potentially be included. Microsoft HealthVault, Dossia, Aetna, IBM, and Google-Health have launched pilot projects that would be ideal tests of integrating information on a national level across stakeholder groups.

President Obama's federal mandate for electronic health records by a target 2015 will incentivize new efforts in agencies receiving federal funds (American Recovery and Reinvestment Act, 2009). Unfortunately, the current mandate does not address consumer access to those records. Developments in government-led health information technology can be tracked at the USDHHS Health Information Technology website: http://healthit.hhs.gov/portal/server.pt

CHALLENGES TO BUILDING A COMPLETE HEALTH RECORD

Challenges of Chronic Disease

Adults are living longer and have high expectations of being well. However, many are living with chronic disease. Quality of life is challenged for some by rehabilitation programs following extensive surgeries, such as coronary artery bypass or hip or knee replacements. In each instance, complex appointments must be juggled, and new routines and medications undertaken. Adults with chronic conditions and older patients with age-related declines often face complications caused by drug dosages, side effects, and interactions with other medications.

Chronic diseases or participation in rehabilitation programs prompted by an acute illness can mean that the individual and family are engaged with multiple health professionals, usually in many settings (hospitals, clinics, rehabilitation services) and possibly tied to multiple pharmacies. Keeping track of laboratory tests, drug prescriptions and regimens, and treatment recommendations from primary care providers, specialists, home health nurses, physical therapists, and other members of the team can be daunting for anyone—let alone a person who is not feeling well. Investments of time can be frustrating as it is hard to know how to collect and sort all of the information. In addition, this traditional perspective does not take into account the other influences on the patient's quality of life such as his or her social roles and network, available capital, and the pressures of daily living.

Challenges of Geography and the Economy

The problems inherent in the diverse healthcare delivery systems of developed nations are multiplied by travel or moving. Well-off boomers may be traveling the globe and even living abroad for extended periods. Many boomers take long trips with and encourage visits from grandchildren whose parents are away on their own vacations. Individuals who migrated to the United States may regularly return to their homeland to secure healthcare services they cannot obtain here. Others may spend time abroad to take care of family members and receive health care during their stay. Other unfortunates will be refugees from war and catastrophe that sweep away health records. In fact, as boomers visit each other, episodes of illness and accidents will occur in settings remote from usual care.

The subprime mortgage problems in the last half of the first decade of the century increased the number of adults of all ages who have had to move and, once again, change healthcare providers. Many boomers will downsize their housing to reflect their postretirement lifestyle and income. Further, shifts in housing can occur, from forced moves to assisted living to a nursing home for one's own or one's partner's needs. Homelessness, an increasing problem for some aging adults (Hahn, Kushel, Bangsberg, Riley, & Moss, 2006), creates innumerable challenges not only in obtaining care but in sustaining any semblance of continuity. Any geographic move, or economic shift, whether short or long term, creates challenges to accessing health information specific to individuals and families. Having quick access to key medical information could minimize misery, save lives, and avoid duplication of costly tests.

Challenges of Aging

This new responsibility for managing one's care puts particular pressure on older adults. Older adults experience new lifestyles as their work and family obligations change; they may have developmental challenges in physical and cognitive changes, and they often face challenges of chronic disease and disability. In addition, after age 65, older adults in America have to negotiate new ways of covering healthcare costs as they enroll in Medicare and, in some cases, lose work-related coverage. Each of these changes creates its own issues with respect to the information required to coordinate health care and maximize opportunities for health-related quality of life.

Collecting information becomes harder when the source of medical cost coverage changes. Very few adults have the same medical coverage from young adulthood to retirement. As jobs change, adults may have to switch providers to fit the new insurance plan coverage. With unemployment, new challenges to obtaining health care and new sets of players are added. Poor or low-income adults may be continually juggling where they obtain health care as moves and economic factors fluctuate. Medicare enrollment creates its own information challenges. In the present system each set of payers has their own system of information collection, storage, and accessibility.

Healthcare Information Fragmentation

Even without changes in coverage or in source of care, information is fragmented in our healthcare system. It is commonplace that each health professional is unaware of the recommendations of other health professionals. This is the usual case, even when the professionals are all in the same medical center. If you add specialists from differing medical centers, occasional forays to an urgent care clinic, pharmacies in the home neighborhood, and pharmacies attached to the hospital or to the clinic, the possibilities for duplication, omissions, and errors multiplies.

Across counties in the United States, public health systems and public hospitals often rely on record-keeping systems that are not readily accessible, even within the system. Public health facilities rarely share a database. Patients may have multiple chart identification numbers within the same system. Even in medical centers associated with major research universities, which could be expected to be the models of cutting-edge practice, access to clinical record information is a problem. The author (and probably most readers) can recount multiple experiences, either as a provider and/or a patient, where departments, close enough to fly a paper airplane of laboratory or x-ray results, could not access chart data critical to clinical decision making. These access limitations constrain health professionals from using their highly specialized human capital (skills, attitudes, information) to accomplish health-related goals for their clients and patients.

Issues with Incomplete Records

The lack of a consumer-controlled central database or repository for personal health information creates multiple problems. For many people, there is a loosely connected or totally disconnected collection of agencies and people who have information and recommendations about how to be healthy or how to recover from illness and accident. In any circumstance, this information patchwork makes for a ragged approach to health care. This fragmentation is a problem as services may be duplicated or contrary, and conflicting advice may be given or incompatible drugs prescribed. This creates burdens for the patient and family, generates unnecessary costs, and sets the stage for waste and fraud.

Tracking Information Sources in a Provider-Oriented Model

The ways our health system collects and controls data are not consumer oriented. Creating an aggregated record for oneself has many dilemmas. To begin with, many consumers do not mentally map the multiple locations within an agency or health service where personal information is collected. These can include registration/admitting, the patient care or treatment area, medical records constructed by clinicians and technicians in laboratory and procedure areas, notes on the clinical interaction taken by both professionals and aides, and patient accounts or billing. Patients often complain about having to repeat key details each time they encounter a new person in the system. It is surprising that consumers continue to tolerate this dysfunctional pattern.

Although the consumer may observe the data being collected in seemingly disparate chunks during a visit, in most agencies in the United States, all of this data is aggregated in a paper or electronic file—in its many repetitive iterations. Access to the file is intended to be granted only to staff in that agency. This agency-specific file is available to patients in most settings only after a formal request. The structure and content of the record is designed to meet the needs of professionals who plan and provide care in primarily discipline-specific, body system structures for an episodic care model. Control over this key human capital resource is maintained by the agency or independent healthcare provider. Concern focuses on the ability or inability of health professionals to access core information.

For each new health contact, providers outside of a specific public or private system, or from other geographic areas or community-based or private facilities, often ask the patient or family to obtain records. With the implementation of the Health Care Portability and Accountability Act (HIPAA) in 2003, patients have the right to their records (U.S. Department of Health and Human Services Office for Civil Rights, n.d.). For an overview see http://www.hhs.gov/ocr/privacy/hipaa/understanding/consumers/consumer_rights.pdf. However, the process is clumsy. The patient has to generate a list of all providers, submit a written request to each, and may be required to pick up the records in person. This often means a trip across town to pick up the records, assuming one has located the gatekeeper who will copy and release the papers. This burden discourages centralizing one's health information.

Historically, only high-risk pregnant women have had an advantage in ready access to portable information for clinical decisions. The POPRAS record system was adopted in many public hospital systems for Medicaid patients to ensure that this potentially mobile group would have continuity of care (Dombrowski, Tomlinson, Bottoms, Johnson, & Sokol, 1995; Perinatal Health Inc., 2007). This standardized format for aggregating data was on special paper (NCR) that made multiple copies. At each prenatal visit, the form was updated. Women were to carry the forms with them everywhere in case of an emergency. This system was in place in many settings across the country. However, the author is unaware of any uses in the private sector or for any conditions other than high-risk pregnancy. A Google and Ovid Medline search resulted in no reports of applications for other health conditions.

Rather, we are trapped in a system that both disempowers health professionals who lack complete information for making clinical judgments and discounts the patient and family roles as informed decision makers about available options. Isolating consumers from their own health data is compatible with the developed world's long-standing hospital-centered system of care, but incompatible with efforts to shift to a system that is distributed and home centered (Kim, Mayani, Modi, Kim, & Soh, 2005). Having a centralized data bank for one's personal health information is an alternative.

OPPORTUNITIES WITH A CENTRALIZED RECORD

Transition from Medical Home to Health Habitat

One early approach was to construct a "medical home" as a central record repository (Deloitte, 2008), A quick review of the American Health Information Management Association (AHIMA) and American Medical Informatics Association (AMIA) (2007) list of "shoulds" for centralized, personal health records reveals a very traditional medical model. As an alternative to a medical orientation, the PHR might better be thought of as a interface for one's *health habitat* (Jordan-Marsh, 2008). Such a habitat would be constructed in a socio-ecological model that considers the individual consumer as an empowered member of a social network in a variety of communities. Data that goes beyond the medical picture might include personal health goals with dates for achieving them, healthy lifestyle diaries, pedometer readings, over-the-counter medications, and whatever the consumer believes is relevant to his or her health. Nurses and social workers might seek information about the composition of the household and the social network. The goal is to take the consumer's perspective on variables that might better explain outcomes than traditional medical data—the personal side of the healthcare equation. Taking a social perspective is part of a global view of personal health records (International Council on Medical and Care Compunetics [ICMCC], n.d.)

Most members of the health team would value information about patient education, how well the patient adheres to lifestyle goals and medical regimens, and inventories of resources and barriers in the physical environment of the patient's home, work, and social life (including religious and hobby settings). Dental records are also useful not only for consumers and caregivers of older adults but for identification purposes as well. Sensors in bed can provide sleep-quality data. With record access in a PHR, clients are able to monitor their adherence to complex regimens in real time. The goal is to create a consumer-centric interactive system (Brennan, 2006) that goes beyond the passive traditional health record designed for physicians and administrators. The real-time data entry is an advantage over the traditional retrospective recall in the clinician's office.

Personal Health Record as Consumer-Oriented Central Record

Centrally available health records are equally important to consumers who want to be in charge of their own health and those who want their healthcare decision makers to have timely access to critical data. *Personal health record* (PHR) is a very common label that has been in use since 1982 (Slezak, 1982). However, the vast majority of articles concerning personal health records have appeared in the last decade. The Indivo website suggests a major development in the field took place in 1994 with the Guardian Angel project collaboration with MIT and Harvard (Indivo, n.d.). The site provides a map of PHR major developments from 1994 to 2009. The WHO endorsement of PHRs (Fisher, Fitton, & Bos, 2007) provides validation for pioneers and innovators.

Unfortunately, there is limited agreement on a definition of the product that will make access to one's own health data possible. How the PHR is defined varies somewhat from the user perspective. There are many complex issues related to the design and implementation of systems that would create a central depository for the health information of individuals. Consumers, payers, policy makers, and healthcare professionals will each have different priorities.

A stepped explanation of PHRs in the form of a tour of key personal health record issues has been provided by the AHIMA at http://www.myphr.org/tour/

tour_page_04.asp. At this site, there is an overview of what is meant by a PHR; there are also explanations of information rights, myths about privacy, free forms to start a PHR, and other relevant details.

The first international portal for patients and public access to personal health records is provided by ICMCC—the International Council on Medical and Care Compunetics (n.d.). This group monitors international developments in the field of personal access to medical records. They provide publication links, news of events, and opportunities for comment related to access to personal health records in the United States and abroad.

IBM (2008) has created a healthcare island that uses a Second Life avatar to explain to consumers how a personal health record could interface with an electronic health record. Consumers walk through the interface potential from home to clinic, emergency room, and hospital. IBM plans to use the island as a continually available sales tool for their records applications.

The most extensive project in terms of support for innovation in developing personal health records has been Robert Wood Johnson Project Health Design. The final report (Robert Wood Johnson Foundation, 2009) provides details of the outcomes of funded projects. The report also has photos of users engaging with their personal health record system. Brennan, Casper, Downs, and Aulahk (2009) describe the successes of the Robert Wood Johnson Project Health Design. Interoperability was a requirement. Providing a graphic interface was common.

Use of graphs is emerging as a core tool for interpreting *data* for consumers to build *information* that can be linked to *knowledge* needed for *wise* choices (see the empowerment cycle in Figure 4.1). Showing peaks and dips and trends over time with built in alerts and links to advice (clinical wisdom) has the potential to *influence* consumers at key transition points to make wise decisions. As the Web evolves (see description of Web 3.0 in Chapter 7, Table 7.6), healthcare professionals and consumers will build links to supportive resources that are tailored to the individual. The links will take into account history and personal preferences in delivering information relevant to the current choice point. This highly individualized Web evolution could become a new source of sociotechnical capital for health.

The following sections in this chapter outline key issues and opportunities to increase consumer ability to use the human capital of information in a personal health record to build health capital. Health capital in this case is having the information required for informed decisions in a systematic format. Health capital is also the perceived capability and willingness to participate in health data collection and partner in decisions. The key criterion is the ability to share that information with advisors and clinicians who are working with the client at the point of care and during follow-up.

Figure 4.1   The Socioecology of Health Literacy: The Empowerment Cycle

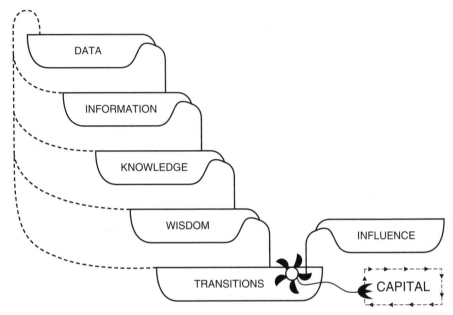

Illustration: Jin DePaul.

Benefits of Personal Health Records and Related Systems

There are benefits of personal health records that will support the agendas of every aspect of the healthcare system. These can be categorized by role group (Table 4.1).

Whether these benefits occur depend on true interoperability, how quickly the record can be populated or filled in during or after a health encounter, how generous the consumer owner is in granting access to data for consultations with providers, and whether the consumer permits, or unwittingly allows, review by employers, policy makers, and researchers.

All expected benefits rely on collaboration among role groups to design systems that monitor changes in data at the individual and group levels. For example, data collectors need to be advised when new data is added, old data hidden, and errors corrected or annotated. This is part of the feedback loop essential to successful implementation (Sarasohn-Kahn, 2009).

Table 4.1   Potential Benefits of PHRs and PHR Systems by Role Group

Roles	Benefits
Consumers, patients, and their caregivers	• Support wellness activities • Manage insurance benefits and claims • Increase sense of control over health • Avoid duplicate tests • Reduce adverse drug interactions and allergic reactions • Support continuity of care across time and providers • Increase access to providers via e-visits • Support home monitoring for chronic diseases • Verify accuracy of information in provider records
Healthcare providers	• Improve access to data from other providers and patients themselves • Improve documentation of communication with patients • Avoid duplicate tests • Improve medication compliance • Increase knowledge of potential drug interactions and allergies • Broaden awareness of full range of providers and services accessed by patient in and out of primary healthcare system
Payers	• Improve customer service (transactions and information) • Track claims and payout data • Promote portability of patient information across plan • Display all insurance plans consumer is eligible for
Employers	• Support wellness and preventive care • Improve workforce productivity • Use aggregate data to manage employee health • Target news of new work-based services
Societal/population	• Strengthen health promotion and disease prevention • Improve the health of populations

(continues)

Table 4.1   Potential Benefits of PHRs and PHR Systems by Role Group (*continued*)

Roles	Benefits
	• Expand health education opportunities • Use aggregate data to track impact of access and reimbursement policies • Provide third-party reimbursement claim data to consumers to limit fraud
Researchers	• Increase timeliness and accuracy of correlative data for studies • Increase accuracy of "self-report" data in general

Source: Adapted from National Committee on Vital and Health Statistics, 2006.

Defining the Personal Health Record

Clarity on what constitutes a personal health record is important to making progress on the difficult issues of privacy and access. Some proponents call for the label *PCHR* to explicitly designate data files (records) that are "personally controlled health records" (Mandl, Simons, Crawford, & Abbett, 2007). The key feature in this designation is that the individual *controls* access, data sources, and any annotations. The Wikipedia note states that a PHR is "*initiated* [emphasis added] and maintained by an individual" (Personal health record, 2010). This author would argue there is considerable merit in allowing the term to also refer to records initiated through a particular institution, agency, third-party provider, or payer if the consumer is in control. However the record is initiated, the contents, links to clinical data sources, and the power granted to the consumer are the core features.

The AMHIA has proposed a PHR definition:

> The personal health record (PHR) is an electronic, universally available, lifelong resource of health information needed by individuals to make health decisions. Individuals own and manage the information in the PHR, which comes from healthcare providers and the individual. The PHR is maintained in a secure and private environment, with the individual determining rights of access. The PHR is separate from and does not replace the legal record of any provider. (American

Health Information Management Association e-HIM Personal Health Record Work Group, 2005, para. 8)

Universally available would imply around-the-clock access. If the individual owns the information, then it is accessible (available) only through his or her gatekeeping actions. Even health professionals might be granted "read-only" access, or they could be granted contributor access, which allows the user to make additions and comments. For some consumers, custodial access is desirable. In this case, if a family member or friend has been granted the privilege of making decisions about care, he or she needs access to the information within the PHR. This *custodian* needs the ability to make decisions about content and how others can access the record for specific purposes.

A critical component is an arrangement where every healthcare provider deposits his or her notes and approves releasing results of any tests and x-rays to be filed in the record. The increasing availability of downloadable software that is populated (automatically filled in from an electronic medical record system) or completed by the consumer and which resides on the consumer's computer is critical to a useful PHR. Such a critical component requires interoperability so that multiple agencies and individuals can contribute to the record without software conflicts.

Most applications offer information in the form of graphs of values that change over time, such as weight and blood pressure or even mood and social interactions. These models might be labeled as comprehensive if the record contains all of the traditional medical elements and allows for personal variations (Table 4.2). The technical aspects important to health professionals choosing or designing a system are discussed in Chapter 5, Devices as Adjunct to Being Healthy at Home, and ethical aspects are discussed in Chapter 7, Consumer-centric Health Technology: Wicked Problems and Delicious Opportunities.

For consumers, content (topics and depth of detail), privacy, methods of adding data, and portability and proprietary status are important considerations. Privacy is the extent to which the sensitive information contained in a PHR can be protected from unwanted and risky viewing by others. Portability is the ease with which consumers can access the record when they change geographic location, providers, insurance companies, and so on. Proprietary control refers to the issue of ownership. It is critical to understand who can grant viewing rights and whether data will be shared with other entities for research or commercial purposes without requesting consumer permission for each incident. These topics are individually addressed after the following overview of the content of a PHR.

Personal health records may be *comprehensive* or *focused*. The two types are illustrated in Table 4.2.

Table 4.2 Personal Health Record: Comprehensive and Focused Applications

Project Title	Audience	Researcher	Location	Platform/Media Type
Comprehensive applications				
Google Health	Any		www.google.com/health	Online PHR Information about conditions Import medical records from participating providers Medicine interactions Physician searches
Indivo	MIT, Harvard students and employees; Children's Hospital Boston patients; other expansions underway to provide service to millions more		www.indivohealth.org	Fully detailed clinical encounters with XML-based storage Patients can subscribe to data updates
Microsoft HealthVault	Any		www.healthvault.com	Online PHR; additionally, can upload data from a variety of health and fitness devices Create emergency document with health information Save health search results and relevant articles

Focused applications

A Customized Care Plan for Breast Cancer Patients	Breast cancer patients	Laura Esserman, MD, MBA Director	Center of Excellence for Breast Cancer Care University of California, San Francisco	PHR component integrates with existing calendars Provides links and prompts to help patients customize and better understand their care
Personal Health Management Assistant	Heart disease patients	George Ferguson, PhD Research Scientist	Department of Computer Science University of Rochester (NY)	Daily check-in (via text or speech) with patients Provides personalized treatment recommendations and collects longitudinal data
Personal Health Application for Diabetes Self-Management	Diabetes patients	Stephanie Fonda, PhD Senior Research Scientist	TRUE Research Foundation Washington, DC	Application that interfaces with gadgets within iGoogle Makes individual recommendations on nutrition, physical activity, blood glucose, self-reported emotional state
Chronic Disease Medication Management	Diabetes patients	John Ralston, MD, MPH Assistant Investigator	The Center for Health Studies, Group Health Cooperative	PHR that records blood glucose, blood pressure, food intake, exercise into cell phone and

(*continues*)

Table 4.2 Personal Health Record: Comprehensive and Focused Applications (*continued*)

Project Title	Audience	Researcher	Location	Platform/Media Type
Between Office Visits			University of Washington, Seattle	transmits it to medical providers who provide feedback and counsel as needed
My-Medi-Health: A Vision for a Child-Focused Personal Medication Management System	Children with cystic fibrosis and their caretakers	Kevin Johnson, MD, MS Associate Professor	Department of Biomedical Informatics Vanderbilt University Medical Center, Nashville	Two-way communication with personal health application Tracks medications, alerts parents when dose is taken, manages refills
Supporting Patient and Provider Management of Chronic Pain with PDA Applications Linked to Personal Health Records	Patients with chronic pain	Roger Luckmann, MD, MPH Associate Professor	Department of Family Medicine & Community Health, University of Massachusetts, Worcester	Touchscreen device prompts user every 2 hours for pain experiences and physical activity Data transferred to Common Platform database for provider analyses
ActivHealth: A PHR System for At-Risk Sedentary Adults	Sedentary adults	Barbara Leah Massoudi, PhD, MPH Senior Research Health Scientist	Research Triangle Institute, Atlanta	Through a Web portal, sensors input information (physical activity and lifestyle) to generate customized plans to increase activity Pedometer and accelerometer

Living Profiles: Transmedia Personal Health Record System for Young Adults	Adolescents with chronic conditions	Christy Sandborg, MD Professor & Chief	Pediatric Rheumatology Lucile Salter Packard Children's Hospital Stanford University School of Medicine	Tap into teen behavior such as texting and music to provide feedback to teen about relationship between behavior and state of health Assist with transition to adult health system
Assisting Older Adults with Transitions of Care	Older adults released from hospital	Stephan Eisenhard Ross, MD Associate Professor	Division of General Internal Medicine University of Colorado at Denver & Health Sciences Center, Aurora	Portable touchscreen computer that a patient receives upon hospital discharge Helps track medication, schedule refills, appointments, etc.

Note: Focused application data compiled from Robert Wood Johnson Foundation.

The comprehensive record is designed as a partner to the medical establishment's electronic health record (EHR). An alternate model is one where consumer priorities and preferences guide design and selection of elements for a specific purpose. These records are consumer focused.

Contents of PHRs

Minimum Elements of a Comprehensive Personal Health Record

The contents of a comprehensive personal health record can be described in terms of the minimum requirements for a PHR to be useful as well as in terms of items selected by the individual to address his or her personal situation. A consensus is emerging on the minimum elements of a PHR (National Committee on Vital and Health Statistics [NCVHS], 2006). These have been revised and presented as model elements in a joint statement from AHIMA and AMIA (see next section). An ideal PHR allows for additional entries as the consumer's needs and interests change.

Model Elements of a Personal Health Record

The joint position statement (AHIMA & AMIA, 2007) reminds consumers that a PHR is broader than the traditional medical record. Commonly agreed on contents are listed in Table 4.3. Perhaps the most critical element is the feedback loop (Sarasohn-Kahn, 2009).

Table 4.3   Characteristics of the Ideal Personal Health Record

- Personal identification:
  - Name
  - Birth date
  - Contact information
- People to contact in case of emergency
- Names, addresses, and phone numbers of health team
- Health insurance information
- Legal documents:
  - Living wills
  - Organ donation authorization
  - Legal representatives
- General information:
  - Height
  - Weight
  - Blood type

Table 4.3   Characteristics of the Ideal Personal Health Record (*continued*)

- A list of significant conditions, illnesses, and surgical procedures:
  - Dates and location of treatments
  - Outcomes
- Current medication and dosages
- Immunizations and their dates
- Allergies or sensitivities to drugs or materials (e.g., latex)
- Doctor, hospital, or other healthcare visits:
  - Reasons
  - Diagnoses
  - Treatments
- Clinical tests:
  - Dates
  - Results
- Pregnancies, including details of pregnancy and birth
- Family/social histories:
  - Conditions
  - Relationships including social network
  - Current status
- Therapy:
  - Type
  - Dates
  - Frequency
  - Outcome
- Vital signs
- Observations of daily living selected by user
- Feedback loop triggered by information patterns

Source: Adapted from AHIMA & AMIA, 2007, p. 24; Brennan et al., 2009; Project HealthDesign, n.d.

There is insufficient data now to appreciate whether an automated algorithm or a connection to a known health professional provides more effective feedback. An automated system that responds using specific rules triggered by reported events (algorithm) could be a very cost-effective strategy. However, the influence accruing from a relationship with a known health professional (personal nurse practitioner, social worker, physician, and so on) may be essential for users to take recommended actions. It will be interesting to see if consumers would interact with an unknown health professional in a commercial application or one sponsored by a credible entity such as the Mayo Clinic or American Diabetes Association. A combination of these approaches is likely to emerge. Until prevention dominates healthcare reform, developing a way to cover costs is likely to be a bigger challenge than developing the infrastructure and response guidelines. An unexplored source of economic capital that may be cost effective would be to engage retired health professionals or those limited by worker compensation restrictions in providing feedback.

Brennan (2006) coaches that the personal health record is a "*system* of tools that documents health experiences, records healthcare encounters, and provides snapshots, even movies of health events" (para. 1). A key component is the ability to support interactions between provider and client around data embedded in the record. These records might be categorized as focused instead of comprehensive. Focused PHRs are not necessarily linked to an EHR. In the Robert Wood Johnson Project HealthDesign grants, applicants were encouraged to develop innovative ways to have the record focus on observations of daily living (Table 4.2) (Project HealthDesign, n.d.). (For fact sheets and podcasts on personal health records and related projects funded by the Robert Wood Johnson Foundation, see Robert Wood Johnson Foundation, 2009a, 2009b). As consumers become more engaged in using PHRs, other elements not envisioned now are sure to be added.

Parameters of Choosing a Personal Health Record

Choosing a Platform

As consumers contemplate adding a PHR to their resources for health management, they need to consider a variety of decisions. The platform and who is providing the service are two factors. Whether information is only accessible with a Web link or is stored periodically on a flash drive or CD is important in terms of convenience, risk, and accessibility.

The joint statement of two prominent professional organizations, the AHIMA and AMIA (2007), is a clearly written, easily understood discussion of potential criteria for a PHR. The position statement notes that individuals could assemble their own PHR with paper files or downloadable software. However, this homegrown record fails the proposed definition that requires universal accessibility. Alternatively, other suppliers of a platform include healthcare providers, insurers, employers, or entrepreneurs. Entrepreneurs range from Google and Microsoft Health Vault to universities (Harvard's Indivo) to commercial entities whose primary product is a PHR (Halamka, Mandl, & Tang, 2008).

Policies for Information Storage and Access

It is important to study policies and practices for storing information—How could your data be used by others? Consumers may want to share information with all or some of their healthcare providers. The ideal is selective access that can be changed quickly and easily. Some consumers will want caregivers, such as adult children, to have access to some or all of the data. Some suppliers will be selling or sharing aggregated, anonymous data for marketing, research, and policy agendas. Consumers will consider whether they want to give permission for each instance or agree on a blanket permission with assurances of *anonymity*. Consumers ideally are reminded, when they are asked to share information, of the difference between anonymity (your name cannot be discovered) compared to *confidentiality* (your personal details are given only to restricted users who promise to protect your privacy).

The joint statement from AHIMA and AMIA (2007) advises that the best record is one that contains clinical information your healthcare providers can use. Important features to consider include: cost; difficulty of updating the record; possibility of having laboratory values, X-ray findings, and other clinical data flow automatically to the record; and the potential for correcting errors.

To be truly a PHR, the record should allow for entering personal observations about daily life or other potentially health-related, consumer-supplied data (Brennan et al., 2009; Robert Wood Johnson Foundation, n.d.). A record initiated by an insurance company may give the diagnosis and medication but lack details of actual lab values and drug doses.

Other desirable features include "ability to exchange messages with providers, schedule appointments, renew prescriptions, enter personal data; decision support (such as medication interaction alerts or reminders about needed preventive services); the ability to transfer data to and from an electronic health record and the ability to track and manage health plan benefits and services" (NCVHS, 2006, p. 15). A controversial element is whether the consumer can choose to hide information from healthcare providers.

Sustaining Privacy and Security

The web of trust between patients and healthcare professionals is protected in a PHR system by requiring identification from provider and patient when the individual account is set up, from the user whenever someone chooses to access the record, and when the account is populated with data (information is added). Access covers both simply viewing the record as well as times when updates or changes are planned. Changes to the record, such as deleting content, adding new laboratory data, new clinical information from healthcare encounters, inserting notes (annotations), or updating any parameters are all instances of times when an identity check is essential. Some systems have relied simply on a user name and password. Others recommend a second form of authentication, such as one tied to a mobile phone (Mandl et al., 2007). In the United Kingdom and elsewhere, fingerprint and a personal identification number (PIN) can limit access.

Some experts are adamant that "privacy myths" are delaying adoption of electronic health records (EHRs) (Manos, 2008, para. 1). The assertion is that it is in the application company's best interest to provide security and encrypted solutions. One marketing vice president maintains privacy violations are more reasonably attributed to easily accessed paper files or to the failure of personnel to follow institutional policies (Manos, 2008). The implication is that breaches of electronic records can be tracked, whereas paper records are easily removed or copied without leaving a trail.

Establishing Responsibility for Security

Consumers, payers, and entrepreneurs developing systems for building and accessing records may find they have different beliefs about who is to be responsible for security. For some advocates, there seems to be privacy protection implied by HIPAA in the United States. However, this federal act does not cover third-party applications (Steinbrook, 2008). The interested reader is also referred to myths about HIPAA (see American Health Information Management Association, n.d.).

Fisher and colleagues (Fisher, Fitton, Poirier, & Stables, 2007), who include the medical director of a private information system, warn that Web access may increase the likelihood that family members, friends, and coworkers may have deliberate or accidental access. Certainly, failure to close an application; passwords that are easily guessed, previously shared, or spied over the shoulder; and outright coercion increase the risk. Fisher et al. (2007) assert that "once the record has been delivered, the patient becomes responsible for its security" (p. 164). However, at least in the United States, multiple instances of entire credit card companies and health record databases being compromised have created a climate of wariness and skepticism on the part of consumers and their advocates.

Each system has to address the security concerns of the experts and users. Consumers may lack the background to evaluate the effectiveness of stated protections. The Personal Health Information Management System (PHIMS) developed at the University of Washington complies with HIPAA regulation by using secure socket layer encryption, encrypted passwords, audit trails, firewalls, integrity controls, automatic logoff, and other strategies to prevent unauthorized access. A universal or widely agreed-on checklist of desirable precautions would be valuable for providers selecting PHR systems and consumers choosing whether to make use of them.

Some patient advocates warn that consumers will have to read privacy agreements very closely. Even then, it may not be clear that third parties can gain access to data through an arcane system of permissions that is not transparent to the consumer. Despite persistent privacy issues there is intense interest in establishing PHRs across the United States (Seidman & Eytan, 2008), and on a world health level (Fisher, Fitton, & Bos, 2007). Many forces are converging to make it happen. At a 2008 conference on health technology, one expert opined that consumers were not as concerned about privacy as were providers, consumer advocates, and government agencies.

However, as telemedicine continues to demonstrate cost-effectiveness, pressure will increase to set up personal health records that can be accessed online.

Capacity for Deliberate Sharing Across Health Providers and Institutions

Experts in constructing personal health records are concerned with interoperability, meaning that a PHR must be designed so that records from different departments within an institution or agency or among institutions and agencies can be shared and that sharing can occur across institutions. Interoperability is a criterion the clinician and the patient should demand. Administrators must support interoperability as necessary but not sufficient for purchase of a system. Interoperability is provided by the computer programmers. If the record is patient controlled, it is critical for consumers to understand the opportunities and consequences of interoperability.

Large companies and healthcare agencies are increasingly providing personal health records as an option. Kaiser, Aetna, and Best Buy are just a few examples. In the early stages, members/employees are usually not required to participate. Individuals sign up or subscribe to gain access. A subscription provides continuous access to specified data from external sources. With a well-designed subscription, healthcare provider notes, laboratory values, x-rays, and prescriptions are all loaded automatically. Without subscriptions, users would have to remember to request that their healthcare information be added to the file. Alternatively, consumers would hand-enter their own data. This would create gaps as the patient or the provider would have to remember to request the file every time something new happens. All of the institutions, laboratories, providers, and possible caretakers involved in an individual's health care should be considered for subscriptions to automatic upload of new data. In a PHR that is controlled by the patient, that person decides who can have access and be subscribed for automatic updates. In a PHR supplied by the insurer or an agency in the healthcare system, ideally, the supplier and the patient would confer and agree on who was allowed access.

Weitzman, Kaci, and Mandl (2009) found that the concept of subscribing is unfamiliar to consumers and may create a barrier to adopting PHRs. Agencies and insurers may have the option for subscribing as a feature in the enrollment process that is revisited at the first personal contact. As personal health records evolve and are linked to EHRs, it is likely that all of the individuals covered by a health plan will be required to *subscribe*. In the absence of this requirement, the healthcare plan will be lacking substantial data needed to evaluate trends and outcomes.

Until all users have broadband access and relevant computer skills, creative solutions will be needed. The healthcare plan administrator could use interviews and paper questionnaires to fill in some gaps in data that comes directly from consumers. Alternatively, free wifi, access through mobile phones, and other innovations may overcome current limitations imposed by the digital divide where some groups are enabled and others decline or are unable to use online resources.

Currency of Information

Currency is a critical descriptor of implementation of a PHR; the consumer and the PHR infrastructure require a systematic approach to populating the record so that providers and consumers can obtain relevant data in a timely fashion. Although some systems are totally controlled by the consumer with gatekeeping functions for every instance of information change, this quickly becomes burdensome even for healthy consumers. Ideally, a protocol is set up at the time of opening the account that is automatically revisited at predetermined intervals. The protocol would include allowing automatic downloading of laboratory data, clinical encounter observations and recommendations, and any other elements of the record without time-specific permission from the record owner. Authentication would be a requirement, but waiting for the consumer to agree to each download would seriously compromise the currency and validity of the record for all stakeholders (see profile of roles in Table 4.1).

Accuracy Issues

Accuracy of the record is a more complex issue primarily because healthcare providers, consumers, and consumer advocates have different sources and levels of *data, information*, and *knowledge*. Consumers may wish to delete or hide certain elements of their health history. An example in the healthcare specialist's office can be refusing to be weighed at the beginning of a visit. An electronic PHR in which the provider is subscribed means the provider can look at last weight, trends, and so on, and be prepared to reinforce, cajole, or lecture the patient about his or her weight. If a consumer is coming to the office for exploration of a symptom that he or she decides is not weight related, may mean that the consumer may not want the topic to arise. Thus, the data is "hidden."

Some providers are "terrified" of the consequences of PHRs (Robeznieks, 2007, para. 3). Concerns include finding the time and reimbursement for reviewing the health records of consumers who have formal access to their records, thus forcing the provider to make clinical judgments based on only the data the patient wants to reveal. Legal liability and professional competence are at issue.

Privacy and Accuracy Tensions

Consumers and their advocates point out that some patients fear being labeled and treated differently based on information that might be prejudicial. Many patients fragment their medical care deliberately so that only one provider is aware of lifestyle habits or preferences they do not wish to reveal. Some examples are history of substance abuse, out-of-wedlock pregnancies, sexually transmitted diseases, gender identity, and more. Some consumers are fearful of a clinician prematurely coming to a conclusion based on isolated data elements in the record and wanting an interview and physical examination before the consumer reveals all of his or her history and data. For patients seeking a second opinion, this may be of equal concern to the patient and the insurance company. On the other hand, if patients are allowed to delete or hide data permanently, the patient may be in a crisis where appropriate treatment decisions cannot be made. Similarly, patients may want to obscure data for a particular time or from an agency or provider and may forget to adjust shields for other situations or when the circumstances change.

One option is to create a flag that reminds the consumer that data has been deleted or hidden and invites an action each time the consumer accesses his or her records. Providers would benefit from seeing the same flag as it would signal them to inquire about the obscured or altered portion of the health record. Some systems, such as Harvard's Indivo do not allow deletion of any content, only the hiding of documents. Furthermore, Indivo does not allow editing of documents that the consumer did not create, but it does permit annotations to provide the consumer's view of the contents. These restrictions, Mandl and colleagues (2007) argue, are critical to sustaining the web of trust. They argue that healthcare providers must have confidence in the accuracy and quality of the data reviewed before making decisions.

Before overreacting to concerns about electronic systems, consumers and their advocates need to appreciate the limits of the current record system. In a paper-based system, it is easy for consumers to mask data by visiting providers in different departments or agencies. Furthermore, when a hospital or clinic paper record is requested, part may be omitted by the medical records department if there is legal action pending. In the future, as new treatments are tried, documentation of efficacy may not materialize as consumers hide some key information from all or selected role groups (see Table 4.1). Data on mental health, substance abuse, and domestic violence are likely candidates for restricted access or total omissions. Anticipated benefits of PHRs may have unintended consequences. Employers might use aggregated data from an employee group (personal information removed) to change benefits offered to the group of employees. Such benefits could include on-site clinics, incentives for lifestyle changes, and reduced options in coverage of specific healthcare procedures or conditions. These changes may be made because a link could not be established between providing a service and changing outcomes, such as absenteeism. Employee groups may disagree with the decision and could argue that they would choose different criteria for retaining or introducing services. Making aggregated reports available to all stakeholders will create capital for wise decisions—an ecological recognition that everything is connected. Sometimes finding the connections requires multiple vantage points.

At present, much information about health conditions, treatments, and medications is mined by researchers and pharmaceutical companies from traditional paper records and source-specific reports. The more PHRs are stored in electronic formats, the more accessible personal health information becomes. An unfortunate side effect of concerns about individual data breaches may be a wave of consumer decisions to limit access to data sharing even when identifiers are stripped. This would severely compromise public health planning and research on health care and treatments (Steinbrook, 2008). Peel, the founder of Patient Privacy Rights suggests *smart consents* (Peel, 2008). Smart consents allow patients to selectively agree to sharing data. Smart consents, Peel predicts, would increase opportunities to participate in research. This level of personal control would take the place of the current *data stewardship* models. In this stewardship model, agency staff, a provider, or a third-party administrator decide on giving access for research or marketing purposes.

Privacy and Proxy Designations

Hiding, annotating, and deleting data may be more of an issue in the case of proxy roles. There are instances where individuals may wish to allow full privileges to the person who is the primary decision maker on their behalf. Individuals who are terminally ill or older adults who have given medical power of attorney and other decision-making controls to adult children are examples. However, those same individuals may wish to limit caretaker access to certain portions of their PHR. Minors are a more complex situation where privacy may be dictated by legal statute, institutional policy, clinical judgment, and the demands of the particular situation. An ideal system would flag or alert both the consumer and the provider when legal statutes or agency policies dictate limitations. Consumers may want to search for PHR applications where sensitive data access is an *opt-in* feature. This feature means the user must choose to share information. The alternative is an *opting-out* application where information is broadcast until the owner declares he or she does not want to share.

Facebook provided a vivid example of the consequences of *opting out* as a default. One Christmas shopping season, many consumers on Facebook did not notice they had to actively block sharing their shopping data—they had to opt out. Facebook planned to increase the effectiveness of its clients' advertising by using the personal endorsements of Facebook participants. If a Facebook user bought something online, it would be posted on the user's Facebook page as a personal endorsement of that product, with the desired result being that the Facebook user's friends would be influenced by the endorsement. However, this meant also that gift recipients prematurely learned what had been purchased for them from their holiday wish list. The happiest consequence is a spoiled surprise; a more tragic outcome is learning that there is another significant other in the buyer's life! Asking if shopping data can be posted was the compromise—an *opting-in* choice. Similarly, if the default on a PHR is revealing all health data unless forbidden, speculation as to why a particular topic is restricted may occur. Also, a stressed or ill patient may be too distracted to thoughtfully decide whether to veil or reveal potentially vulnerable areas of information.

Blanket Consents as System Norm

The debate about privacy in third-party online applications is intense. However, many consumers forget that most healthcare providers and agencies now require that the consumer sign a blanket consent that gives wide-ranging permission for data sharing. There is no option for restricting data or permissions in the paper-and-pen world of contemporary health care. If a patient refuses to sign, no care will be provided until an administrator agrees to negotiate an alteration to the institutional agreement.

Reading Privacy Statements

For any third-party offering, it is especially important to review the privacy policy. Many make vague statements that claim conformance with HIPAA and all applicable laws. Related concerns are: Where is the company based, and to what extent are they are mandated to follow US laws with respect to medical information? To state that a company was founded in the United States is not to state that it is an American corporation. Reading privacy documents and "About" pages on a website may provide useful cues to the potential users.

Following the announcement of Google Health and Microsoft's Health Vault, a number of cautionary blogs appeared (ha.ckers.org, 2008; Hamilton, 2008). However, before deriding these third-party agencies, self-designated patient advocates need to review privacy practices of major medical centers. See the USC Notice of Privacy Practices at http://policies.usc.edu/hipaa/privacynoticeengl041403.pdf and the privacy practices pertaining to Beth Israel Deaconess Medical Center, Harvard Medical Faculty Physicians Group, and Medical Care of Boston at http://www.bidmc.org/PrivacyStatement.aspx (University of Southern California, 2003; Beth Israel Deaconess Medical Center, 2009).

Some medical centers with electronic records do assist patients by allowing them to audit who has examined their records (Rubenstein, 2008). Rubenstein recommends tracking the "Explanation of Benefits" section on statements mailed from (or posted by) insurers as a check on fraudulent use of insurance. Rubenstein also recommends websites designed for consumers that provide information on privacy law, give tips on dealing with medical identity theft, and one that offers a tool kit. The tool kit provides forms and information for preventing and responding to privacy problems (see Patient Privacy Rights, www.patientprivacyrights.org). Other resources include forms to request medical records and lists of restrictions on use of medical data. Under the "Policy" tab, this site also provides information on current legislation. Another resource is the World Privacy Forum (www.worldprivacyforum.org), which links the viewer to a wide range of privacy concerns that go beyond health.

Breaches of Privacy

Breaches of privacy are not limited to electronic personal records. In April 2002, several hundred patients were sent unsolicited samples of Prozac weekly through the mail, along with instructions to discontinue their current medication and begin taking the new medication the next day (Dyer, 2003). These instructions arrived on letterhead, in some cases signed by their physicians. Lawsuits have been filed against the drug's manufacturer, Eli Lilly, whose sales representatives planned the mailings; the pharmacy chain that filled and mailed the prescriptions, Walgreens; as well as three physicians who signed blank letterhead and allegedly provided a targeted list of patients taking other antidepressants. This action raised privacy concerns about who has access to a patient's medical records (Dyer). In 2008, the UCLA Medical Center was formally reprimanded when staff at many levels were found to have viewed records of celebrities and fellow personnel. In some cases, tabloids took advantage of this "reliable source" (Associated Press, 2008). So, refusing to participate in a personal health record system will not necessarily protect one's personal health data. In each of these cases, a personal health record was not the point of entry.

Ownership and Control

As indicated earlier, many consumer advocates, including entrepreneurs in the field, are campaigning for a platform that would provide consumer-centric data. Some definitions of a personal health record, according to AMIHA and AMIA (2007), distinguish PHRs from EHRs on the element of consumer control. Control means both gatekeeping access and monitoring accuracy, but it also includes entering data and comments that are specifically tailored to the interests and needs of the specific client and his or her family. Given the nascency of PHRs, many users will have a hard time imagining how the different features of a PHR might be useful to them.

Increasingly at issue is the question of who will hold the accumulated data in a personal health record. Wolter (2007) advocates a model from financial banking where a neutral third party holds the record on behalf of the consumer. The Health Record Banking Alliance is a nonprofit corporation that has proposed a set of design principles related to ownership and control of the records and to the operation of health record banks. The model is useful because users are accustomed to the familiar steps of opening an account, making deposits, creating audit trails, and establishing consumer ownership of the information "asset." Ball, Costin, and Lehmann (2008) compare the PHR to an ATM card. Consumers are able to access both their personal information and a variety of healthcare related services, for example, making appointments, refilling prescriptions, and downloading required documentation of vaccinations. Wikipedia offers the model of a credit report where you can get a record from different sources: entrepreneurial groups, employers, health insurance companies, hospitals, and so on. Issues of transferability arise—thus the value of the bank metaphor.

One feature of the UK National Health Service that consumers in the United States may want to request is called Copying Letters to Patients (Fisher, Fitton, Poirier, & Stables, 2007). This feature allows patients to see the letters written on their behalf. In the United States, this might include worker compensation letters, temporary disability statements that are not work related, and communication to specialists or other members of the health team. The WHO recommendations on PHRs (Fisher, Fitton, & Bos, 2007) also make the case that seeing letters is an important dimension of understanding one's healthcare issues.

Government Initiatives

The National Health Information Network (NHIN) is a key component of the US strategy to improve the American healthcare system. At the Department of Health and Human Services website on health information technology, consumers and experts alike can access current information about the Network and its progress (http://www.hhs.gov/healthit). Recently, the NHIN celebrated a successful test of interoperability across systems of electronic health records (EHRs). The goals of the NHIN are to have health information be tied to the consumer wherever the consumer receives care, to support clinical decision making, and engage in other information-related exchanges that will support health at the community and individual levels. The Network strategies include:

- Developing capabilities for standards-based, secure data exchange nationwide
- Improving the coordination of care information among hospitals, laboratories, physicians offices, pharmacies, and other providers
- Ensuring appropriate information is available at the time and place of care
- Ensuring that consumers' health information is secure and confidential
- Giving consumers new capabilities for managing and controlling their personal health records as well as providing access to their health information from EHRs and other sources
- Reducing risks from medical errors and supporting the delivery of appropriate, evidence-based medical care
- Lowering healthcare costs resulting from inefficiencies, medical errors, and incomplete patient information (USDHHS, n.d.)

CONSUMER ENGAGEMENT IN DESIGN

Just as there is no universal definition of a personal health record, there is even less agreement on the features or components of such a record. Failure to achieve consensus is a reflection of the newness of the PHR. However, it is also attributable to limited consumer engagement. Morales Rodriguez, Casper, and Brennan (2007) note that consumers are not routinely engaged in most product development until the system is finished. At that point, satisfaction surveys may be conducted. Morales Rodriguez et al., propose that the development and acceptance of personal health records and related products would be advanced by engaging consumers early in the design and evaluation of products intended for their use. Morales Rodriguez and colleagues in the Project HealthDesign (2007) funded by the Robert Wood Johnson Foundation and the California Health Care Foundation all argue for the use of user-centered design (UCD). In this formal approach, the focus is on the target population and "what they will do with the product, where they will use it, and what features they consider essential" (Project Health Design, 2007, pp. 44–45). What is unique to this design is that consumers are consulted throughout the development of the product or tool. Perhaps in the future, just as consumers watch for the UL (United Laboratories) holographic seal on electrical appliances, they will also look for a UCD logo on electronic products and tools.

The benefits of advocating user engagement in the development of a product may quickly make sense to engineers and product designers. However, consumer engagement in policy setting about health information technology and related access and reimbursement is controversial. First, consumers are rarely engaged in health technology developments until the later stages when satisfaction and intent to use are primary variables (Morales Rodriguez et al., 2007). One legitimate dilemma is in choosing the consumers to engage. Professional organizations and government groups are a common source of requests for representation, but their interests can be very narrow. In some instances, federal groups, such as AHRQ, have engaged health professionals with a family member affected by the disease or policy issue.

Features of Interface for Older Adults

One examination of PHRs for older adults focused on medication use (Daly et al., 2008). Both older adults and physicians participated in a focus group. The PHRs known to these individuals were not attractive. The data entry was seen by patients as busywork. Patients had concerns about the computer environment—their skills and privacy. Older adults were concerned that physicians would be typing during a visit and not listening. Physicians were concerned about reliability of the data and the interface with the EMR. Benefits agreed on were the information sharing, especially for older adults who were highly mobile, for encounters with new physicians and healthcare professionals, and in emergencies. PHRs were seen as good for conditions that were very complex and for conditions where self-care management was required. Nonetheless, their summary was that barriers outweighed benefits.

Kim et al. (2005) designed a personal health record application for a predominantly low-income, elderly, or disabled public housing population (see discussion of outcomes below). Kim et al. included uniformly structured Web forms with consistent options for interaction responses for each category of health information. This strategy is used to build confidence for naïve users. In addition, each category of health information was visible in as few screens as possible, requiring only a vertical scroll. To accommodate the slower motor–vision synchronization of older adults, response timings were designed to account for extended reaction time. Font size flexibility is another key feature for older adults. Ensuring that these needs are met requires consumer participation in the early design stages. Providing coaching on the new literacies required for eHealth will be an equally important strategy (see Chapter 2, Literacy for an Age of eHealth).

Mass Collaboration Opportunities

The transparency afforded by the Internet can allow a wide range of consumers to become aware of the opportunities available to engage in the dialogue around health care. New strategies might be developed for building the same "mass collaboration" in health care as Tapscott and Williams (2006) describe are evolving in the field of manufacturing. Those who are formally designated as consumer representatives or even liaisons (NCVHS, 2006, p. 4) might have the responsibility of "taking the pulse" of the groups they represent. Both qualitative and quantitative strategies can be employed, ranging from classic focus groups, to monitoring designated blogs that appear after key documents are posted for public comment, to performing surveys such as those facilitated by websites such as Survey Monkey (www.surveymonkey.com).

Once consumers are named as members of boards and committees, multiple barriers to sustained participation may arise. Some barriers are specific to being a consumer whose work is not healthcare oriented. Time taken to participate in focus groups and attendance at policy review meetings can create stresses on the job or home life. Just as physicians are concerned about being reimbursed for reading PHRs, reimbursing consumers for participating in policy making is a legitimate issue. Most professionals who are committee and panel members are encouraged to participate by their employers and receive rewards of professional advancement and enhanced credibility in their field. These supports shift the perspective and meaning of decisions and recommendations. Some consumers lack the vocabulary, credibility, and communication strategies needed to be heard in discussions.

INNOVATIVE PERSONAL HEALTH RECORD APPLICATIONS

Numerous PHR applications have emerged, some from government-funded projects, such as Indivo from the National Library of Medicine; some from healthcare management groups, like Kaiser; others from third-party entrepreneurs such as Google Health and Microsoft Health Vault, and some from competitions funded by private foundations such as the Robert Wood Johnson Foundation. The term *PHR* in most of the Internet sites and literature implicitly means a very comprehensive repository of information specific to an individual. However, more limited applications also use the term *PHR*. A notable variant is described by the focused applications in the Robert Wood Johnson Foundation's Project HealthDesign (2007).

Other *focused* applications are evolving from consumer organizations or third-party groups with very limited goals. For example, see the set of applications in Table 4.4, which are limited to physical fitness for purposes of illustration and brevity. Other consumer designed and commercially prepared single-focus applications are expected to emerge continually as smart phones and inexpensive sensors proliferate with infinite potential for innovative applications.

Third-Party Platforms

Government-Funded and Supported Comprehensive Applications

Indivo is a Web-accessed implementation developed at Harvard University with initial funding from the National Library of Medicine and the Centers for Disease Control and Prevention (Children's Hospital Informatics Program, n.d.; Weitzman et al., 2009). Indivo is notable for using public, open source standards and being free (Mandl et al., 2007). The Indivo personally controlled health record (PCHR) is designed around an ecosystem approach to integrating health-care information and patient-driven applications to "improve the quality, effectiveness, and convenience of the healthcare system" (Mandl et al., Conclusion, para 1). Individual projects and sites offer this approach to their collaborators. Indivo has multiple partners using the software platform (Indivo, n.d.). Some of these partners include Dossia and the Massachusetts Department of Public Health (see website for current information).

Another major partnership is underway in South Carolina where Medicare patients are invited to use a free electronic personal health record called MyPHRSC (South Carolina Nurses Association, 2008). This electronic record is filled in automatically with the past 2 years of Medicare claims history when a person registers at https://www.myphrsc.com/. The personal history of diagnoses, clinic visits, and hospitalizations are all provided to users. Registered users are required to enter medications, allergies, and healthcare services from non-Medicare sites on their own initiative. There is a place for adding user-generated notes as well. The record is intended to streamline claims information and provide continuity of care. MyPHRSC is notable in that it is usable across different fee-for-service provider systems. The needs and skills of senior consumers were taken into account in the design. Participation is optional for beneficiaries. Access is controlled by the consumer who determines whether the provider may view the file. An alternate to granting access is printing out information from the record.

Table 4.4 Tracking Health and Fitness with Technology: Features and Parameters

Company/ Website	Features	Cost	Physiological Parameters	Graphs/ Tables	Social Networking	Computer Skill Level	Self-Report	PHR
AARP www.aarp.org/ health	Boomer-friendly health tips, articles, etc. Step Up to Better Health: enters steps per day from pedometer and tracks progress on great American trails, such as Route 66	No cost; must have pedometer	Allows you to calculate your BMI (not automatic)	Provides tables that track and summarize your walking information	Sole Mates: allows you to share progress with friends and family	Basic Internet skills. Very thorough demo on how to use the program	Yes	No
iPod + Nike www.apple. com/ipod/nike	Transfers workout data to the Internet when you plug in; also tracks your run in real time Compares and analyzes runs (speed distance, calories burned) Connects with other runners around the world—challenge anyone to a virtual race	No cost for service; iPod Nano starts at $149; sensor is $29	Provides calories burned (automatic)	Graphical interface allows you to view performance history, set goals	Allows you to challenge other users around the world	Basic computer skills Transfer of information from iPod to computer is automatic	Information transferred from iPod, not self-entered	No

Revolution Health www.revolution health.com	Diet and fitness plans from partner, SparkPeople Articles, tips, links, expert-led groups	No cost	Allows you to calculate your BMI (not automatic)	Tracks information that user enters and tracks changes	Online health communities, user-created profiles, blogs, etc.	Basic Internet skills	Yes	Personal Health Portfolio (user maintained)
Pod Fitness www.podfitness.com	Custom audio workouts based on user's fitness level, goals, and equipment. Uses mixes of user's music and instruction provided by fitness experts and celebrities	$59.85 per quarter (13 weeks) Must have mp3 player	None	Tracks the programs you have used	No	Download and install program, basic mp3 technology	Self-report of fitness level	Compatible with Microsoft Health Vault
President's Challenge www.presidents challenge.org	Provides different exercise programs for different ages and activity levels Sets realistic fitness goals and provides ideas to get active	No cost	Allows you to calculate your BMI (not automatic)	No graphical interface; can review progress through activity log	Can join/create groups with family and friends	Basic Internet skills	Yes	No

(continues)

Table 4.4 Tracking Health and Fitness with Technology: Features and Parameters (*continued*)

Company/ Website	Features	Cost	Physiological Parameters	Graphs/ Tables	Social Networking	Computer Skill Level	Self- Report	PHR
Online Fitness Log www. online fitnesslog.com	Tracks nutrition and exercise information Customizable for user's diet and exercise regimen	No cost	Calculates calories consumed/ expended Calculates basal metabolic rate	Tracks information that user enters and tracks changes Sorts graphs based on multiple fields	Online community forum	Basic Internet skills	Yes	No
Wii Fit www.nintendo. com/wiifit	Control on-screen avatar with movement on balance board with 40+ activities (strength training, yoga, aerobics, balance games)	Wii balance board: $89.99 Wii console: $249.99	Calculates BMI (automati- cally weighs you)	Tracks your "Wii Fit Age" and BMI over time	Can create profiles for up to eight users, allowing for competition	Basic skills to install and use game console	The game weighs the user and tracks usage; may also self- report other fitness activities	No

Trimble GPS Pack www.trimbleoutdoors.com/GPSpack.aspx	For use with compatible cell phone Fitness training and tracking, geocaching application, outdoor trip planning and navigation	$6.99 per month, plus cost of compatible GPS-enabled cell phone and service plan	Calculates calories burned	Tracks your route, records distance, time, pace, calories burned, allows you to view recent sessions and weekly log from handset and Internet	Can share workouts with others via the Internet	Cell phone application, basic Internet skills	System records user's information	No

My Health eVet is a portal provided by the Veterans Health Administration (n.d.). According to the MyHealth eVet Virtual Tour transcript, there are multiple features. The personal health record has a section for tracking health statistics that provides graphs, stores personal information for registration and emergency contacts, and a section with information about providers and care locations (Get Care). Get Care records the individual's care providers, treatment facilities, and health insurance information and supplies a means of communicating with providers. There is a prescription refill section and a place labeled Research Health that provides information about common conditions and VA health programs. A social information site focuses on the veteran community with news and events and information on volunteeering. This personal health portal was recently linked to the EHR of the Veterans Health Administration services (ihealthbeat, 2007).

Commercial Applications Internal to Agency or System

MyChart from Epic Systems Corporation has the potential for building widespread application as many medical centers use this company's EHRs. They can include the PHR function if they choose (Epic Systems Corporation, 2009). This is an example of a PHR system provided by a healthcare agency or group where the consumer has a prior relationship. Consumers may trust these applications more as they are internal to their chosen healthcare providers. However, it is not clear to what extent the applications feature the interoperability required to interface with other healthcare providers and Internet-available gadgets and features.

Kaiser Permanente's *Myhealthmanager* is a very successful model. It is directly linked to Kaiser Permanente's HealthConnect, an electronic health record used by all of the interdisciplinary provider teams, labs, and pharmacy. In this model, consumers view the same clinical record their healthcare provider sees. In addition, interactive tools encourage communication (Kaiser Permanente, n.d.). The goal is to create a central resource for consumers. It is not clear how consumers would add variables and measures of interest to them. See Microsoft partnership below.

Commercial: External and Third-Party Platforms

Microsoft, Google, and IBM

Comprehensive personal health records will be an attractive entrepreneurial offering now that the government has mandated electronic health records by 2015.

Among the groups making entries in this area are Microsoft, Google, and IBM. Microsoft posts generic ads on its site; Google has stated they will not post any ads. No information was available from IBM at the time of this writing.

Microsoft and Google Partnerships

Two major healthcare leaders have bought into the information repositories offered by external groups. The New York-Presbyterian Hospital has decided to work with Microsoft's HealthVault in a patient-controlled database, and Cleveland Clinics is working with Google Health (Lohr, 2008). These changes are transformative and offer business opportunities for groups new to health, and cost and efficiency savings for employers (Mandl & Kohane, 2008). For example, Microsoft's HealthVault allows consumers to consolidate and store health records from multiple sources to be shared with healthcare providers of their choosing (Microsoft, 2009). This program directly competes with Google Health and Indivo.

Kaiser presently offers a personal health record with a smooth flow of information from laboratory, X-ray, and other departments directly to an online access point. Anecdotally, the transfer is quite prompt, the files provide access to a glossary to explain terms, and normal values are provided. The ability of the patient to add material has been limited. This electronic record has been predominantly a consumer "window" into his or her own health data. In 2008, the Kaiser healthcare system experts decided to pilot partnering with Microsoft to test the potential for the system. Employees will be allowed to use HealthVault in the Northern California Kaiser system. If this is successful with employees, and the partnership is cost-effective, it will be opened up for patients (Neupert & Silvestre, 2008).

Focused-Specialty PHR Applications

Some digital information resources, such as those funded by Project HealthDesign's initial focus on urgent needs such as hypertension or diabetes management, have a high likelihood of motivating both consumer and health professionals to participate. Successful users of these products may be more willing to engage later in a more comprehensive personal health record system and to request that all of their healthcare providers subscribe. Project HealthDesign programs and the websites of family and friends are examples of narrowly focused personal health records for specific, limited purposes.

Project HealthDesign is an initiative funded by the Robert Wood Johnson Foundation. Its goal is to "create the next generation of personal health records

(PHRs) and PHR systems" (Project HealthDesign, 2007, p. 1). The projects are characterized by attention to the details of daily living as a way to facilitate health-related decisions and empower patients (Brennan & Downs, 2009). Nine interdisciplinary teams were funded, and they have developed the following projects (Brennan & Downs, 2009):

- A customized care plan for breast cancer patients: The University of California, San Francisco, Center of Excellence for Breast Cancer Care intends to help breast cancer patients better understand and proactively coordinate their care. This is predominantly a calendaring program that merges doctor's appointments, diagnostic tests, and treatment projections with patients' personal calendars.
- Personal health management assistant: A University of Rochester team is building a conversational interface using speech and text to check up daily with patients with heart disease. Information is collected and a personalized treatment plan is generated from computer interpretations of the data shared. A focus on observations of daily living provides longitudinal data to supplement guideline-based care.
- Personal health application for diabetes self-management: TRUE Research Foundation and the Diabetes Institute at Walter Reed Army Medical Center is the design team. Their program will collect data on nutrition and diet, daily activity, prescribed medication, continuous blood glucose data, and self-reported emotional states. The PHR will analyze, summarize, display, and make recommendations based on observations specific to daily living—data provided by the patient. Linking with Google gadgets is a unique feature that extends its usefulness.
- Chronic disease medication management between office visits: Creating an interface for a mobile phone so that adult diabetics can share data with their healthcare provider anytime, anywhere, is the goal for the Group Health Care Cooperative at the University of Washington. Blood glucose, blood pressure, food intake, and exercise levels will be uploaded wirelessly. Providers will synchronize data with the agency's electronic record and provide feedback and counsel as needed.
- My-Medi-Health: A vision for a child-focused, personal medication management system. This application from Vanderbilt University Medical Center has a child-centered reminder system for children with cystic fibrosis. The goal is to track at home and school whether medication doses were taken and to manage refills in an application with age-appropriate "skins."
- Supporting patient and provider management of chronic pain with PDA applications linked to personal health records: Throughout the day this PHR collects pain and activity data in an interactive diary format on a

handheld device. Providers and patients will use a menu to choose their preferred analysis and display modes.

- ActivHealth: A PHR system for at-risk sedentary adults. This is a networking Web-portal application developed by Research Triangle Institute International and the Cooper Institute that will use observations of daily activities to generate a customized plan to change daily routines. Biosensors will be used to validate self-reporting.
- Living profiles: Transmedia personal health record systems for young adults. This application from the Art Center College of Design in Pasadena, California, is designed to facilitate the transition from the pediatric to the adult care system for adolescents with a chronic illness. Strategies to improve communication and taking responsibility for health include texting, graphics, and music. Data will include observations of daily living, mood, medication reminders, and calendaring to build knowledge of the relationship between behavior and health.
- Assisting older adults with transitions of care: The team at the University of Colorado at Denver and Health Sciences Center is developing a portable touch-screen computer to simplify medication management by using ambient computing (bar codes) to assist with scheduling prescriptions, ordering refills, preparing for visits, and more. Reminders and alerts will be included. In addition, medications will be linked to Medline Plus to ensure availability of information on the purpose, side effects, interactions, and other aspects of medication and its self-management.

A review of these applications highlights the underlying model of opportunity-based interaction with the healthcare provider or parent/caretaker. The Google, Microsoft, and Indivo applications, on the other hand, in their first iterations were predominantly consumer tools. New links create potential for interaction with healthcare professionals. It remains to be seen how Kaiser and Cleveland Clinics adapt their pilot affiliations with these two mega offerings. The Kaiser MyHealthManager application specifically promotes provider–client communication. However, there does not seem to be a feature for consumer-initiated observations.

Low-Risk Family-Oriented Health Information Sites

A partner or an alternate version of a PHR would be a site that is designed to post information simply for friends and family. This would be especially useful in the perioperative period, or as a pregnancy comes to term. This sharing website could also be helpful in the case of an extended illness characterized by peaks and valleys—remissions and relapses. The idea is that one does not have to repeat basic information and incidents over and over for each concerned relative or friend. Retelling the details and stories can be exhausting to the family member who is expected to provide updates. Also, by limiting data and information to transitions in health status on a restricted website, risks of breaching privacy are contained.

CaringBridge offers websites for patients and families experiencing a healthcare crisis, and has hosted nearly 86,000 individual users (CaringBridge, 2009). Another resource that provides free patient websites, blogs, and community is CarePages (CarePages, 2009). These two sites have endorsements from external reviewers. They have received more than 542 million visits, and those visitors have written over 13 million guest book entries of support and encouragement (Charities Review Council, 2007).

Some healthcare organizations, such as ProHealth, actively encourage families to use CaringBridge. The ProHealth Web page summarizes that Caring-Bridge is free and secure and an important way to "stay connected with friends and loved ones during challenging health times....CaringBridge is the oldest, most widely used online resource to support families when someone is receiving care or facing other health challenges" (ProHealth Care, 2009, para. 1–3). This service is supported by sponsor fees from hospitals and from user donations. A search for *Caring Bridge* turned up appeals in memory of a loved one. CarePages provides a similar service that is supported by advertisements and hospitals that pay fees to post a link on the hospital website.

Stand-Alone Applications

Pocket MD has recently been advocated by Crystal Cruises. The cruise line recommends purchasing the service from mypocketmd.com/crystal. This record system service contacts designated physicians to get all of the information consumers authorize. Data is loaded onto a credit card-sized memory chip. Consumers are given a choice of two plans, which allow only two physicians and limited updates. Customers of Crystal Cruises pay more and get unlimited physicians and updates for 1 year. The company allows password protection but points out that this would defeat its major benefit in case of an emergency away from home. This creates risks if the memory chip is lost. If this application succeeds commercially, other variations are sure to follow.

Everyday Experience with PHRs

The primary question with respect to PHRs is the ease with which prospective users can access the record, find desired information, and post desired information. If the interface is too complicated, features fail to engage the user; if the interface proves unstable, all other issues fade in importance. PHRs vary from all previous health records in that the user can use observations of his or her own daily life to live healthier (Brennan, as cited in Project HealthDesign, n.d.).

Being able to use a PHR effectively calls for literacy that goes beyond basic skills for health information and Internet use. Core PHR tasks identified by Baur and Kanaan (2006) are:

- Navigating websites and other applications
- Seeking out information
- Entering data
- Comparing two or more pieces of information
- Reading charts and graphs
- Writing messages
- Analyzing reports
- Reading textual information

In addition, the consumer is called on to

- Synthesize information comparisons with personal goals to set priorities.
- Adapt recommendations for health actions to personal situation and data.
- Observe and record actions and outcomes using questions provided or self-designed.

Marketing

With respect to older adults, targeted marketing will be important so that prospective users are willing to try out the PHR. For some users, endorsement by their own healthcare provider will be pivotal. For others, the availability of around-the-clock technical assistance will be very attractive to reluctant users. Individuals with chronic illnesses or multiple acute problems involving multiple health providers may seek out this resource in hopes of improved management of their care. In general, principles of ubiquitous computing and universal design are likely to be compelling approaches. Setting out to design a system intended only for older adults is unlikely to become successful. The boomer/zoomer generation is sensitive to any approach that seems patronizing (Harwood, 2007).

The PHR can be a central resource in empowering patients if it is seen as part of the socioecological framework (see Figure 4.1). A key implication is that information within the record needs to be specifically referenced in patient–provider visits and in the interim linked to feedback between patient and provider. Records must also provide information that increases the ease of managing healthy lifestyle changes and chronic conditions. Individuals who desire better access to information for healthcare decision-making need substantive coaching until using the PHR becomes routine. Similarly, health professionals will need coaching on how to integrate the PHR reports into conversations with patients. A key strategy is to signal the importance of the *data* entry and resulting *information* as an *influence* on professional recommendations at the point of *transitions*. Healthcare professionals can give weight to the *knowledge* available through the PHR by coaching patients to make use of the graphs and links. New assessment tools that inventory available and potential sources of capital will increase the impact of the PHR on care decisions, attitudes, and willingness to acquire new skills. The healthcare professional can reinforce the power of considering the entire *health habitat* as context for health: the range of work, play, and daily living settings and roles and variations of *capital* and potential influences in each. These variations form the frame for patient and family selection of variables personal to their situation to be constructed in the PHR.

Relevant steps in terms of the everyday experience are detailed in Table 4.5.

Table 4.5   Everyday Experience Notes: Phases* of Consumer Engagement with PHR

Phase I: Getting started: Making choices, setting priorities
- Choosing a purpose for engaging with a PHR
  - Monitoring key vital signs and lab reports
  - Observing trends for vital signs and lab values (e.g., graph)
  - Documenting personal observations (Downs, 2006)
  - Providing emergency data while traveling
  - Coordinating multiple providers and agencies
  - Sharing information around a health incident or hospitalization with family and friends
  - Facilitating coordination when multiple family and friends provide support
  - Medication and appointment reminders
  - Insurance claims, reimbursement tracking
  - Appointment setting
  - E-mail provider
  - Measure vital signs, pressure sores, etc. with peripherals
- Assessing preferences for platform
  - Wallet-sized CD
  - Flash drive
  - Web-based stand-alone
  - Combination of device storage and Web access

Table 4.5   Everyday Experience Notes: Phases* of Consumer Engagement with PHR (*continued*)

- Querying interoperability—sharing capacity across health contacts
  - Laboratories, clinics, EHR, pharmacy compatibility
  - Personal observation upload capability
- Assessing risk comfort
  - Employer provided
  - Third party (e.g., Microsoft, Google, IBM, Dossia, Indivo)
  - Healthcare agency provided or linked
  - Self-contained storage device from personal computer
  - Consequences of allowing others "custodial" status, decision-making role
  - Insurance linked
  - Ability to block specific types or items of information by provider or shared user (family, etc.)
- Examining skill level required and training available
- Reviewing presentation style
  - Google menu, Microsoft buffet
- Choosing method of populating record
  - Third party obtains records and enters
  - EHR flow from healthcare agency with option for personal categories and entries
  - Totally self-entered data
  - EHR from agency only

Phase II: Deciding on system, application, and signing up

Phase III: Testing the system
- Online models
- Fill-in capability: You start typing, system completes word
- Viewing data from external sources
- Sending and receiving messages
- Adding read-only for trusted confidant who comments on data available

Phase IV: Reinforcing adherence to provider recommendations, regimens, personal goals
- Integration with primary care provider visits
- Moderator monitored: VHA, cardiac rehabilitation
- Social networking: Within family, across health goals or disease groups
- Signaling diversions from normal or set goals, missing data queries

Phase V: Collaborating
- Persuading others to try system for their records
- Enrolling caregivers, family members as partners in your health goals

(*continues*)

Table 4.5   Everyday Experience Notes: Phases* of Consumer Engagement with PHR (*continued*)

> - Joining linked support groups
> - Adding gadgets that extend usefulness
> - Adding new categories of information to own record
> - Blogging on problems, suggestions, work-arounds
> - Joining interest group relevant to the PHR system itself

*Labels for phases adapted from Rogers, 1995.

Intense effort is required to persuade naïve clinicians and consumers of the value of the PHR. Equally intense training for integrating the record into routine health care and daily life will be required.

Ease of Use

For older adults, perceived ease of use will vary widely depending on the preexisting Internet-related skills of the individual. For those who have used interactive applications with success for other purposes, there may be greater willingness to try several PHR applications and make a choice based on personal preferences. One trade-off for designers will be richness of features versus simplicity of use. The approach taken by Microsoft HealthVault and Google Health is to offer a basic product with optional add-ons. The gamble is whether the basic product offers features seen as essential by the individual consumer and their health professional. Researchers at the University of Rochester are developing a voice-activated application using natural language to conduct a daily checkup for heart disease patients (Project HealthDesign, n.d.).

Defining ease of use may vary with the experience and preferences of the user and his or her coach or caretaker. Google Health is a menu-driven setup that eases the user into the many options. The screen presentation is simple with a lot of white space. Microsoft HealthVault, on the other hand, uses more of a buffet presentation. Multiple options are laid out as soon as you open the page. For some older adults, this will be confusing as the product labels may be unfamiliar, and the names are not necessarily intuitive. To be competitive, each PHR provider will be scanning the market and seeking feedback to update their interface and features. Coaching older adults to engage in social media to provide information on their experience will expedite the process. In this consumer-empowered era, it is difficult to underestimate the power of online sharing of experiences linked to brand names.

OUTCOMES

There are relatively few reports of results for EMRs or PHRs. The detailed review of EHRs by Häyrinen, Saranato, and Nykänen (2008) found that the role of patient-entered data in the EHR has not been taken into account. Ball et al. (2008) writing from the IBM Center for Healthcare Management observe that the PHR is dependent on the EMR. They observed that PHRs create new challenges for consumers by demanding new roles and relationships. They observe that the new tools change the clinician's workflow and thought flow. As we gain more information about consumer participation, outcome studies should be monitoring for changes in patient thought flow and workflow in their self-care activities.

One outcome study is the PHIMS[1] installation in a low-income public housing site that has a predominantly older and disabled population (Kim et al., 2005, 2009). Although age distributions were provided, there was neither assessment of cognitive or physical disability in the user population nor of educational level or previous computer experience. Access was through an Internet connection in a group computer room with graduate nursing assistance one morning a week. The project was successful in getting 24 out of 180 residents to participate over a 4-month period. Information update events were recorded, primarily on the day assistance was available or the following day. Satisfaction surveys were uniformly positive with all but one respondent able to enter data without the graduate assistant. Participants were convinced that the personal health record would improve their health status and relationships with medical personnel. Those who brought printouts to medical encounters had positive experiences. The availability of free access and onsite, in-person technical support overcame the digital divide for some residents. However, sustained participation was low (Kim et al., 2009).

An application for patients with heart failure provided online Web access to records, an educational guide, and a messaging system (Ross, Moore, Earnest, Wittevrongel, & Lin, 2004). The randomized controlled trial intervention lasted for 12 months. The group using the Web-based record was superior in their general adherence to recommendations and were more satisfied with

---

[1]The Personal Health Information Management System (PHIMS) was developed at the University of Washington.

patient–doctor communication. A key finding was that this information-centered application resulted in better informed patients but no difference in health status. The authors concluded that revisions were needed to make the information more relevant and more empowering.

Another small qualitative study in Norway by Wibe and Slaughter (2009) found that there were emotional consequences of granting access to records. These were especially negative when the patient found a discrepancy between clinician notes and his or her recollection of the encounter.

The World Health Organization recommendations draft states in section 3.21: "We know that informed patients have both better outcomes and use health services less" (Fisher, Fitton, & Bos, 2007, p. 312). This WHO document and the ICMCC website provide a detailed list of positive outcomes associated with the PHR and granting access to health records. These are aggregated in Table 4.6. Specific reference citations to support these conclusions are not given. As indicated earlier, documentation is difficult to find. The ICMCC and WHO authors

Table 4.6   Positive Outcomes of PHRs for Consumers

- Shared decision making is increased
- Trust is enhanced when record matches or enhances patient recollection
- Practical advice is available and retrievable by patients
- Outcomes have improved for cardiac patients
- Patients feel empowered to make decisions about their health
- Consultations are more efficient with and on behalf of patient
- Health promotion behaviors are increased
- Confusion about instructions is minimized
- Care pathway changes are rapid
- Caregivers and advocates provide better support with shared access
- Shared data supports patients with mental health issues in participation
- Incorporation of alternative treatments and over-the-counter drugs is improved
- Information seeking by patients is enhanced with well-chosen links
- Unnecessary appointments are minimized
- Test results are reused and not redone for missing paper slips
- Record accuracy is improved as patients monitor information errors
- Care fragmentation is minimized as patients monitor coordination
- Sensor use may increase as results are linked to record and decisions
- Portability is independent of geography

Source: Adapted from ICMCC, n.d., and Fisher, Fitton, & Bos, 2007.

have access to a wide variety of sources that, when aggregated, may account for their confident summary. Certainly, the literature on eHealth implies these benefits will accrue with full implementation of linked EHRs and PHRs.

Meaningful Use as Outcome

Although meaningful use was to be a definitive criterion for electronic medical records, little progress has been made (for updates see http://meaningfuluse. org). Brennan made the case, in testimony to Congress (*Incorporating patient-generated data*, 2010), that the peersonal health record is a critical component of meaningful electronic records. She stated that meaningful use standards should include:

1. "Health information technologies and policies that enable information selected and gathered by patients to be integrated into clinical care.
2. Health information that is accessible to patients in a computable form.
3. Health information for patients must be actionable." (*Incorporating patient-generated data*, 2010, pp. 3–4)

It is critical that both consumer advocacy groups and health professionals participate in the dialogue about meaningful use. Those with special interest in the topic will want to confer with their congressional representatives and be systematic about following the discussion.

SUMMARY

There is worldwide interest in the adoption of personal health records linked to electronic health records created by providers and their administrative agencies. The potential of these records is sufficient to attract major players outside the healthcare system such as Google, IBM, and Microsoft. Controversies exist as to what extent the client will actually control the record. Control refers to the ability to grant and withhold access to information, to amend the record including adding measures personally selected by the consumer. In particular, the client would be able to create entry categories to track daily life observations that can provide context for clinical data.

These daily observations are expected to be very useful in empowering clients undertaking lifestyle change or attempting to manage chronic illnesses. Unfortunately, there is very little data on the impact of using these records.

Agencies offering the personal health record have not had an overwhelming response. Studies with multiple stakeholders using or planning PHR implementation vary in the conclusions to be drawn. One focus group study (Weitzman et al., 2009) found that benefits outweighed barriers. However, another focus group with older adults and their care providers led to the conclusion that barriers outweighed benefits (Daly et al., 2008).

However, acceptance and outcomes are as yet unclear given the limited implementation of personal health records. What is needed is consumer and provider experience in a socioecological approach that takes into account the wide range of environmental variables that affect health behaviors and health services. The combinations now emerging with feedback loops occuring with personal health care records linked to electronic health records may create a dramatic shift in both acceptability and implementation.

The construct of a health habitat is proposed to structure a record that has a socioecological, culturally competent foundation. Offering a personal health record where everyone and everything is connected may be the key to the extravagant expectations of consumers for improved adherence, better outcomes, and cost savings.

REFERENCES

American Health Information Management Association. (n.d.). *HIPAA myths and facts.* Retrieved on November 8, 2009, from http://www.ahima.org/pdf_files/HIPS_Mythsfootnotes.pdf

American Health Information Management Association & American Medical Informatics Association. (2007). The value of personal health records: A joint position statement for consumers of healthcare by the American Health Information Management Association and the American Medical Informatics Association. *Journal of AHIMA, 78*(4), 22.

American Health Information Management Association e-HIM Personal Health Record Work Group. (2005). The role of the personal health record in the EHR. *Journal of American Health Information Management Association, 76*(7), 64A–64B-D.

American Recovery and Reinvestment Act of 2009. H.R. 1. 111th Cong. § 3001 (2009).

Associated Press. (2008). *UCLA fires workers for snooping in Spears files.* Retrieved June 6, 2008, from http://www.msnbc.msn.com/id/23640143

Ball, M. J., Costin, M. Y., & Lehmann, C. (2008). The personal health record: Consumers banking on their health. *Studies in Health Technology & Informatics, 134,* 35–46.

Baur, C., & Kanaan, S. B. (2006). *Expanding the reach and impact of consumer e-health tools: Executive summary, a vision of e-health benefits for all* (Electronic No. 2006). Retrieved June 16, 2010, from http://www.health.gov/communication/ehealth/ehealthTools/summary.htm

Beth Israel Deaconess Medical Center. (2009). *Privacy statement.* Retrieved November 6, 2009, from http://www.bidmc.org/PrivacyStatement.aspx

Brennan, P. (2006). *Re: PHRs: They're hot, they're sexy, but what are they exactly?* [weblog comment]. Retrieved June 16, 2010, from http://rwjfblogs.typepad.com/pioneer/2006/12/phrs_theyre_hot.html

Brennan, P. F., Casper, G., Downs, S., & Aulahk, V. (2009). Project HealthDesign: Enhancing action through information. *Studies in Health Technology & Informatics, 146*, 214–218.

Brennan, P. F., & Downs, S. J. (2009). Project Health Redesign. Rethinking the power and potential of personal health records. *Round one final report*. Retrieved November 7, 2009, from http://www.projecthealthdesign.org/media/file/Round%20One%20PHD%20Final%20Report6.17.09.pdf

CarePages. (2009). Retrieved on November 9, 2009, from http://www.carepages.com

CaringBridge. (2009). Retrieved on November 9, 2009, from http://www.caringbridge.org

Charities Review Council. (2007). *Review: CaringBridge*. Retrieved June 16, 2008, from http://www.smartgivers.org/SmartGiversReview/421529394.html?view=2

Children's Hospital Informatics Program. (n.d.). *Indivo: The personally controlled health record.* Retrieved November 7, 2009, from http://indivohealth.org

Daly, J., Doucette, W., Eichmann, D., Farris, K., Gryzlak, B., Hourcade, J. P., et al. (2008). PHRs for medication use: Views from elders and their physicians. Paper presented at the AHRQ annual meeting. Retrieved November 9, 2009, from *ahrq.hhs.gov/about/annualmtg08/090908slides/Chrischilles.ppt*

Deloitte. (2008). *The medical home: Disruptive innovation for a new primary care model.* Washington, DC: Author.

Dombrowski, M. P., Tomlinson, M. W., Bottoms, S. F., Johnson, M. P., & Sokol, R. J. (1995). Computer-generated admission forms have greater accuracy. *American Journal of Obstetrics and Gynecology, 173*(3, Part 1), 847–848.

Downs, S. (2006, December 14). *PHRs: They're hot, they're seky, but what are they exactly?* Robert Wood Johnson Foundation. Retrieved June 16, 2010, from http://www.rwjfblogs.typepad.com/pioneer/2006/12/phrs_theyre_hot.html

Dyer, O. (2003). Drug company and pharmacy send unsolicited samples of Prozac to Florida residents. *British Medical Journal, 327*(7421), 950a.

Epic Systems Corporation. (2009). Personal health records (PHRs) and portals. Retrieved November 7, 2009, from http://www.epic.com/software-phr.php

Fisher, B., Fitton, R., & Bos, L. (2007). WHO recommendation on record access (draft). *Studies in Health Technology & Informatics, 127*, 311–315.

Fisher, B., Fitton, R., Poirier, C., & Stables, D. (2007). Patient record access: The time has come! *British Journal of General Practice, 57*(539), 507–511.

ha.ckers.org. (2008). *Google health*. Retrieved June 6, 2008, from http://ha.ckers.org/blog/20080521/google-health

Hahn, J. A., Kushel, M. B., Bangsberg, D. R., Riley, E., & Moss, A. R. (2006). Brief report: The aging of the homeless population: Fourteen-year trends in San Francisco. *Journal of General Internal Medicine, 21*(7), 775–778.

Halamka, J. D., Mandl, K. D., & Tang, P. C. (2008). Early experiences with personal health records. *Journal of the American Medical Informatics Association, 15*(1), 1–7.

Hamilton, D. (2008). *Google health privacy: All talk, no teeth?* Retrieved June 6, 2008, from http://industry.bnet.com/healthcare/2008/05/22/google-health-privacy-all-talk-no-teeth

Harwood, J. (2007). *Understanding communication and aging: Developing knowledge and awareness.* Thousand Oaks, CA: Sage.

Häyrinen, K., Saranto, K., & Nykänen, P. (2008). Definition, structure, content, use and impacts of electronic health records: A review of the research literature. *International Journal of Medical Informatics, 77*(5), 291–304.

Health Information Technology: For the Future of Health and Care. (n.d.). US Department of Health and Human Services. Retrieved August 5, 2010, from http://healthit.hhs.gov/portal/server.pt

IBM. (2008). *IBM opens new 3D virtual healthcare island on second life.* Retrieved October 17, 2008, from http://www-03.ibm.com/press/us/en/pressrelease/23580.wss

Ihealthbeat (2007). VA adds HER data to veterans PHR. Retrieved June 16, 2010, from http://www.ihealthbeat.org/Articles/2007/1/25/VA-Adds-EHR-Data-to-Veterans-PHRs.aspx?topic=ehrs%20and%20phrs

Incorporating patient-generated data in meaningful use of HIT. Hearing before the HIT Policy Committee, Meaningful Use Workgroup. (2010, April 10). (Testimony of Patricia Flatley Brennan). Retrieved June 30, 2010, from http://www.rwjf.org/files/research/phdtestimonyapril2010.pdf

Indivo. (n.d.). Retrieved June 16, 2010, from http://www.indivohealth.org

International Council on Medical and Care Compunetics. (n.d.). ICMCC record access. Retrieved June 16, 2010, from http://recordaccess.icmcc.org

Jordan-Marsh, M. (2008). Health habitat aspects of software as a service (SAAS/WEB2.0) reinforcing diabetic self-confidence: The PHRddBRASIL case. *DESAFIO International Symposium: Diabetes, Health Education and Guided Physical Activities,* 39–42.

Kaiser Permanente. (n.d.). *My health manager.* Retrieved November 7, 2009, from http://info.kp.org/richmedia/experience/index.htm

Kim, E., Mayani, A., Modi, S., Kim, Y., & Soh, C. (2005). Evaluation of patient-centered electronic health record to overcome digital divide. *Conference Procedings IEEE Engineering in Biology and Medicine Society, 2,* 1091–1094.

Kim, E., Stolyar, A., Lober, W. B., Herbaugh, A. L., Shinstrom, S. E., Zierler, B., et al. (2009). Challenges to using an electronic personal health record by a low-income elderly population. *Journal of Medical Internet Research, 11*(4), e 44.

Lohr, S. (2008). *Google offers personal health records on the Web.* Retrieved June 9, 2008, from http://www.nytimes.com/2008/05/20/technology/20google.html?_r=3&scp=2&sq&oref=slogin&oref=slogin

Mandl, K. D., & Kohane, I. S. (2008). Tectonic shifts in the health information economy. *New England Journal of Medicine, 358*(16), 1732–1737.

Mandl, K. D., Simons, W. W., Crawford, W. C., & Abbett, J. M. (2007). Indivo: A personally controlled health record. *BMC Medical Informatics and Decision Making, 7,* 25.

Manos, D. (2008, April 21). Vendors, stakeholders aim to dispel privacy myths about EHRs. *Healthcare IT News.* Retrieved July 1, 2008, from http://www.healthcareitnews.com/news/vendors_stakeholders_aim_dispel_privacy_myths_about_ehrs

Microsoft. (2009). *Welcome to Microsoft HealthVault.* Retrieved on November 7, 2009, from http://www.healthvault.com/Industry/index.html

Morales Rodriguez, M., Casper, G., & Brennan, P. F. (2007). Patient-centered design. The potential of user-centered design in personal health records. *Journal of AHIMA, 78*(4), 44–46.

National Committee on Vital and Health Statistics. (2006). *Personal health records and personal health record systems.* Washington, DC: U.S. Department of Health and Human Services.

National Health Service. (2009). *HealthSpace.* Retrieved on November 9, 2009, from http://www.connectingforhealth.nhs.uk/systemsandservices/healthspace

Neupert, P. & Silvestre, A. (2008, June 9) News Conference Call—Microsoft HealthVault & Kaiser Permanente Pilot Program. Retrieved June 16, 2010, from http://www.microsoft.com/presspass/press/2008/jun08/06-09HealthVaultConCall.mspx

Peel, D. (2008) A plea for using smart consent tools. GHIT notebook. *Government Health IT*. Retrieved September 30, 2008, from http://www.govhealthit.com/blogs/ghitnotebook/350512-1.html

Perinatal Health Inc. (2007). *POPRAS III: Problem oriented perinatal risk assessment system*. Retrieved June 16, 2008, from http://www.popras.com/About%20PHI.htm

Personal health record. (2010, June 23). In *Wikipedia, the Free Encyclopedia*. Retrieved July 1, 2010, from http://en.wikipedia.org/w/index.php? title=Personal_health_record

ProHealth Care. (2009). *Stay connected with CaringBridge*. Retrieved November 7, 2009, from http://www.prohealthcare.org/services/RegionalCancerCenter/caringbridge.aspx

Project HealthDesign. (2007). *Designing PHRs for Living: Project challenges experts to create personal health records that people want and need in their daily lives*. Retrieved November 7, 2009, from http://www.rwjf.org/files/research/projecthealthdesign092007.pdf

Project HealthDesign. (n.d.). *E-Primer 3: Health in everyday living*. Retrieved October 25, 2009, from http://www.rwjf.org/files/research/phdprimer3.pdf

Robert Wood Johnson Foundation. (2009a). *Pioneer*. Retrieved November 7, 2009, from http://www.rwjf.org/pioneer/search.jsp?typeid=115

Robert Wood Johnson Foundation. (2009b). *The power of personal health records*. Retrieved November 7, 2009, from http://www.rwjf.org/pr/product.jsp?id=32412

Robert Wood Johnson Foundation. (2009c). Waste in US health care spending: Potentially avoidable complications, chronic condition care. Retrieved November 7, 2009, from http://www.rwjf.org/pr/product.jsp?id=47129

Robert Wood Johnson Foundation. (n.d.). *Health in everyday living. E-Primer 3: Project Health Design*. Retrieved October 25, 2009, from http://www.rwjf.org/files/research/phdprimer3.pdf

Robeznieks, A. (2007). Getting personal. Legal liability, patient-data overload among issues making physicians uneasy over emergence of personal health records. *Modern Healthcare, 37*(21), 40–42.

Ross, S. E., Moore, L., Earnest, M. A., Wittevrongel, L., & Lin, C. (2004). Providing a web-based online medical record with electronic communication capabilities to patients with congestive heart failure: Randomized trial. *Journal of Medical Internet Research, 6*(2), e12. Retrieved October 25, 2009, from http://www.jmir.org/2004/2/e12

Rubenstein, S. (2008). *Are your medical records at risk?* Retrieved June 6, 2008, from http://online.wsj.com/article/SB120941048217350433.html

Sarasohn-Kahn, J. (2009) Participatory health: Online and mobile tools help chronically ill manage their care. Sacramento, CA: California Healthcare Foundation. Retrieved October 30, 2009, from http://www.chcf.org/documents/chronicdisease/ParticipatoryHealthTools.pdf

Seidman, J. & Eytan, T. (2008). Helping patients plug in: Lessons in the adoption of online consumer tools. *California Health Foundation*. Retrieved July 1, 2008, from http://www.chcf.org/topics/view.cfm?itemid=133659

Slezak, L. (1982). Marketing forum: Pocket-size personal health record. *Journal of the American Medical Record Association, 53*(2), 44–46.

South Carolina Nurses Association. (2008). *Medicare to test an electronic personal health record (PHR) in South Carolina*. Retrieved June 6, 2008, from http://findarticles.com/p/articles/mi_qa4103/is_200806/ai_n25418937

Steinbrook, R. (2008). Personally controlled online health data—The next big thing in medical care? *New England Journal of Medicine, 358*(16), 1653–1656.

Tapscott, D., & Williams, A. (2006). *Wikinomics: How mass collaboration changes everything*. New York: Penguin Group.

U.S. Department of Health and Human Services. (n.d.). *Nationwide Health Information Network*. Retrieved October 12, 2009, from http://healthit.hhs.gov/portal/server.pt?open=512&objID=1142& parentname=CommunityPage&parentid=1&mode=2&in_hi_userid=10741&cached=true

U.S. Department of Health and Human Services Office for Civil Rights. (n.d.). *Your health information privacy rights*. Retrieved November 7, 2009, from http://www.hhs.gov/ocr/privacy/hipaa/ understanding/consumers/consumer_rights.pdf

University of Southern California. (2003). *Notice of privacy practice*. Retrieved June 6, 2008, from http://policies.usc.edu/hipaa/privacynoticeengl041403.pdf

Veterans Health Administration. (n.d.) My HealtheVet. Virtual tour transcript. Retrieved June 16, 2010, from http://www.myhealth.va.gov/mhv-portal-web/ShowDoc/BEA%20Repository/multimedia/ MHVVirtualTour_transcript.pdf

Weitzman, E. R., Kaci, L., & Mandl, K. (2009). Acceptability of a personally controlled health record in a community-based setting: Implications for policy and design. *JMIR: Journal of Medical Internet Research, 11*(2), e14. Retrieved June 16, 2010, from http://www.jmir.org/2009/2/e14

Wibe, T., & Slaughter, L. (2009). Patients reading their health records—What emotional factors are involved? *Studies in Health Technology and Informatics, 146*, 174–178.

Wolter, J. (2007). Working smart: In confidence. Health record banking: An emerging PHR model. *Journal of AHIMA, 78*(9), 82–83.

CHAPTER 5

Devices as Adjunct to Being Healthy at Home

SHIFTING HEALTH PARADIGM

Devoting an entire chapter to devices is consistent with the paradigm shifts occurring in health care, and in particular, disease management. The new millennium in health care quickly led to consumers recognizing that "managed care means—you manage your care!" For most consumers this meant negotiating for appointments, desired treatments, medications, and services, and following instructions from experts. Only recently are payers, providers, and healthcare systems recognizing that engaging the consumer as an active partner is key to changing health status and managing costs (Dishman, 2007). This approach has three key changes: a shift in time frame, a shift in the "geography" of interactions between consumer and healthcare providers, and new capacities for tracking and monitoring health behaviors and clinical conditions. The opportunities for interaction are discussed in Chapter 7. The key aspects with relevance to appreciating devices is that a device can collect and transmit information 24/7 and can operate wherever the user is located. Patients and those interested in wellness no longer have to accommodate the weekday, daylight hours preferred by health professionals for appointments. Increasingly, health-related data collection that used to require a visit to a medical facility can be done remotely.

This chapter focuses on the devices or gadgets that support the interface for both telehealth (provider-driven delivery) and self-care eHealth (consumer-driven engagement). The extent of this shift is shown in reviewing the monograph *Expanding the Reach and Impact of Consumer e-Health Tools* (Baur & Kanaan, 2006). The report was compiled to define the state of the science and potential of practice. The extensive review of e-tools listed only two instances where Internet applications were linked to a device that collected biomedical data such as blood pressure or blood glucose. Applications were rapidly emerging, but they were poorly known and not widely studied in trials.

A major factor in this paradigm shift is the emergence of what is called Health 2.0 and the emergence of Health 3.0 (Ricciardi, 2009). In this digital revolution, Health 2.0 facilitated online health empowerment and collaboration for individuals. Now, Health 3.0 makes possible direct, automated connection between an individual's sensed physiology and his or her Health 2.0 tools and communities (David O'Reilly, as cited in Ricciardi, 2009). The connection is accomplished by means of various devices.

Another critical aspect of the paradigm shift is underway with respect to "assistive technology" or devices. In the past, a standard definition implied that "assistive devices" were a resource for people not able to function normally (Lauer, Rust, & Smith, 2006). For many people, much health-related technology was specific to being handicapped or old. Today, adults of all ages and conditions use devices to support mental and physical health and create a quality of life that minimizes stress and maximizes entertainment. For the purposes of this chapter, devices will be limited to those that enable digital interactions, data collection, signaling, or analysis.

Demand for and willingness to pay for devices is expected to escalate given the upcoming population explosion of older adults (Vanderheiden, 2007). Conditions are such that the desire to "age in place" has intensified as more than a personal preference but an economic imperative. Shifts in the economy and ever-increasing complications of air travel have made it more difficult for adult children to fly in and check on aging parents.

Trends Increasing Attractiveness of Digital Devices

In each case, new designs are emerging that will benefit not only those with disabilities of any source (age, injury, birth, chronic illness) but adults of any age with specific preferences for digital engagement as well. We can reasonably expect new attention to "universal design" and "ubiquitous computing," as described by Vanderheiden (2007). A variety of social and economic trends, melded with advances in science and technology, create a new and evolving context for considering the role of technology in health-related quality of life. Several trends are rapidly multiplying the urgency of having health professionals be knowledgeable in this area. First, there are new options for individuals across the life span related to specific advances in miniaturization and portability. Specific developments identified by Vanderheiden (2007) include agreement on international standards for remote controls and advances in natural language capacity. Increasingly, individuals can control appliances and sensors by speaking a simple request or command. As devices become more portable and less obtrusive, individuals are more willing and able to leave home knowing they are supported. Those who are new to the use of devices in clinical practice may still encounter peers who are reluctant to incorporate technology in their care plans. In some cases, the concern that accepting this technology will make the client housebound is a specific rationale. In other cases, confidentiality and privacy issues predominate.

It may be useful to refer to the Unified Theory of Acceptance and Use of Technology (UTAUT). Given the issues inherent in the discontinuance of device use, health and social welfare professionals can increase intention to use new devices and support required behaviors by applying the UTAUT. This model was an adaptation by Venkatesh, Morris, Davis, and Davis (2003) that expanded the original Technology Acceptance Model (TAM) developed by Davis in 1989; it has become well disseminated across a wide range of technological applications, as shown by thousands of results on searching Google Scholar for UTAUT.

Table 5.1 presents relevant consumer queries for each of the core components of the model.

Table 5.1   Unified Theory of Acceptance and Use of Technology: Consumer Queries

Dimension of Experience	Consumer Query
Performance expectancy	How much will this device help me do a task better or faster? How soon will I experience results?
Effort expectancy	How hard will it be to figure out how to use this device? Will the experience of using the device be easy and pleasant once I learn the basics?
Social influence	Are other people whose opinion I value using this device? Will people admire me for using this device? Will I have different relationships with people if I use this device?
Facilitating conditions	What kind of training and support is available if I use this device? Will those resources cost money? Are they easy to access 24/7? Will this device work with or replace other devices I am using now?
Mediating factors	Experience with similar devices, gender, age, voluntariness of use

Source: Adapted from Venkatesh et al., 2003.

The user-centered questions assist potential users of technology and related coaches in making decisions. Organizing queries in terms of the consumer needs provides a context to assure the wary that a particular technology will be selected on the basis of the situation, the characteristics of potential users, and the various sources of capital available to them. In a subsequent section of the chapter, these dimensions will be expanded in terms of the everyday experience of potential users of technology.

DIVERSE AUDIENCE FOR HEALTH TECHNOLOGY ASSISTIVE DEVICES

Older adults are not the only potential market for digital devices to support health. The National Center for Chronic Disease Prevention and Health Promotion (2009) at the Centers for Disease Control and Prevention (CDC) reported on chronic disease prevalence using available statistics for 2005. More than half of Americans lived with at least one chronic condition that year. This trend becomes more salient as we note that the CDC summarized 75% of the 2005 $2 trillion medical care costs as attributable to chronic disease. These statistics on specific conditions give a new perspective on spiraling healthcare costs (see Table 5.2).

Table 5.2   CDC Chronic Care Costs, 2005

Chronic Condition	Cost Estimate per Year
Pregnancy-related conditions: predelivery	$1 billion
Diabetes direct and indirect costs	$174 billion
Arthritis medical care and lost productivity	$128 billion
Smoking, direct and indirect costs	$19 billion
Cancer	$89 billion
Dental services	$98.6 billion
Heart disease and stroke	$448 billion (2008 projection)
Obesity	$117 billion (2000 data)

Source: Adapted from National Center for Chronic Disease Prevention and Health Promotion, 2009.

Dunbar-Jacob, an expert on lifestyle change and adherence to regimens, noted that in the United States, there is very little clinical support for the individual with a chronic disease (Dunbar-Jacob, Schlenk, & Caruthers, 2002). On average, she summarizes, individuals get only *1 hour* of health system contact spread out over *1 year*. Most chronic conditions, she reminded the audience, require complex self-care plans with multiple regimens related to nutrition, medication, physical activity, and monitoring of biomedical parameters such as blood pressure and blood glucose. Given the complexity of self-care for chronic illnesses, it is not surprising that few individuals have their disease under control. Devices that facilitate interaction between the patient, provider, and caregivers are expected to improve chronic care management and cut costs (Dishman, 2007).

Simultaneously, life spans are increasing around the globe, with individuals less likely to die of communicable diseases or traumatic injuries. Many military personnel are returning from combat with injuries that require new dependence on devices. The complex limb replacements and other bionic appliances are beyond the scope of this book; however, other consequences of combat injuries and post-traumatic stress syndrome mean that younger adults will be interested in a wide variety of devices formerly geared to older adults. Many individuals with disabilities, severe injuries, older adults, and their family "caresharers" place a high priority on community dwelling even during rehabilitation. Both recovering and aging "in place" then, are levers for accepting new technology for independence.

Equally important is appropriate interdependence. Families with complex demands for time and scheduling, individuals with complex chronic illnesses, individuals coping at home after surgery or with trauma-related early discharges all have needs for devices with digital capacity or adaptive capacity so that digital applications are accessible. "Young and old alike aspire to long lives full of warmth and meaning. The myth is that aging is mainly the concern of old people. The reality is that aging touches, changes, and influences everyone and everything" (Bill Thomas, as cited in Brown, 2008, para. 21).

Potential Contribution of Digital Devices

Digital health technology devices have the potential to sustain or increase participation in work, home, recreational, and community activities. Devices can decrease risks and improve safety at home or in other environments. Devices can enhance coping and adaptation to stressors in the environment, as well as stressors created by health-related goals and conditions. Technology devices can promote and sustain the social interaction and communication central to health and self-care; awareness of the potential of assistive devices is essential to any discussion of health technology.

Digital devices can also create new problems when cost limits choice, installation is complex, technical support is scarce, or when the device fails unexpectedly. Privacy issues are also important. These "darker" aspects of technology will be discussed separately. For this book, *digital* devices are the focus.

Digital devices can be as simple as a gadget* attached to a computer site, a PDA, or mobile phone, or as complex as the housewide systems often called "smart home" or "intelligent home" (in the UK and Europe) and wearable technology. These topics will be discussed in subsequent sections. Gadgets or widgets that are software applications linked to other programs to increase versatility were covered in Chapter 3.

Interplay of Health System Costs and Gaps in Resources

Frost and Sullivan (2006) describe a market rich with potential for expanded device distribution. They note there are cost-of-care increases taking place against a global imbalance between aging adults and the workforce participation needed to cover costs for health (Frost & Sullivan, 2006). They describe a dilemma in the developed nations of disconnections between hospital care availability and next-stage community resources. For example, increasing expectations (and costs) for intensive care are challenged by the shortage of intermediary care facilities. This gap slows discharges from acute care facilities; further, the imbalance does not take into account the global shortage of nurses and the lack of most healthcare professionals' readiness to care for older adults, "wounded warriors," and the growing population of adults with Alzheimer's disease.

Universal Design and Ubiquitous Computing

The issue of ubiquitous computing and universal design is paramount. This model assumes that features designed to support needs specific to particular disabilities may have value for everyone. It is a philosophy that calls for building in features with new applications and devices rather than modifying existing devices, buildings, and so on.

Embracing universal design calls for products that provide flexible interfaces able to meet multiple demands. The core idea is that individuals with disabilities, whether attributed to birth defects, injuries, or age, need not buy special products; products are adaptable to their needs. This approach has multiple

---

*Gadget here means a small electronic device, hardware, sometimes called a gizmo.

advantages. First, many adults are reluctant to embrace any device that singles them out as handicapped, disabled, or perhaps the most dreaded—old. Obtrusiveness or any overt signals of being "helped" are deadly to adoption. There is much discussion in the rehabilitation and health technology community that many devices prescribed to assist adults languish in closets, never adopted for routine use (Martin, Kelly, Kernohan, McCreight, & Nugent, 2008).

Universal design is built on the assumption that digital resources can benefit everyone—regardless of handicap or age. Ubiquitous computing means that access to digital resources is not tied to a physical location. Devices are mobile, and distance from home base is no longer an automatic limitation.

Vanderheiden (2007) summarizes advances that make new expectations possible. He highlights changes in microphone/earpiece capacity such that background noise is filtered; portability and miniaturization that makes discretion possible—even to blending devices into clothing; and chips that permit speech recognition and digitization in very inexpensive applications. Bluetooth and phase array microphones have brought hands-free capacity that both healthy teens and arthritics have adopted with pleasure. In Vanderheiden's lab, progress is being made in using the power of thought to move a cursor on a computer screen to select letters, words, and actions. This is another application with universal computing appeal. It would be ideal for quadriplegics and a boon to the busy mother monitoring dinner preparations and a clutch of lively children.

As we become immersed in the new millennium, the economy and the promise of technology that is the "can't do without" of the younger generations suggest that assistive technology may become mainstream. Examples of this approach are the "curb cuts" in sidewalks that were installed for people in wheelchairs but are used—without thinking—by teens on skateboards, mothers with strollers, and delivery agents with carts.

Indeed, leading experts on smart homes (Davidoff, Lee, Zimmerman, & Dey, 2006) make the case that a busy young family with multiple obligations may thrive best in a digitally connected, intelligent home. A smart home has alarms, sensors, and interactive programs that create the "intelligent" network. These interconnected features can benefit all consumers if they are tied to surveillance resources.

Usability: Human Rights Aspects

Fostering a philosophy that health technology designs begin with the expectation of universal appeal calls for early engagement of users. This approach will increase the usability and thus adoption of new devices. Usability is a technical criterion for evaluating new devices that will be discussed in the "Everyday Experience of Digital Devices" section of this chapter. However, it is also "An ideology: the belief in a certain specialized type of human rights" (Nielson, 2005, Usability as Ideology section, para. 1):

- The right of people to be superior to technology—If there's a conflict between technology and people, then technology must change.
- The right of empowerment—Users should understand what's happening and be capable of controlling the outcome.
- The right to simplicity—Users should get their way with computers without excessive hassle.
- The right of people to have their time respected—Awkward user interfaces waste valuable time.

Stakeholders

Understanding core issues in device use requires attention to five stakeholder groups: (1) device users, (2) significant others (family, friends, caregivers), (3) health and welfare agency representatives, (4) payer groups and investors, and (5) device and software designers. Each of these groups can influence the assessment of need for, acquisition of, adaptation to, and sustainability of digital devices. The value of a device may vary with the stakeholder as well. The human rights specified above should apply equally, if differentially, to the different stakeholder groups. Dialogue among these groups may advance health technology implementation. Engaging each group early in the process, especially users, can avoid costly delays and "re-dos" (Morales Rodriguez, Casper, & Brennan, 2007).

User Issues

These are dealt with in depth in the "Everyday Experience" section of the chapter. It is critical that there is collaboration among the stakeholder groups, with the user at the center. One issue with individuals who feel an imbalance of power is the phenomenon of preference uptake versus preference suppression. In particular, with older adults or those with significant disability or emotional fatigue, it is easy for other stakeholders to ignore the wishes and preferences of the user. The convenience of the social network members or significant others may take precedence. Alternatively, agency representatives, including the health professional, may go with what is expedient or familiar. Many features of devices can be assessed for availability of choices that are acceptable to the primary user.

For example, the ability to tailor the device interaction to personal preferences and needs is key. Ideal adjustments include the ability to choose for displays a large or small font, and background and foreground color adjustments. Other useful options are control of the pace of information (all available at once or a small amount at a time), and auditory, visual, or tactile interaction (Braille display device, touch screens). The software could include a feature advising users of device flexibility and providing hints as to why a choice might be helpful to the viewer. This coaching is important as most sites do not provide this ability to tailor their display. As devices become more widely used, color, footprint (space required), and other design choices will become selling points. Consumers need assistance to appreciate the potential value of such choices and the steps to take to accommodate their preferences. An online experience in learning about alternative devices is provided at SNOW Chat and Learn (2008). Demand for options will spur development of choices. Conversations with health professionals, starting discussions on social networking sites, and blogging are all ways to quickly create demand.

Issues Involving Significant Others

Family, friends, and caregivers may call attention to technology that they believe would enhance the quality of life for the potential user or family members. In some cases, the goal may be very altruistic and in others, a recommendation to explore the potential of a device may be to free up the user or caregiver for other priorities. When a friend or family member persistently promotes digital devices in the face of reluctance or outright resistance, it is often useful to explore the motivation. Significant others may similarly discourage exploration of devices because the perceived dollar cost is burdensome, or the process of acquiring, installing, and learning to use the device is anticipated to require large investments of time and energy on the part of those around the potential user.

When a device empowers a previously limited person, the new capacities may change relationships. These changes, if unanticipated, may create serious disruptions in role expectations, such that a spouse, for example, who has become the major source of information, navigation support, nutrition, or any other life-enhancing function may feel superfluous. Alternatively, new capacities may increase the disruptions in the lives of significant others who may now be expected to monitor new data, respond to e-mails, phone calls, and instant messaging. As data is shared across the social network, competition among family members may emerge (Morris, Lundell, Dishongh, & Needham, 2009). At times of *transition*, it is especially important to pay attention to the wide range of *influences* that can facilitate or unduly pressure individuals or families to adopt specific options promoted by others.

Agency Representatives

In this category are providers and case managers, eligibility workers, and others who act on behalf of the consumer or user. In some cases, there may be incentives to promote one product over another. Sometimes, these incentives are material and benefit the professional in the form of money, discounts, trips, or other favors. Increasingly, however, professional groups and agency infrastructures are taking the position that accepting any reward or incentive to recommend a product is unethical.

Another dilemma with some health professionals is a tendency to define *user centered* as meaning independent of social or economic capital. The individual's expressed or projected preferences are the focus without attention being paid as to how they will be implemented: It is important to take a socioecological perspective, to create a person–environment fit consistent with available resources.

Payer Groups

Payer groups may be the most difficult to work with, and in many instances, health professionals and savvy consumers find a way to circumvent rules. Technology is widely believed to reduce costs. However, as Wielawski (2006) has noted, often the up-front costs are born by parts of the system that do not reap the benefits. Some payers have experienced extensive fraud or seen devices purchased and not used. This has created a reluctance in some places to approve reimbursement for some devices and related services. In some instances, individuals are not compensated for items like a multifunction cell phone if it is also a mainstream consumer item. This may lead to the ridiculous situation in which a patient cannot afford a cell phone in any case and is locked out of the technology that might enable greater self-sufficiency and a healthier lifestyle.

Investors are part of the financial loop as well. As noted in Chapter 4, new partnerships are emerging as the viability of the market for consumer-oriented health technology becomes more attractive. It is not clear to what extent Internet-facilitated *mass collaboration* (see Tapscott & Williams, 2006) will play a role in shaping the dialogue among stakeholder groups.

Device Use by Older Adults

Most older adults said they would use health IT devices if they were available, according to a survey by AARP and the American Association of Homes and Services for the Aging (Barrett, 2009). Sixty percent of older adults said they would use a personal emergency response system, while 47% said they would use telephone-based monitoring. In addition, 40% said they would use an electronic pillbox, and 38% said they would use an Internet-monitoring system that would let them communicate with their care provider. The survey found that 84% of respondents said home safety devices would make them feel safer, while

82% said the devices would give their family and friends more peace of mind. However, 81% of older adults said the devices cost too much to install, and 79% said the devices cost too much to maintain. Eighty-four percent of respondents said they would be willing to pay less than $50 per month to use home safety devices, while just 11% said they would be willing to pay $51 to $100 per month to use such devices. The December 2007 survey, which was commissioned and funded by the Blue Shield of California Foundation, included 907 adults ages 65 to 98.

Complex Capital Demands in Choosing a Device

Engaged consumers, their families, and providers must assess health, human, economic, and sociotechnical capital in choosing devices and evaluating their impact. *Human capital* addresses literacy skills essential to selecting, learning, using, and adapting health technology devices (see Chapter 2). A survey of older adults and their caregivers was conducted by Knowledge Network for Blue Cross in December of 2007 (Barrett, 2009). Telemedicine and telepharmacy were well accepted by the older adults. Other technology of interest are devices that maintained social contact, promoted safety in the home, and promoted personal health and wellness. But again, responses to this survey captured the dilemmas of this new field. More than 80% of the older adults said that they would feel safer at home with supportive technology; they acknowledged that their family and friends would have greater peace of mind if such devices were installed. However, concerns about the cost of installation and maintenance were high. Caregivers reported they would find technology useful in meeting *their* challenges but predicted that it would not be easy to persuade older adults to use the items.

Time Frame as Adoption Parameter

Devices can save time but they also have built-in time costs. An important dimension of preparing consumers for adoption of a device is a clear assessment of match between a device's functional demands and the consumer's needs and preferences. Review of literature suggests that individuals define "functional time frame" from their own perspective (Pape, Kim, & Weiner, 2002). In practical terms this means that some devices that researchers and providers expect will increase independence may not be adopted by users. The example given by Pape and colleagues is a device that allows independence in dressing. However, the effort and time required to use the device were judged sufficiently burdensome that potential adopters preferred to be dressed by someone else. This dilemma has multiple implications. One is related to the learning curve demands for any device.

Equally important is the trade-off in time between the new technology and alternative resources. And sometimes, the potential consumer does not have a future vision equal to that of the inventor or the health professional who sees the risk of failure to adopt the device as increasing dependence.

On the invention side, the imperative is to engage potential users early in the process of development (Morales Rodriguez et al., 2007). On the provider side, framing the potential of the device in terms of its match with client priorities becomes critical.

Increasingly, consumers need to learn how to make trade-offs of time, independence, and cost related to devices. In many instances, these decisions will be complicated by the arcane system of reimbursement in contemporary American health care. A recurring issue identified in implementing the chronic care model (Wielawski, 2006) is that cost savings are often recouped well down the line from where costs were incurred. Intense interdisciplinary collaborations are required to develop new policies at government and insurance levels, as well as at the point of care. Too often interdisciplinary collaborations have meant that clinicians confer with each other and policy makers operate remote from consumers and their families and are isolated from the community resource people who implement policies.

Innovations in Costing

The heterogeneity of the needs of those who use adaptive technology creates great challenges in bringing cost-effective products to market. A wikinomics (Tapscott & Williams, 2006) approach has been initiated where those with adaptive needs look out for each other and collaborate to take advantage of what is available but not widely known about or accessible. Users and their social networks are key players in overcoming barriers to customizing applications for accessibility. Open source licensing is critical; the assumption is that prosecution is a real and critical barrier for those who adapt proprietary technology to increase accessibility.

Privacy and Security of the Device

A recurring concern about devices is their capacity to gather very personal information. The risk is that this important form of capital might be misused. Some potential misuses of personal information include:

- Perpetrating fraud, such as ordering supplies, billing for services for nonexistent needs, or diverting supplies
- Using personal information to access other financial resources by knowing the user's name, address, phone number, and identifying details

- Spreading one's personal information as gossip that might be injurious to one's social or work relationships
- Gleaning details to market products whether of excellent relevance or dubious value

The dilemma is that devices specific to health technology are most effective when integrating a wide variety of information-gathering tools. Motion detectors, physiological sensors, video surveillance, gadgets connected to personal health records, and integrated networks of smart or intelligent homes create a web of information that sustains health, alerts to potential health problems, triggers events, and simultaneously creates a sieve of vulnerability.

Many adults, frustrated with fragmented healthcare systems, accept these risks, which include family and caregivers having access to data about an individual's health that prompt assumptions about competence or judgments about choices. These assumptions and judgments may prompt actions that compromise independence and create stress and tension. Similarly, information about social relationships, sexual preferences, financial status, and habits may become available and may be used to compromise, defraud, or embezzle funds. A sensitive and well-networked system easily provides information about the presence of people in the house, and their level of activity—useful for burglars.

Safeguards are important when health professionals recommend information-gathering devices. Cress (2009) observes that professionals who endorse monitoring as a strategy take responsibility by ensuring informed consent and assessing continued consent.

Also, the client needs to be clear about what is in device-related documents. For example, the health record often documents the recommendation for access, the instructions for protecting privacy and security, lists surrogates who are designated to make decisions for impaired participants, and specifies who will control access to the resulting data and what reports will be generated and disseminated. Adults naïve to the potential of security breaches and their consequences may require coaching in choosing login and passwords so that they are not easily guessed by family members, salaried caregivers, and others with intimate knowledge of family matters.

Finally, coaching on selecting and interacting with technical assistance staff may be required to protect users of networked technology. The potential privacy and security risks of losing a device are as important as discussions of the risks of hacking. Many individuals store passwords, pin codes, and identification on cell phones or PDAs in quickly accessible files. Consumers and health professionals can be taught a routine way to disguise stored passwords and to name the file in a way that is not obvious and is encrypted. Unless absolutely necessary, a master file should not be stored on a portable device, however veiled. Most consumers need coaching on encryption and recovery of encrypted files.

DEVICE CONTINUANCE AND ADHERENCE: HEALTH CAPITAL

With respect to devices, adherence or continued use is a persistent problem (Martin et al., 2008). Lauer et al. (2006) found adherence rates of 8% to 75% documented in the literature. This corresponds with Verza, Carvalho, Battaglia, and Uccelli (2006), who reported 37.5% with the majority of devices abandoned immediately for the multiple sclerosis population under study. Lauer and colleagues note that *abandonment* is a common label given to failure to continue use of a device. This term has both negative and misleading connotations. Reports of high *abandonment* of devices creates a perception that that money has been wasted. Some conclude that the device was poorly designed, or that the consumers did not made a "good effort."

With respect to technology for health, it is very important to assess both the individual and family history of device exposure, trial, use patterns, and expressed reasons for discontinuation. Reasons will give insight into strategies for introducing new devices or reconsideration of previously attempted devices. Sometimes a device is no longer used for very logical reasons that do not reflect on the device or the user. Therefore, the ATOMS project team (Lauer et al., 2006) proposes adding *positive discontinuance* as an evaluation category. This terminology could be important as policy makers review expenditures on devices. The goal is accurate reflection of the role of devices in achieving health outcomes.

With digital devices, three compelling reasons may account for potentially *positive discontinuance*. They fall into the ATOMS (Lauer et al., 2006) model of better equipment and alternative solutions but add the dimension of the social network. These rationales include better equipment becoming available, advances in interoperability requiring change to synchronize a particular device with others, and changes in social network preferences. As social networking becomes a more central part of planning and evaluating health outcomes, the device preferences of individuals in a user's social circle will weigh heavily. If the technology in use by family member or key friends has features missing in the patient's device, this may prompt discontinuation of current devices. Compatibility of features is important for the everyday experience of connecting with one's social network. In addition, members of the social network can provide technical support if a device puzzling the patient user is known to them.

Rapid advances are being made with respect to multifunction devices and the improvement in their size and usability. As smart home technology becomes more available and the use of electronic medical records with personal health record options increases, new devices may be required for compatibility. As family and friends change their devices, others in the social network may also switch for simpler communication, cost savings, and reliance on those people for technical assistance. With digital technology, analysis of previous experiences with devices can save time, money, and facilitate motivation.

CATEGORIES OF ELECTRONIC ASSISTIVE TECHNOLOGY (EAT)

There is a broad range of devices and electronic assistive technology (EAT) that use information and communication technology as their core component that are available to foster appropriate independence and interdependence. Devices may operate in a stand-alone intelligent capacity to access, operate, and control appliances. Multiple device integration may create an environment that is technology enriched. EAT can support users in meeting their everyday needs at home, and in addition can send information to providers to enable better decisions about care (Martin et al., 2008).

Alwan and Noble (2008) suggest that there are three key purposes for health technology devices: The first is based on the relationship between the individual and the environment (safety), the second on oneself (physical and mental wellness), and the third on others (social connectedness). They propose that technologies can be evaluated based on their value proposition to each stakeholder in the care process (see Appendix 5-A). Tables demonstrating this framework, with specific applications to safety, physical and mental wellness, and social connectedness, are provided in Appendix 5-A.

Statistical and computational intelligence paradigms are emerging to assist consumers, health providers, and other stakeholders to use the data to make decisions about intervening or, alternatively, about achieving "peace of mind" (Tyrer, Aud, Alexander, Skubic, & Rantz, 2007). A key objective is a responsive system designed so that "simple events will not cascade and catastrophically spiral out of control" (Tyrer et al., p. 4045). This overview of health technology is compatible with Carle's label for caregiver-shared technology as "nana technology," by which he means "technology designed, intended, or that can otherwise be used to improve quality of life for seniors" ("Professor Says Much," 2006, para. 4). Carle further defines five categories for the technologies that are being produced or developed by companies such as Intel, GE, Philips, and Kimberly-Clark, among others ("Professor Says Much," 2006). These categories apply equally well to any health technology for adult consumers:

- Health products, such as robotic medication dispensers designed to reduce errors. Gadgets or widgets linked to health-specific websites might be classified here but given their intangible nature, they are discussed in Chapter 3, in the context of Internet resources.
- Safety products, such as wireless sensors that can track movements, location, and identify falls
- Cognition products, such as computer software programs that quiz elderly residents or patients regularly and send the data to a healthcare professional or family member
- Lifestyle products that provide a convenience factor for seniors, such as mailbox sensors that alert the user that mail has been delivered

- Whole-house/whole-facility products that provide overall home monitoring and management (the smart home or domotics)
- Adaptor devices, such as digital and physical products that enable Internet interactions or use of other digital applications where vision or coordination compromises facility (joystick, touch screen)

This model overlaps the Alwan and Noble (2008) framework of safety and wellness but does not address social connectivity. Alternatively, Carle did not address differential value to various stakeholder groups. Cress (2009) provides a view of technology in terms of how it supports the long-distance caregiver (Table 5.3).

Table 5.3   List of Technologies of Use to Long-Distance Caregivers

Type of Technology	Technology/ Organization	Web Link for Further Information
Home monitoring/ health security system	Examples: • Rest Assured • Xanboo • AT&T Remote Monitor • Quiet Care • Grand Care	www.restassuredsystem.com www.xanboo.com www.attrm.com www.quietcare.com www.grandcare.com
Electronic pillbox	Example: • Epill.com	www.epill.com
Telehealth monitoring	Example: • iCare Health Hero	www.healthhero.com/ partners/partners_icare.html
Secure online personal health record	Example: • LifeLedger	www.elderissuespro.com
Virtual Web meeting place for friends and family	Examples: • CarePages • CaringBridge	www.carepages.com www.caringbridge.org
Video conferencing for caregivers	Examples: • Caregiver Technologies • Virtual Interactive Families	www.internetvisitation.org www.vifamilies.com

Table 5.3   List of Technologies of Use to Long-Distance Caregivers (*continued*)

Type of Technology	Technology/ Organization	Web Link for Further Information
Affordable teleconference link	Examples: • freeteleconference. com • conferencecalls unlimited.com	www.freeteleconference. com www.conferencecalls unlimited.com
Vlogging (video blogging)	Example: • Virtual Families and Friends	www.jimbuie.blogs.com/ virtualfamilies1
Computer-based video conferencing software (do-it-yourself)	Example: • Skype	www.skype.com
Web TV	Webtv.com	www.webtv.com
Printing mailbox (receives and prints e-mails and attachments)	Presto	www.presto.com
E-mail without computer or Internet access	My Celery	www.mycelery.com
Easy-to-use cell phone	Jitterbug	www.jitterbugdirect.com
Digital photo frame and automatic picture updates	CEIVA Digital Picture Frame and Picture Plan	www.ceiva.com
Industry organization	Examples: • Home Care Technology Association of America • American Telemedicine Association, home telehealth and remote monitoring special interest group	www.hctaa.org/aging.html www.atmeda.org/ICOT/ sighomehealth.htm Buyer's guide: www. atmeda.org/news/ 2006buyersguide definitions.htm

(continues)

Table 5.3   List of Technologies of Use to Long-Distance Caregivers (*continued*)

Type of Technology	Technology/ Organization	Web Link for Further Information
Corporation conducting research	Intel Research	www.intel.com/research/ prohealth/dh_aging_in_ place.htm
Nonprofit organization supporting development and implementation of technology for older adults	SmartSilvers Alliance	www.smartsilvers.com Product list: TechEye for the Older Guy (and Gal!) network.smartsilvers.com/ index.php?option=com_ myblog&Itemid=56

Source: Cress, 2009.

An alternative view is presented by Dishman, Matthews, and Dunbar-Jacob (2004) in the definitive monograph *Technology for Adaptive Aging* (Table 5.4).

This classification is driven by the actual mechanism or core technology that accomplishes the task. For consumers and practitioners, the overview intended for long-distance caregivers provides a quick introduction to the possibilities. Most are equally useful for any age consumer and caregivers at any distance. As a care plan shapes up, the Alwan and Noble (2008) model is useful in sorting priorities for safety, wellness, and social connectivity. The tables provided in the chapter appendix set out useful details in terms of function of the technology as well as potential value, and the reader can easily search for updates using constructs presented there.

The classifications presented by Dishman et al. (2004) in Table 5.4 are very useful for interdisciplinary collaborations on new applications of existing technology or visioning new technology. Many adults with complex responsibilities for others, including children, would find most of the functions accomplished by these technologies to be very valuable.

Sensors as the Catalyst for Health Technology Applications

Sensors add a layer of connectedness. Tyrer et al. (2007) have succinctly described the tripartite aspects of sensors. These include the information, interconnection, and longitudinal analysis capacities that allow for early detection of

Table 5.4   Selected Technologies and Their Roles in Telehealth

Technology	Role in Telehealth
Information Issues and Resources	
Bodily diagnostics, biosensors	Real-time and store-and-forward clinical information (blood pressure, etc.); medication adherence
Ambient displays, actuator networks	Smart home resources: consumer and caregiver feedback; social network monitoring
Personal health informatics	Storehouse for health information; allows visualization of long-term trends
Activity sensors, behavioral diagnostics	Observations of daily living; build patterns of activities for alerts to changes
Interfaces	
Adaptive, distributed interfaces	Interface tailored to user; activate system without computer link
Remote community and collaboration	Social support links
Information fusion, inference engines	Alarm/alert for deviations from patterns that require contact or action
Wireless broadband	Connectivity more convenient than cabled link
Agents, assistants, coaches, companions	Interpret device feedback, weigh choices in face of alerts/alarms, cognitive and social stimulation

Source: Adapted from Dishman et al., 2004.

improvements or declines. A brief overview of sensor capacities will set the stage for learning about emerging technologies (see Table 5.5).

There are a variety of sensors that provide motion, location, and activity information; sensors are available to monitor physiologic and medical conditions; and

Table 5.5   Sensor Overview

Purposes:
- Detect changes in patterns that signal improvement or early failings.
- Signal need for urgent or emergency help.
- Integrate with websites or mobile units to promote communication.
- Have ubiquitous monitoring for peace of mind for older adult and family.
- Keep an inventory of supply levels for medications and other resources.
- Coach and monitor exercise effectiveness and participation in games.

Information potentials:
- Physical: Motion, location, activity
- Physiological/medical: Pulse, temperature, sweat, blood chemistry
- Social: Telephone or Web interaction counts or identification
- Memory support: Monitoring cooking steps, adherence to regimens
- Communicate safety issues: Stove use, fire, unsecured doors

Communication:
- Devices and protocols networked to connect to computers
- Statistical and computational paradigms for analysis
- Applications for interaction with emergency rescues, providers, and social network

Monitoring target examples:
- Restlessness as indicator of disturbed sleep
- Gait changes as indicator of drug side effect or physical debility
- Extended bedrest as indicator of depression or physical debility
- Pill counts as indicator of adherence or side effect issues

Source: Tyrer et al., 2007.

a variety of communication devices and protocols are available to interconnect these sensor systems with computers. Finally there are a variety of statistical and computational intelligence paradigms that will help make sense of the data.

Indeed there is much that technology can do for the elderly. Ubiquitous monitoring in space and time can provide urgent or emergency help rapidly. Longitudinal assessment of the data can provide a means to detect early failings for an appropriate intervention. Access through websites or other means of communication can extend the caregivers to include loved ones.

Social Alarms as Sensor Application

Social alarm is the label given in Europe to those devices or networks of devices that act to improve the quality of life with respect to safety. There is some evidence they are more widely used in Europe than in the United States, but it is nevertheless interesting. Three levels or generations have been identified (Frost & Sullivan, 2006, Market Sector section, para. 2–4):

- "First-generation alarms: These devices consist of a simple telephone unit and a pendant with a button that can be triggered when help is required by the user. The monitoring center receives the call, which displays the caller's identity and location, thereby enabling care staff to provide immediate response based on the level of urgency. The decision about urgency is made by the user. This requires that the user be alert on some level and is most suited for physical problems or panic.
- Second-generation alarms: This segment, otherwise known as "telecare," refers to the use of sensors such as smoke, fire, and flood detectors, among others, which enable the care staff to respond to a crisis by providing immediate response in case of emergencies.
- Third-generation alarms: This refers to a more advanced type of telecare service, which collects activity data automatically through various sensors on a continuous basis through the detection of various movements such as opening of doors, cupboards, flow of water, and the use of electrical appliances. Widely used sensors include front door open/close detectors, fridge open/close detectors, pressure mats, bed/chair occupancy, and electrical usage sensors."

RFID (Radio Frequency ID Devices) as Coordinating Sensor in Smart Home

In the smart home or intelligent house, radio frequency ID (RFID) devices are emerging as potential sensor, inventory control, and data-collection devices. They can be active or passive, and they can be ingested, implanted, or simply attached, depending on the application and the needs of the individual. A major advantage of RFIDs over bar code bands is that RFIDs do not require a line-of-sight connection; clothing, bed coverings and nonmetallic surfaces are not barriers to reading information. Vilamovska et al. (2009) summarize that RFIDs process information faster than bar codes, can read at wider ranges, and have greater memory capacity.

Using sophisticated systems, people can have a home device accessible from their place of work to see which grocery items are needed, or a home device could be programmed to alert the owner when a supply of something is running low. These systems can be used to generate shopping lists that feature frequently enjoyed items or items that need to be replaced. The systems can also manage collections such as books, records, and films. Currently, RFID applications are in limited use. However, it is anticipated that this responsive technology will be widely disseminated in consumer health technology in the future.

The RFID can be used for tracking, identification and authentication, automatic data collection, and transfer and sensing. A detailed state-of-the-art report done for Rand Europe by Vilamovska et al. (2009) provided the details for the following overview. Vilamovska and colleagues anticipate that RFIDs will advance home-based patient care management, as noted above. The sensing and data collection functions that can be facilitated by both active and passive RFIDs will also be important adjuncts. Some of the applications include collecting and transferring data on vital signs, sensing wetness for bedridden or paralyzed patients at risk for pressure ulcers, and monitoring compliance with medication regimens.

Treatment-Based RFIDs at Home

It is not clear how soon treatment-based applications in place in hospitals could be used in home settings to track information, such as an inventory of key health supplies, healing after surgery, handwashing practices, neuromuscular stimulation, and assistance for the visually impaired. Identification and authentication of medications, biometric data, and progress is an important application in the institutional setting. As older adult couples live at home together with comorbidities and various declines associated with aging, a way to distinguish and track these data for each person will become very important.

In their report, Vilamovska et al. (2008) note that while existing wifi may seem like an appealing choice, it does have limitations. They further note that wifi is less secure and has inferior error protection and location accuracy. They conclude that a combination of bar codes, RFIDs, and wifi may be the best design strategy. Infrastructure costs, ease of installation, and public acceptance were cited as probable factors in the ultimate success of these applications.

RFIDs—Controversy and Best Use

The RAND report by Vilamovska et al. (2009) indicated that organized opposition to RFID technology has emerged in the United States. The VeriChip, while touted as a resource in emergencies, says the opposition, can be easily spoofed. Vilamovska et al. (2009) recommend that its use be limited to providing positive identification rather than serving to provide authentication for access to resources. A number of concerns have arisen related to more widespread use of RFID technology. Some of these identified by Vilamovska et al. in the RAND report (2009) include privacy violations and security issues, but there are other fears from some religious groups linking the technology to evil and from others who fear ubiquitous surveillance. These are detailed for RAND by Vilamovska et al. (2009). The RAND group also noted that other controversies are whether the technology is sufficiently advanced, the business case known, and operational and managerial challenges overcome. In their review they note that sensing capacities, tracking and identification, data collection and health infrastructure applications have been successfully implemented. Vilamovksa and colleagues emphasize that these issues will need to be addressed in a convincing manner so that RFID can become more accepted as technology advances and telehealth applications become more available. RFID controversies are an instance where taking a socioecological perspective will be invaluable. Sorting out the beliefs and expectations developed from various sources of influence of all of the stakeholders at each point of transition and appreciating the capital available to each group will be a powerful strategy. Promoters of RFID use in telehealth cannot rely simply on providing information and expecting that to lead to acceptance.

SENSOR APPLICATIONS: CONSUMER-SELECTED BODY COMPUTING

Next-generation health care is increasingly mobile and, as it becomes more truly consumer dependent, it will revolve around new technologies that do not require proactive intervention from the wearer or health professional (Barrett, 2009). In some cases, the technology captures data and analyzes patterns that trigger interventions, such as glucose monitoring with patterns that indicate that the person needs to take predetermined steps to reestablish desirable levels. Alternatively, a caregiver may be alerted that a family member is not following his or her usual pattern of activities and needs to be checked. This ubiquitous computing works with devices that can be worn on the body. Some are embedded in clothing and others are attached, making health care very mobile (Table 5.6) What is highlighted here are devices that are targeted to consumers who will select one based on their own health goals or their wish to provide remote monitoring and support for a family member. There are even more highly sophisticated devices intended to link patient and health professional for continuous and intermittent monitoring, but they are not described here.

Wearable Embedded Technology

Smart fabrics and interactive textiles with embedded sensors are creating new potentials for monitoring health status. These new monitoring options have

Table 5.6   Emerging Wearable Devices: Embedded or Attached

Clothing Embedded	Body Attachments
Game and Internet interface • Exploding and vibrating vests • Air puffs for game events • Foldable textile keyboards (Smart Fabrics, Australia)	*Monitors: clinical alerts, activity* • Activity type, duration • Sleep–awake state • Daily living patterns of movement • Falls • Heart rate, respirations (Bodymedia, Humana, Sony W710i phone)
Lifestyle • T-shirts that signal wireless hot spots • Luminous bedclothes to read by • Sleeve controls for electronics (ski parkas) • Shoe insert sensors for steps, duration (Nike iPod) • Mattress piezoresistors for sleep states	*Eyewear* • Oakley audio glasses, sunglasses with built in earplugs and MP3 player • Designer glasses with video display wireless connection to pocket browsers, GPS, media players (Lumus-Israel) • Contact lens with telephone display on retina (U. Washington)
Power generators • Energy-capturing knee brace	*Wrist-mounted device* • Stress meter, gathers information about environment; conducts interviews about person's current well-being • Displays of sport monitoring
Remote controllers • Sleeve controls for electronics (ski parkas)	*Cameras* • Camera with social programming for autistic adults: monitors attention being paid by listener. Autistic adult gets feedback to change conversation. • Necklace camera to monitor pill adherence, cooking steps if interrupted
Physiological sensors • Immunosensors in dressings to detect healing (Biotex) • Oximetry sensors on shirts for breathing • Strain sensors for muscle movements	*Computer strap-on* • Allows wide gestures to control program actions; useful for construction, emergency workers

Table 5.6   Emerging Wearable Devices: Embedded or Attached (*continued*)

Clothing Embedded	Body Attachments
Movement sensors • Support for poststroke patients with upper-limb impairment, detects accuracy of exercises and can be used in home or at the hospital	

Sources: Felong, 2008; Curone et al., 2007; Tellzen, 2008.

implications for improving cardiac rehabilitation through managing vigorous exercise. Current options are measuring body temperature, heart activity, and body inclination, signaling a risk for falls. On the horizon are biosensors that collect sodium potassium and chloride levels from perspiration. Other developments with implications for telehealth at home are probes to measure the conductivity of perspiration, immunosensors integrated into dressings to detect specific proteins indicating progression of healing, and probes for oxygen saturation around the thorax. Under trial is a passive system that will not require a battery, thus reducing user burden. The systems are currently targeted for people with diabetes and obesity, as well as athletes and firefighting and rescue teams.

The availability of this level of information in real time may extend an older adult's ability to continue to be engaged in such demanding occupations as rescue, firefighting, and sports. Continuous monitoring can dampen risk and encourage engagement of experienced individuals in settings where age has traditionally been the criterion for retirement. One dilemma noted by Luprano (as cited in European eHealth News, 2008) is the lack of clinician experience with continuous remote monitoring and the lack of data on the relationship of real-time indicators to acute and chronic illness decisions. Progress on these fronts can be checked at the BIOTEX website http://www.biotex-eu.com/html/public.html where PDFs from presentations are posted. A related overview of recent papers on wearable sensors can be found at http://www.artificialvision.com/newpubs/wearable_sensors.

Wearable Attached Devices

Wearable digital devices that track the user's health at all times of the day or night are one of the latest trends. Some of these devices even have the capability of sending data to other devices. A Bluetooth-enabled biosensor wristwatch from Exmocare tracks the pulse of the wearer and monitors heart rate changes as well as skin conductance. As if these features are not enough to make it an excellent lifesaver, it can also monitor the location and the activity level of the user through an accelerometer and GPS. Eyewear, minicomputers hung on the belt and run by gestures are also in the mix (Ross, 2001; Tellzan, 2008).

Another company that is currently developing wearable technologies for health is BodyMedia. Their SenseWear armbands track levels of physical activity, energy used, number of steps taken, and sleep and awake states. This device creates easy-to-understand graphs on a computer. The computer display is complemented by a wrist device for immediate feedback.

SENSOR APPLICATIONS: SMART HOMES

Rialle, Duchen, Noury, Bajolle, and Demongeot (2002) introduced the concept of the health smart home. The underlying concept is sometimes referred to as *domotics*, a term found in European and American writings. Domotics is a contraction of the words *domus* for house and *robotics* for automation (Tonet et al., 2008). Domotics can contribute to a better quality of life and can be useful for disabled and elderly people to increase their independence and autonomy. Domotics can be applied to safety and remote surveillance, to household appliances, and to the control of doors, windows, lights, indoor climate, and multimedia and communication devices.

The concept of environmental control is interesting also for other habitats, like an office, a car, or outdoor environments. Aldrich (2003) proposes five classes of smart homes based on the level of complexity and capacity to gather data, analyze patterns, and trigger actions independent of human intervention.

Pangher (2008) lists these core issues: (1) Who is going to pay for the technologies and consumables? (2) Who is going to maintain the protocols in the data analysis? and (3) Who is liable if systems are not successful and result in health damages? These issues have not been addressed in the highly enthusiastic reports of smart home applications.

Other considerations in smart home design and selection are based on experiences at Georgia Technology University (Davidoff et al., 2006). It is key to recall that while families are *plural*, most systems are singular in their setups and programming. The *thermostat predicament*: rules don't always agree. This refers to when family members have different ideas on the ideal temperature, and the smart system is unable to resolve the dilemma. Families perceive chores as activities, not procedures—the core of a programmed smart home. Many tasks are device and/or location independent. Ownership of chores can be ambiguous—and very important. The house plays a role in family and individual self-definition. Given these principles, it is not surprising that there are constraints in development and dissemination of smart homes.

The Oatfield nursing homes are models of creative ways to aggregate digital devices to support graceful aging (Lundberg, 2007). In presentations on their experience, the representatives claim that the older adults are quite willing to participate in the tracking of their movements and gathering other information on daily life patterns. Residents agree to wear a badge that tracks their location. In case of a fall in a stairwell, this is very helpful. If a resident leaves without signing out, the system sends an alert. Residents can be weighed in bed before arising. All of this information can be tracked centrally by staff. Residents can choose whether they allow family members to monitor as well.

Research on Smart Homes

Two extensive reviews have been done of the research on smart homes (Chan, Esteve, Escriba, & Campo, 2008; Demiris & Hensel, 2008). An extensive discussion of the prototypes is provided by Chan et al. Demiris & Hensel summarize that functional monitoring seems to be most prevalent. Functional variables include activities of daily living such as meal intake, gait, level of activity, and emergency notifications. Traditional physiological measures such as pulse and blood pressure were not as common as anticipated. Demiris and Hensel suggest that the technology may not be sufficiently advanced for the restlessness of "well" residents. Social interaction measures were even less common. Attention to applications emerging after these reviews (See Morris et al., 2009), suggests that previous examples may not have been sufficiently interactive or game-like. Finally, smart home sensors focusing on cognitive or sensory applications were least common. These would include reminders, task instructions, and supports for individuals with hearing, vision, or other deficits.

Most problematic is the failure to find any evidence that experiencing a smart home environment changes any health outcomes or has an effect on acute episodes or delays nursing home placement (Demiris & Hensel, 2008). Chapter 7 addresses a wide range of factors that affect smart home implementation and impact in the context of the move to telehealth.

Intel is taking leadership in partnering with manufacturers and distributors (GE, in particular) to increase the rapidity with which innovations become available. Their methodology embraces user-centered design. Dishman (2007) describes a model where ethnographic methods are used to observe interactions with available technology in natural environments.

Dilemmas of Personnel Shortage: Robots as Alternative

In recent years, even robots have become attractive as potential health resources, particularly for older adults. Roy and Pineau (2007) launch their discussion by noting that the nursing shortage creates a critical issue in coping with the aging population. They go on to present technologies of robotics and artificial intelligence (AI) as a resource. They make clear that robots will not replace humans but could increase their effectiveness. In addition, robots have more patience with slower-paced clients.

Roy and Pineau (2007) also make the case that robots work well with low-cognition tasks, those that may precipitate caregiver burnout. Low cognition tasks make few intelligent demands, have a cycle of repetition, and are predominantly mechanical. Roy and Pineau list reminders, physical assistance, and monitoring as examples of such tasks. Robots could assist with sensing tasks when mobility limits use of fixed devices, as well.

Robots for in-home use have for some time been a focus of the work being done at the School of Nursing at the University of Pittsburgh in conjunction with Carnegie Mellon and the School of Engineering at the University of Southern California. Judith Matthews from the University of Pittsburgh (personal communication, October 2, 2003), who directed the Nursebot project, indicated that older adults were quite receptive to the robots in her project and questioned their absence during any researcher visit. Roy and Pineau (2007) conclude that commercially viable robots are limited by provider reluctance to accept them and their high costs; providing a sense of presence, and a way to communicate will be easier than a cost-effective robot able to provide manipulation assistance. They also conclude that commercially viable products have begun to appear on the market. However, they do not indicate a source.

Declines of Aging and Illness Relevant to Devices

Hearing Loss

Hearing acuity decreases progressively, which begins for most people in their 40s (Berk, 2004). However, there is rising concern that many young adults have altered acuity related to use of music devices that deliver sound at decibels that create damage over time. In addition, any adult using these devices with ear buds may miss traffic noises that signal a need for special attention to road conditions.

Visual Dilemmas

Around age 50, adults need more light in order to be able to read (Charness & Schaie, 2003). In some cases magnification is required that goes beyond what contact lenses and corrective lenses can provide. There is a major market for devices to enhance vision. These devices are designed to support reading medication labels, menus, and price tags; to support writing tasks and hobbies; and to support meaningful attendance at shows and conferences. Many of these devices are expensive and not very portable. One vision enhancer, for example, is described as "light" and weighs 1.3 pounds. In 2008, the basic unit cost more than $1500. As with all devices, the risk is that adults and their "helpful" family members may find advertisements and stories that advocate the potential of these devices and make a purchase without an expert assessment of their actual value to the eventual wearer.

Devices Enabling Driving

An emerging issue with high emotional content is related to driving automobiles and minimizing distractions. These are sensory and cognitive dimensions that are relevant to all ages. Sensory dimensions include visual, auditory, and psychomotor capabilities. Visual abilities begin to decline at age 20 (Meyer, 2004). An excellent discussion of the specific issues can be found in Meyer's NRC report. Interestingly, this summary suggests that the "increase in accident rates for older drivers could be due to greatly increased accident risk for a fairly small group of older drivers who suffer from dementia or severe sensory problems (of which they may not be aware)" (Meyer, 2004, p. 265). Thus, making the case that increasing driving safety with facilitative devices could have universal value.

Many people discuss the need to support the older driver giving attention to reduced reaction time. Some strategies focus on minimizing distractions. However, distractability and the condition of multitasking is a life span issue. Again, using the universal computing construct (Vanderheiden, 2007), designers and health professionals can promote adaptations to current automobile design that benefit most drivers. Many new automobiles are moving devices to control radio and other features to the steering column to minimize the time, visual distraction, and motions required to activate phone and entertainment devices.

Decreased flexibility in the neck area can limit ability to see an object behind the car when backing up or changing lanes (Meyer, 2004). Toyota is one manufacturer offering a "universal design" feature to improve visibility in this area as a standard feature. Offered as a "glamour" perk ostensibly to show the technical leadership of Toyota cars, this is a valuable safety device.

Anyone whose driving reaction times are affected by stress or age-related slowing is a target consumer. Emerging resources developed under the SPARC (Strategic Promotion of Aging Research Capacity) initiative in Britain include windshield displays of approaching traffic signs and audible feedback on speed (Musselwhite & Haddad, 2008). In both cases, the objective is to minimize the need to look at the roadside or dashboard instead of the road itself. The SPARC study led to a paradigm shift from previous design strategies that take control from the driver. These included systems that automatically limited car speeds or regulated distance between the subject car and the vehicle in front. The goal is to prolong safe driver behavior that supports continued independence.

Medications and Driving

Given the increase in chronic conditions for American adults and the dominant paradigm of medicating these conditions and their symptoms, the likelihood of impaired driving skill has escalated. Regularizing the use of alerting devices that detect somnolence would be a valuable innovation in preventing accidents at any age (NHTSA, n.d.). In the meantime, health providers can include questions in their assessments that cover driving habits and incidents. (This prompts a recommendation for exploring indirect questions such as quality of car insurance coverage and experience in making claims.)

Game Devices

The equipment needed to play health or serious games might also be considered in the category of devices. The gaming aspect is covered in Chapter 6. However, the equipment itself bears discussion in this context. Attention to devices specific to gaming will become increasingly important in telehealth. For example, PlayStation may become a key tool in participating in eHealth (e.g., Altizer, 2010; Lalley, 2006). Adapting game consoles would be part of ubiquitous technology, which is so promising in terms of minimizing stigma and increasing adoption of new health technology innovations. Playing digital games may require use of trackball, Wii remotes and elaborate controllers, special interface pads, "guitars," and other peripherals. These in turn may require adaptations for adults with chronic illness or declines specific to aging.

It is readily apparent that users must follow manufacturers' recommendations for securing remotes and be reasonable about the time they allocate to game playing. Au's (2009) extensive review of the literature, presented at the 2009 Games for Health Conference, suggests minimal cause for alarm to date. Pacemakers are not at risk when reasonable care is taken. Light fixtures and TV sets apparently are more likely to be damaged than game players injured. Some spectacular cases seem to point to more of a media overreaction than a significant health problem. Some conditions that did turn up in the Au review, however, include repetitive stress syndrome, lateral epicondylitis (tennis elbow), rashes and bumps, eyestrain, photosensitive epilepsy, motion or simulation sickness, addiction, and physiological stress with some psychological stress. Addiction, Au concludes from the literature, was related more to preexisting conditions than game playing per se.

Cell Phones

Increasingly, Americans are going mobile for a wide range of digital activities (Horrigan, 2007). Nonvoice data activities are used by 58% of Americans. This includes texting, e-mailing, taking a picture, looking for maps, and recording video. This Pew Internet survey found a sharp reversal in attitudes, with respondents now most likely to nominate the cell phone as most difficult to do without. This is compared to the 2002 choice of a landline phone as truly necessary. Advances in mobile phone technology are opening the door for health technologies that are convenient and easy for users. A glucose monitoring cell phone application has been tested with adolescents that is equally relevant to adults (Marrero, 2009). A blood test is done with special strips and then read using a port on an adapted cell phone. The results are then uploaded to a site trending findings and are available to the health professional.

Fox (2008) observes that Health 2.0 is creating new ways to reach populations previously not connected to online resources. She notes that cell phones are a venue more relevant for African American and Latino adults than are the Internet, TV, or landlines. The development of Health 3.0 will enhance the potential of cell phones as well as the Internet.

DEVICES PROMOTING ADHERENCE TO DRUG REGIMENS

Among the devices that adults might find useful are options for taking medications on schedule. Adherence to drug regimens is a major and persistent problem for adults (Ryder & Brue, 2008). Consequences of failure to follow the prescribed regimen include unexpected drug interactions, readmission to hospital, failure to resolve symptoms, and conditions such as pain, infection, and restricted mobility. Many options have evolved using timers and announcements (e-Pill Medication Reminders, 2009). Of particular relevance here are devices linked to the Internet or mobile phone. Choosing a drug reminder device, with good prospects for continuing consumer use, calls for attention to variables affecting relevance of any adaptive device.

Available Pill-Monitoring Devices

The e-Pill website features multiple versions of pill-monitoring devices from electronic to paper systems (e-Pill Medication Reminders, 2009). Several connect to a phone line that alerts caregivers or providers to a failure to respond to prompts (e-Pill Medication Reminders, 2009). However, these devices are not truly digital in nature, they are not networked, nor do they build a database of patterns and trends.

A digital device not featured on this site is MedSignals (www.MedSignals. com) (Figure 5.1).

Figure 5.1   Example of Web-Connected Medication Reminder Device

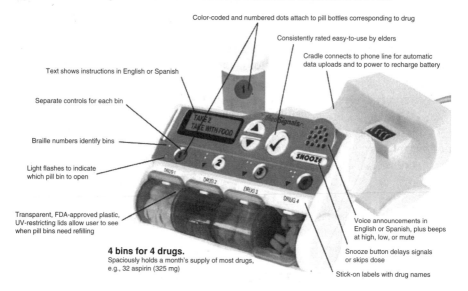

Color-coded and numbered dots attach to pill bottles corresponding to drug

Consistently rated easy-to-use by elders

Cradle connects to phone line for automatic data uploads and to power to recharge battery

Text shows instructions in English or Spanish

Separate controls for each bin

Braille numbers identify bins

Light flashes to indicate which pill bin to open

Transparent, FDA-approved plastic, UV-restricting lids allow user to see when pill bins need refilling

Voice announcements in English or Spanish, plus beeps at high, low, or mute

4 bins for 4 drugs.
Spaciously holds a month's supply of most drugs, e.g., 32 aspirin (325 mg)

Snooze button delays signals or skips dose

Stick-on labels with drug names

Source: Reproduced courtesy of MedSignals.

This device is an example of a new generation of networked adaptive devices that support adherence across the life span and aging in place. The company has reported three studies that demonstrate improved adherence and consumer satisfaction. A randomized crossover study with culturally diverse older adults (Ryder & Brue, 2008) demonstrated improved adherence in the number of pills taken and on-time doses. A phase 1 randomized crossover trial demonstrated improved on-time adherence for antiretroviral medications with adults (Brue et al., 2007) (Figure 5.2).

MedSignals had planned a 12-medication device but found low consumer interest:

> Instead we found they wanted two or three devices scattered in various rooms, enabling them to have their pills in proximity when they needed them. We instead built two or three to daisy chain in one version or to Bluetooth to a command unit in another configuration. Lately, we've also introduced the first of the Vital Signals line, [which are] Bluetooth-enabled. Our new weight scale was just released in Bluetooth that reports to a MedSignals device that is Bluetooth-capturing. (V. Brue, personal communication, August 25, 2009)

Figure 5.2   Adherence Patterns to Medications with MedSignals Device

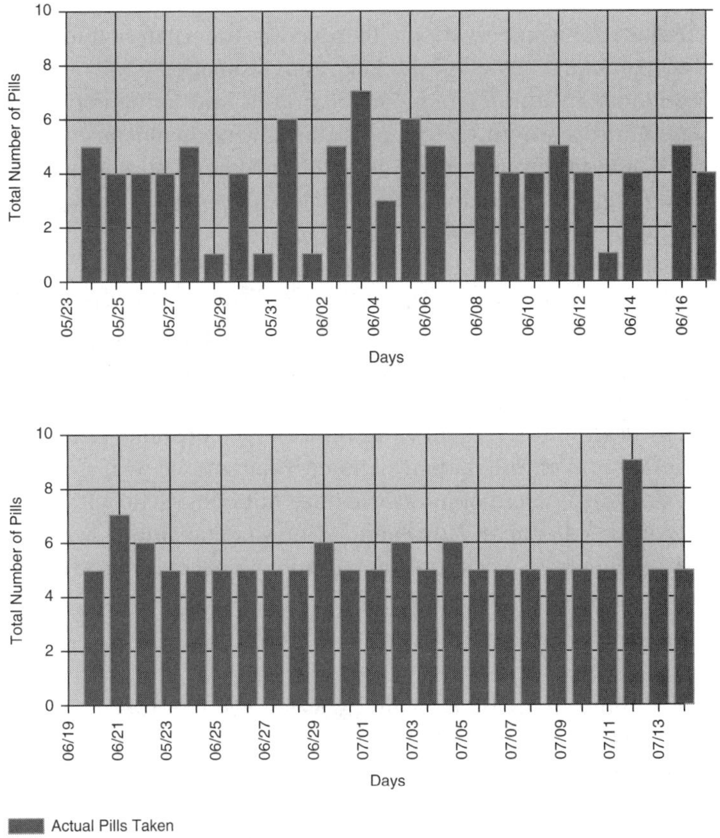

Actual Pills Taken

Comparing the difference that MedSignals makes, the illustration (above) depicts daily medication use records before and after MedSignals was activated. The illustration represents one subject's record across time in a recent clinical trial of elders using MedSignals. Above, the patient receives no beeps or alerts but the masked device monitors every lid opening. Below, the alerting features were activated and the participant shows significantly improved adherence and doesn't miss a day.

Source: Ryder & Brue, 2008. Used with permission.

A very promising system with good preliminary data from a randomized control trial for improving outcomes are Glow Caps (Cella, 2010). This system includes behavioral reminders, engages the social network, and provides feedback. It relies on sensors on pill bottles with a flasher device and back-up phone calls and e-mails.

Medication/Treatment Communicating System as
Health Capital Resource

A key feature of any medication adherence system is an online link that can be shared with case managers, physicians, and designated family members. The current MedSignals version can be set remotely, and uploads data using the home phone and Bluetooth technology. Caregivers, health providers, and/or researchers can monitor patterns. This real-time data feature can be important in spotting emerging cognitive issues signaled by repeated failure to respond appropriately, anticipating potential clinical problems related to medication errors, and alerting case managers to unanticipated admissions to healthcare facilities with prolonged failure to respond. As companies work to integrate medication adherence systems with personal health record systems such as Google Health and Microsoft HealthVault, the potential promise of personal health records may be realized more rapidly (see Chapter 4, Personal Health Records). The health professional working with the consumer patient will want to explore influences on the patient's choice. Charismatic websites or insistent significant others may have opinions that are not congruent with abilities and preferences of the consumer. However, at times of transition, such as immediately after discharge from a hospital, temporary options may need to be accepted that are not the consumer patient's first choice.

Adherence Communicating System as Research Capital

In addition, for researchers testing interventions, a networked reminder system will provide tracking of the fidelity of the intervention. It is rare that studies of innovations in behavioral therapy, trials of one new drug, or tests of health promotion strategies collect data on patterns of treatment adherence in real time that yield the most relevant explanation of results.

Study participants who improve on clinical outcome measures may be demonstrating a halo effect due more to better adherence to preexisting medication regimens than use of a new drug, new lifestyle habits, or counseling experiences. Conversely, participants in studies may believe that the activities or medications of the study protocol diminish the need for adhering to prestudy medication regimens. Simply abjuring participants to "continue with your usual medications" may be insufficient coaching. Therefore, failure to achieve study outcomes may be more related to changes in "unrelated" medication patterns than to the study protocol. A networked pill-communicating system would provide continuous data to put these potential patterns in perspective.

Future Developments in Medication Communication Devices

Liquid medication dispensers are rare, but becoming more available. A pouch system linked to a handheld device is an option for mobile consumers. Taking medication multiple times a day creates problems in terms of memory burden and keeping track of device location, and also carries a stigma for consumers engaged in activities outside the home. Ryder and Brue (2008) have tackled these issues in several ways.

The tracking problem is addressed by creating electronic, networked devices for adults and children that have GPS capacity. A tracking function might be equally useful in cluttered households. Neon colors were used for associated pouches that proved attractive to the children and served to reduce stigma. Adults also might wish artistic license in choosing the pouch appearance. The reminder protocols may be convertible to mobile phone applications. Linking medication communicating systems to mobile phones is in the spirit of ubiquitous and universal computing that minimizes stigma.

Over time, medication communication devices will become more intelligent. Burg (2009) describes plans for devices that have a physiological module and an ingestion module. He notes that current dispensers are based on a calendar that imposes a rigid routine, and this may account for adherence issues. This dual system would recognize physiological conditions or lifestyle "events" that may signal a change in medication timing.

Burg (2009) notes that the properties of a medication (physical, chemical, and biological) relate to the physiological condition of the body. Timing of meals is a major variable. Exercise or rest events are also important. Some medications should be taken on arising and others at time of sleep or prior to vigorous exercise. Changes in a physiological parameter, such as blood pressure or blood glucose level, may trigger a change in medication alert. When these changes occur has ramifications for fixed-time medications. Burg proposes a system that can recognize the potential of interaction between fixed-time medications and event-based medications and adjust dispensing accordingly. In his system, the programming would be set up to assign priorities to medications. Thus, a medication to be given at mealtimes might require adjustment of fixed-time medications when mealtime changes. Similarly, medications responsive to cardiac events would be given priority.

In a truly innovative adaptation, Burg (2009) proposes that a medication-communicating device could be connected to smart home networks and medical sensors. Motion detectors would track movement of the user, including operation of appliances that signal rest or meals. He proposes GPS links that would signal that the user is at a restaurant or heading away from a dispenser at a critical time. Finally, he hypothesizes that contact, motion, and photo sensors could detect the opening of microwave, refrigerator, and food cupboards signaling a meal event. Finally, Burg proposes that multiple benefits can be anticipated—for example, more effective medication action, fewer side effects, decreased drug–drug interactions and allergic responses, and accommodation to personal preferences and lifestyle variations.

EVERYDAY EXPERIENCE OF DIGITAL DEVICES

Individuals, families, and caregivers are confronted with an ever-increasing array of devices to promote sustained ability to live with dignity and to manage shifts in abilities and the burden of chronic illness. An "everyday experience"

Table 5.7   Everyday Experience as Factor in Device Adoption

Meaning to individual if device is adopted:
- Enjoyment of device interaction
- Importance of supported activity
- Contribution to level of desired independence and control
- Time/energy freed for personal priorities
- Message implied about physical, social, and emotional health status
- Preferred self-image in context of cultural norms
- Functionally defined time frames (idiosyncratic)
- Financial commitment: reimbursement prospects and related sacrifices
- Evidence of effectiveness: research, testimonials, professional endorsements, personal experience

Installation and learning curve: Effort expectancies
- Complexity and burden of choosing from alternatives
- Installation options and burdens
- Availability of on-site setup
- Training requirements
- Degree of intrusiveness: space allocation, socioemotional impact, financial

Performance expectancy variables
- Usability or user-friendliness of the interface
- Effectiveness given user vision, coordination, cognitive status
- Literacy demands: linguistic, numeracy, verbal, visual
- Privacy protections and risks
- Reliability of performance: self-healing systems, power failure protection
- Interoperability with devices and interfaces currently in use

Sustainability over time: Facilitating factors
- Efficiency and effectiveness of completing target tasks
- Integration with health habitat: self-care, agency practices, provider links
- Congruence with anticipated meaning
- Cognitive load: instantaneous, cumulative

Table 5.7   Everyday Experience as Factor in Device Adoption (*continued*)

- Comfort and physical demands: fatigue, capability stretch, portability
- Robustness to noise: mental, technical, auditory
- Obsolescence curve
- Access to technical support: 24/7, platform (live, chat, e-mail), language
- Social network engagement: invited, required
- Continued economic feasibility
- Evidence of effectiveness of device
- Payment process burden: self-pay or reimbursement requirements

Source: Adapted from Pape et al., 2002; Tonet et al., 2008; Venkatesh et al., 2003.

approach takes into account the meaning of each device, installation and learning curve or effort expectancies, performance expectancy variables, and factors that facilitate sustainability over time (see Table 5.7).

Reviewing in advance four everyday experience aspects of device adoption may increase the likelihood of sustained, effective use. The goal is to minimize abandonment or "discontinuance" of devices that have continued potential and for which the expense of dollars and effort have been incurred. The meaning of the device to the individual, the installation and learning curve effort, performance expectancy, and factors affecting sustainability over time are variables worth considering. The list of factors related to device adoption has been accumulated on the basis of a review of the literature and the author's experiences at a professional and personal level.

Meaning to the Individual

- Contribution to level of desired independence and control
- Time and energy freed for personal priorities
- Enjoyment of device interaction
- Message implied about physical, social, and emotional health status
- Preferred self-image in context of cultural norms
- Functionally defined time frames (idiosyncratic)
- Financial commitment: Reimbursement potential and related sacrifices
- Evidence of effectiveness: Research, testimonials, professional endorsements, personal experience

Devices may come into play for a variety of reasons—it can be a need or desire experienced by the consumer or a recommendation by a family member, caregiver, or a healthcare professional. In any case, it is individuals who make sense of the device from their unique perspective and circumstances. One assessment is the contribution to the level of desired independence and control. Devices that are very complex to operate or have a steep learning curve may create such a strong initial frustration that adoption is unlikely. Mobile phones with multiple options but complex operating instructions are one example. However, if the phone provides a reminder system that decreases reliance on others, this barrier may be willingly surmounted. So understanding the consumer's level of desired independence is critical.

It is useful to appreciate that consumers may be very eager to be independent in managing basic activities of daily living, but minimally motivated to acquire independence in interfacing with digital devices. Older adults, in particular, may be content to let someone else manipulate interaction with electronic devices, including computers. Such individuals may be willing to give up control over small details, such as choice of browser, access device (voice, mouse), and more critical aspects such as privacy and confidentiality. The technical assistant may gain access to passwords and personal information that create an unintended vulnerability.

In building the case for adopting a new device, information on how use of the device will free time and energy for other activities that are a high priority can be motivating. The advocate (family, caregiver, provider) may have a priority for improved blood sugar control or less frequent middle-of-the-night appeals for assistance. If these are not priorities for the consumer, there is a risk of discontinuance. Linking device use to personal priorities is key.

Closely related to this dimension is enjoyment of device interaction. Enjoyment of the interaction is a function of the usability. Another important dimension of adopting and continuing the use of a device is the message implied about physical, social, and emotional health status.

The case of the hearing aid provides a useful example. A leading expert, Dr. Robert Jackler, chair of otolaryngology at Stanford University School of Medicine, noted that adopting a hearing aid means you "lose 30 IQ points and age 20 years" (as cited in Fuoco, 2006, para. 2). However, he and other experts cited in the news article suggest that as Bluetooth, MP3 players, and other devices become prominent, the stigma of a hearing aid will diminish.

A properly designed earpiece for a hearing aid could link socioemotionally to technology embraced by young adults. These shifts in social image of device use are closely related to understanding the individual's preferred self-image in the context of cultural norms.

For some adults in the American consumer culture, affiliating with images of younger people fosters attempts to adopt new technology. Some devices, such as those used in Wii gaming, have had great appeal across the life span. However, some of the Wii games have been associated with injuries, for older adults in particular. Margo Apostolos (personal communication, October 10, 2009), professor of dance at the University of Southern California and consultant on dance medicine, notes that some older adults feel compelled to compete with younger players and sustain injuries of overcompensation for diminished abilities and sustained overexertion.

Another dimension to consider is the functionally defined time frame, which is idiosyncratic to the person and device. Time has the dimension of minutes passed and perceived interval elapsed. In some cases, devices save time in accomplishing routine tasks and free up time for more pleasurable occupations. Many adults summarize their lives as "too busy" to take on another thing and that specifically includes learning to use a new device.

Appreciating not only minutes saved but the perception of newly available time can be meaningful for consumers and those with whom they interact. For example, Intel's Proactive Health Lab (Intel, 2007) identified the potential of sensors to provide peace of mind for caregivers who could nap or do other activities while counting on monitoring devices for safety alerts.

Financial Commitment

Financial commitment is another swing vote factor in adoption of a device. Cost of devices relates to purchase, installation, maintenance/subscription, and payer. For some devices the initial outlay can be quite expensive, especially if the individual is buying multiple devices to sustain a particular level of independence.

Some digital devices require a subscription in addition to initial installation costs. For example, the MedSignals device (https://www.medsignals.com/HowToOrder.aspx) with only six medications is $49 for the device and setup, and requires a $29/month subscription to the online service. The Bodywear fit sensor for calculating calorie burn, number of steps, and minutes exercised has an Internet analysis feature also and requires initial device purchase, a monthly subscription and, for on-the-spot readings, an extra wrist display.

Reimbursement for costs incurred is a major factor. At present, programs are not reimbursed by insurance plans or Medicare. (See the tables on the barriers/benefits matrix in Appendix 5-A.) The companies offering the devices suggest that savings are sufficient to justify reimbursement. See https://www.medsignals.com/Providers.aspx for the rationale and links to relevant studies supporting cost savings.

Similar cases for cost savings are being made for digital games by promoting the "game-care" revolution (Brown, 2008). As these devices build links to personal health records (see Chapter 4) adopted by consumers, their cost-effectiveness may become more accepted.

For providers, the evidence of effectiveness based on research may be the critical element. However, in many instances, this data is lacking or is scattered.

Joseph Kvedar (2009), a well-known expert on connected health, summarizes the dilemma:

> The question we should be asking is not whether it is valuable, but rather how does it compare to other monitoring tools such as phone-based outreach (disease management) and intensive clinic-based monitoring. These questions should form the substrate for the next wave of research on telemonitoring. (Kvedar, para. 8)

For consumers and professionals, testimonials and professional endorsements can be very motivating and supersede ambiguous or conflicting research if the source is respected. Dishman (2007) suggests that trust is built when a device is supplied by a well-known brand or has third-party certification. Personal experiences with similar devices, whether satisfactory or frustrating, can be a lever in making a case for considering a new device or updated version.

Installation and Learning Curve: Effort Expectancies

- Complexity and burden of choosing from alternatives
- Degree of intrusiveness: space allocation, socioemotional impact, financial demands
- Installation options and burdens
- Training requirements

Complexity and Burden of Choosing from Alternatives

Once an individual is persuaded to try a new or updated device, the next level of variables that affect actual adoption relates to the installation requirements, including the learning curve. The decision-making process requires a review of alternatives. In some cases, this is a choice of continuing with the present situation with no facilitating devices or examination of potential resources. The healthcare provider may recommend some products and services. Alternatively, the consumer, caregiver, or family members may share informal referrals from their social network or experience. Some of the involved stakeholders may receive information from newsletters or magazines, support groups, or from surfing the Internet.

For some individuals and/or families, the complexity and burden of making choices may be overwhelming. There is the issue of the range of items, a concern about whether choices have been exhaustively reviewed, and then matching preferences with availability. For some stakeholders, press releases and stories of ongoing research may create problems as highly desirable options may not yet be available to the public. Joining condition-relevant online groups (see http://www.patientslikeme.com) and subscribing to newsletters may provide advance notice of new products or may lead to invitations to test pilot versions. However, in many instances, an overview of the elements of meaning, effort, performance, and sustainability as a first step may help to narrow options (refer to Table 5.7).

Intrusiveness as Influence

Intrusiveness is a decision factor that does get attention in the literature (Dishman, 2007; Vanderheiden, 2007). Intrusiveness has multiple dimensions. There is the literal issue of space allocation—the footprint—or physical area required to add the device to one's life. This is an issue: whether the user must carry the item on his or her person, attach it to an existing device, or give it table, wall, or floor space. The individual may have multiple constraints with respect to finding a place for the device.

Assessment of demands of interacting with the device in relation to its location is critical. Common kitchen wisdom has a role here—if the appliance is not visible or if other items have to be moved to access it, use is unlikely. Manufacturers enticed cooks to put blenders—and later, chopping machines—on the counter to increase routinizing use. This maxim motivates designers to develop devices that operate passively. This means that the device is somewhat "intelligent" and requires only installation, calibration, and occasional monitoring. Information is gathered without a human interface and actions are triggered based on data.

Intrusiveness is also related to the extent to which others in the environment are cued to a disability (Vanderheiden, 2007). For this reason, some assistive devices are packaged as jewelry or built into glasses or clothing that provide a hidden display of information. The rapid advances in the capacity of mobile phones and the associated Bluetooth technology have contributed to minimizing alerting other people to diminished capacities that are supported by devices. Universal design and ubiquitous computing advances has meant that clever digital jewelry, wearable computing, and multifunction cell phones are sought by people of all ages and capacities. Socioemotional intrusiveness is equally important. To the extent that the device signals illness, weakness, or disability, full adoption is at risk. In some cases, minimizing size is key, in other instances adding color and aesthetic dimensions highlights interest and can be a conversation starter over stigma.

Designers overcome dilemmas of stigma by universal computing and user-centered designs (Morales Rodriguez et al., 2007). Universal computing is a strategy where digital devices and applications are designed to benefit all potential users. Designs are not targeted to the "old" or "disabled," but to anyone who might enjoy the enhancements to their lives. User-centered design is a strategy that brings potential consumers into the process much earlier than has happened in the past. Morales Rodriguez et al. propose that early engagement enhances the product design, builds a marketing advantage, and speeds adoption by wider audiences. Participant evaluation of smart home installations indicates that some older adults found the technology was not intrusive (Demiris, Oliver, Dickey, Skubic, & Rantz, 2008). Too often, family members and professionals make decisions about the intrusiveness of technology without giving older adults the opportunity to make decisions for themselves.

Financial Demands

Financial demands can be an element of intrusiveness if the consumer must make multiple payments, is pestered by frequent calls to upgrade for new features, or payers change reimbursement plans. Reimbursement from Medicaid or private insurance for expenses may have eligibility issues and process issues. If the paperwork is complex, and monthly maintenance or a subscription is required, the burden may be discouraging.

In some cases, it is not easily apparent that a monthly maintenance or subscription is required. In other cases, it is easy to misconstrue costs. For example, one major body sensor site offers a package price that makes it look like one is acquiring an annual subscription bundled into the initial cost. Instead, by paying the package price, one gets a discount for a year and a monthly cost is incurred—albeit "reduced."

Installation and Maintenance Options and Burdens

Installation and maintenance options and burdens can make or break the adoption process. Too often devices have such complex setup requirements that users return or shelve the device. Horrigan (2007) in a Pew Internet Study reports that even individuals who consider themselves somewhat tech savvy require assistance. Here, the Intel design principles (Dishman, 2007) are key for those developing or recommending new devices—keep it simple and build on the way existing devices work (Table 5.8).

Table 5.8   Health Technology Design Principles: Intel

1. *Create nonintrusive technology.* Intel's research found that technologies such as alarms and security cameras are quickly abandoned by users because they disrupt people's normal routines and make them feel uncomfortable at home.
2. *Provide enough (but not too much) support.* Help users to accomplish tasks without making them reliant on technology for things they could do themselves.
3. *Build on existing metaphors of how things work.* People are more likely to use new technology if it comes in the form of a familiar device, such as a remote control.

Table 5.8   Health Technology Design Principles: Intel (*continued*)

> **4. *Keep it simple.*** Use one-mode/one-function devices when possible (e.g., a wall-mounted CD player that plays when a user pulls a string).
>
> **5. *Foster trust.*** A device from a well-known brand or with independent, third-party certification will have a greater chance of being adopted.
>
> **6. *Adapt to changing needs.*** As people age and change, so do their needs (in the case of Alzheimer's disease, needs can change weekly or even daily). Technology should adjust in response.
>
> **7. *Don't stigmatize.*** Design devices that anyone, not just an older or disabled person, might use. (For instance, Intel designers are experimenting with a pill box and reminder system disguised as jewelry.)
>
> **8. *Facilitate, don't replace, social connections with technology.*** Focus on concepts that foster connection, rather than technology that replaces social interaction (e.g., virtual worlds).

Source: Dishman, 2007. Used with permission.

An example is the model of the remote control adopted for the Wii compared to the complex, multifunction, winged structure controller device for the Playstation. Setup instructions that provide a "quick start" minimize installation burdens. For some devices, availability of onsite setup is key. In this case, a technician from the company or healthcare agency or someone in the social network comes to the place where the device will be used. Alternatively, the device may be brought to a central location where installation takes place and the features are demonstrated. This option is so attractive that one cruise line offers an electronics concierge (Associated Press, 2009).

It is key that the user "returns the demonstration." Too often the technical expert whizzes through the process, holding the device and "showing" the user. As the advocate for the consumer, the health professional might "prescribe" three trials as part of the setup. In some cases, it is helpful to have the user him- or herself write down what to do if the device does not function as expected. Similarly, agreement on where the help line phone number will be kept should be determined and who in the social network will have the backup number.

Training Requirements

Training requirements are poorly understood with respect to technology for adults. Understanding the interaction between humans and adults as an information process provides a useful framework (Czaja et al., 2006). In this model, tasks related to device use can be analyzed in terms of the abilities required (Table 5.9).

The selection of the device itself requires the ability to choose from among competing options. In some cases, adults with minimal technical literacy or experience may opt to defer this choice to an "expert."

The next step is to search for the relevant operating instructions and display the information; this requires good working memory and both field scanning and focused attention. Ideally, the instructions are in a preferred language, supported by graphics that cue steps in sequence and are quickly mastered without recourse to a complicated manual. It is interesting to note how many of the device-based games, such as Wii, have minimal printed manuals and rely on verbal and visual cues given after turning on the application.

Selecting responses to proceed with installation and use or to customize an application may require some motor coordination. Beginning use of the device will require recalling commands and procedures, working memory, and having some linguistic literacy. Deciding on next steps, or termination, will require filtering noise, recognizing loops and endings, and coping with unanticipated or undesirable events.

Table 5.9 Human Technology Interaction: Information-Processing Tasks and Abilities

Tasks	Abilities
Choose appropriate device	Choosing among competing options
Search for relevant operating information	Working memory
Display information as needed	Attention: focused and field scanning
Select responses	Motor coordination
Recall commands and procedures	Linguistic literacy
Execute response	Visual literacy
Decide on termination or next steps	Filtering noise: auditory, cognitive, fatigue Recognizing loops and endings Coping with unanticipated or undesirable events

As adults and younger people interact around technology, it becomes clearer that differences in their introduction and experience can be vast in their implications. Aarsand (2007) discusses intergenerational differences as both a challenge and resource. For example, it is clear that older adults usually approach playing games in terms of clock minutes elapsed, and children think of their interaction with games in terms of achieving levels of accomplishment. Individualizing training for adults might consider whether the adult learner would commit to achieving a level of success, rather than setting a time commitment.

Alternatively, the coach would look at the requirements of the device and its tasks and suggest one task or level. For example, "In this session, let us focus on adding new names to the directory in your social alarm system." Device coaches often fail to set and agree on objectives for a session. Also, there is a great temptation when the learner achieves one goal to slip in another. The risk is that the adult learner will feel overwhelmed and end a training session in frustration rather than triumph over mastering a task. Proposing a break to walk around with long looks into the distance allows relaxation of eyes and limbs and enjoyment of success. Scheduling of the next session can be renegotiated.

Coaches who are experts might keep in mind the risk that the learner believes he or she needs to please or compete with the coach. These expectations could lead to sustained participation past the point of mental or physical fatigue. A coach who calls for a break for him- or herself models good practice and grants permission for calling a halt.

One question that arises is how to organize training. The goal is to have safe, efficient interaction with the myriad of technological advancements that are part of accomplishing activities of daily living, communicating with family and friends, and managing the increasing expectation of self-care for chronic illness. Hickman, Rogers, and Fisk (2007) note that training programs are differentially effective for younger and older adults. Their work suggests that the goal is to be able to use the system without instructional materials and to develop skills and insights that generalize to other tasks. Hickman et al. discuss two strategies: *guided action training* and *guided attention training* (Table 5.10).

They found that overall, *guided attention training* was better than *guided action training* for both younger and older adults.

Performance Expectancy Variables

Another dilemma is the pattern of advertisers who market devices as "easy"—having minimal demands on the user—when inventorying steps reflects the opposite (Rogers, Mykityshyn, Campbell, & Fisk, 2001). The expectation set by

Table 5.10   Approaches to Technology Training for Adults: Action and Attention Models

Guided Action
Strategy is to tell which steps to perform and in what order.

Training terms:
• Click, press, wait, click up arrow to X position, click choice A, click finish or done
Situation:
• Best when step-by-step instructions available or actually attached to device
• Suited to situations where interaction with the device is temporary (e.g., diagnostic procedures, determining preference for one device over another)
Benefit/risk:
• Reduced demand on working memory capacity
• Risk is that task is not learned but simply performed in steps

Guided Attention
Strategy is to coach on where to focus attention, but this requires active determination of what to do for each step.

Training terms:
• Select the appropriate tool, adjust and select type or level, complete task
Situation:
• Instructions are lost or need retrieval
• Suited to tasks where generalization will promote independence in adopting other devices
Benefits/risks:
• Older adults increase accuracy and completion time
• Younger adults increase task completion
• May benefit older adults more than younger
• Demands working memory capacity

Source: Adapted from Hickman et al., 2007.

the promotional materials, the researchers argue, leads potential users to blame themselves when things go wrong. Variables to consider are:

• Tasks or links the device will accomplish, trigger, or manage
• The usability or user-friendliness of the interface
• Accommodation for user vision, coordination, cognitive status
• Literacy demands: linguistic, numeracy, verbal, visual
• Privacy protections and risks
• Reliability of performance: self-healing systems, power failure protection
• Interoperability with devices and interfaces currently in use

Figure 5.3   User-Design Experience

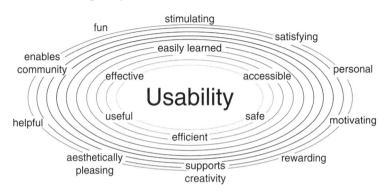

Source: Dishman, 2007. Used with permission.

Performance expectancy is a dimension of the UTAT model (Venkatesh et al., 2003) that speaks to what the user anticipates will be his or her experience in using the new device. This encompasses the tasks the device will accomplish or facilitate, or the links the device may trigger or manage. Some devices will actually do a task, such as reading blood glucose level, counting steps or minutes, or taking photos. Other devices such as the laser-guided walker (Matthews et al., 2007) assist the individual in the task of safe locomotion. Usability or user-friendliness has been elegantly defined for Intel by Dishman (2007) (Figure 5.3).

At the core, the device should be functional: effective, easily learned, useful, efficient, accessible, and safe. The affective dimensions include a user experience that is fun, stimulating, satisfying, personal, motivating, rewarding, aesthetically pleasing, supports creativity, is helpful, and enables community. The health professional or social network supporter who knows the user well can use these indicators to assist the potential user in choosing among alternatives and perceiving the learning curve demands as worth the effort. These user-centered indicators would be useful review criteria for experts creating lists of devices for comparison purposes. In preparing for this book, the author found multiple instances of presentation of the functional aspects in the device literature. However, the affective dimensions are rarely addressed in the professional literature on devices linked to digital technology.

Responsiveness

An indicator of performance is responsiveness or *accommodation* to *variations in visual acuity, coordination, and cognitive status.* As adults age, the size of font for labeling features becomes more important. The ability to select a font or built-in font can be critical if the user cannot easily memorize the position of buttons or keys. Coordination becomes a factor as devices become more miniaturized and ability to activate features is more difficult, especially when tremor is present. One implication of declines in cognitive status (working memory and executive function) is changed ability to learn new multi-step skills. Health professionals will want to assess the demands of potential devices in the context of the abilities of users. Some devices require more extensive working memory than others, since activating features require multiple steps, such as for digital devices that monitor blood glucose levels.

Literacy Demands

A persistent challenge in reducing disparities of the digital divide is the complex literacy demands of emerging devices. Literacy is discussed in detail in Chapter 2. One overt feature is the extent to which users with different linguistic literacies can interface with the device. As adults suffer symptoms of chronic disease or declines related to aging, the likelihood of having a caregiver or assistant with limited skill in the dominant language of the country increases. This is particularly the case in the Western world where immigrants take on minimum wage jobs, such as nursing assistants and home health aides. The ideal device would be functional for multiple language users.

Increasingly, numeracy is a form of capital required for self-management of rehabilitation from injury or surgery, prevention of deterioration with chronic illness, and health promotion lifestyle changes. Abilities such as tracking time and number with medication doses, tracking treatment regimens, interpreting patterns of responses, setting schedules, and other numeric skills are increasingly important.

Verbal literacy has also gained in importance. Individuals and their significant others and caregivers need to be articulate in written and spoken communication as the demands on health professionals' time increases. The ability to read, comprehend, and apply messages related to installation, maintenance, and use of devices, as well as related decision parameters, is of central importance as self-care expectations mount across the life span.

Finally, there are new demands for visual literacy (Metros, 2008). Digital devices often require interfacing between a website and the device. To get maximum performance, skills identified by Metros are required (see Chapter 2 for details). For example, the user must be able to decode and interpret visuals, since the instructions that accompany a device increasingly use visuals to minimize the demands of linguistic compatibility. The consumer may be viewing visuals posted by other users to document their experience with a device. Becoming an informed critic who can judge accuracy and validity of an image increases functionality and impact of web-linked devices. In some cases, "consumer" patients may be asked to supply meaningful visuals to document their current situation and progress.

Privacy Protection and Risk for Consumers

Consumers are admonished to be careful about privacy protection and risk as they navigate the digital world. Devices that do passive monitoring can lull the user into decreased vigilance. Whether active or passive, it is important that the user and social network appreciate the risks to confidentiality and to impartiality of relationships when device-gathered data is freely shared on social networking sites. Health professionals who request or require that patients post data gathered by devices to the Internet have a responsibility to explain risks and to provide coaching on setting and reviewing privacy statements periodically.

Consumer willingness to share device data should vary with their ability to manage their own care. As consumers gain independence after traumas, hospitalizations, and other debilitating episodes, transparency in privacy settings may no longer be appropriate; the number of people with access to data and the frequency of data sharing may become more restricted.

The meaning of HIPAA compatibility needs to be carefully explained. For example, devices that purport to assist travelers by compressing data on portable devices can be "compatible" if the user gives permission to transmit the data to the device. How protected the data will be if the device is lost or information uploaded to commercial websites is not clear from the "compatibility" label (see Chapter 4). Performance expectancy is also assessed by how vulnerable the individual will be in a power failure—what backup is provided and how dependent is the backup on consumer monitoring of battery power or other actions such as activating online backups? An ideal digital device will be protected in a self-healing system. This kind of system reads patterns or breaks and automatically implements fixes.

Interoperability with devices and interfaces currently in use is a goal with paradoxical consequences. On the one hand, consumers, professionals, and members of the social network would value the ability to exchange data that is not hampered by variations in browsers, operating systems, or other parameters of a device and its data functions. On the other hand, the Intel design principles (Dishman, 2007) would caution against building ever-increasing complexity at the cost of compatibility (refer to Table 5.9).

In some cases, consumers will be tolerant of stand-alone functionality if the device truly provides passive monitoring or duplicates only one or two features of another device. To some extent this may be a function of generational cohort. The iPod Touch device, for example, is highly popular, but it is not a cell phone. Thus, users must carry two devices. For younger people, this trade-off may be acceptable. For older adults, learning two systems may be sufficiently stressful to impede sustained use of a new device.

The issue of browser incompatibility cannot be ignored. Safari, preferred by MAC users, and Mozilla Firefox, preferred by tech experts, simply do not interface with some Web-based applications. In some instances, it is not obvious to the new user of a device with a Web link that the browser is the issue. In some cases, the device company offers a work-around. However, often the user must adapt to the company's default.

Sustainability over Time: Factors Facilitating Continued Use

- Efficiency and effectiveness of completing target tasks
- Evidence of effectiveness of device
- Aesthetic dimensions or usability
- Integration with health habitat: Self-care, agency practices, provider links
- Congruence with anticipated meaning
- Cognitive load: Instantaneous, cumulative
- Comfort (physical demands): Fatigue, capability stretch, portability
- Robustness to noise: Mental, technical, auditory
- Obsolescence curve
- Access to sociotechnical capital (technical assistance): 24/7, platform (live, chat, e-mail), language, and costs of access
- Social network engagement: Invited and required
- Continued economic feasibility
- Limited need for intervention by others
- Payment process burden: Self-pay or reimbursement requirements

Sustainability of adoption over time is essentially a composite of the everyday experiences previously discussed. However, it may be useful to examine these from the perspective of having made the decision to use the device, installed it, and being in the phase of mastery verging on routine use. The consumer has the device in place, can use core features, and has practiced use extensively. It is not possible to rank the indicators that might universally predict or compromise sustainability as these will be highly individualized and sensitive to the context of *influences*, especially during *transitions*.

Efficiency and Effectiveness

Efficiency and effectiveness of completing target tasks and evidence of effectiveness of device are closely related but different aspects of sustainability. In the first case, the user develops a perception of how convenient the device is for the completion of the desired task and how well it works. To some extent, this can be highly subjective, and effectiveness, in particular, can be highly influenced not only by functional usability but by affective dimensions of usability (refer to Figure 5.3).

A device that is fun, builds community, and supports creativity, for example, might be rated highly by the user. However, with respect to health applications, evidence of effectiveness will need to be congruent with functional standards for achieving health promotion goals and managing rehabilitation or chronic illnesses. In this case, the consumer, his or her caregivers, and family will have an advantage if they work out outcomes and evidence in advance with the relevant health professional.

For those who are targeting increased physical activity, this might call for a device that documents minutes expended and pulse rate in a format that is interoperable (can be shared) with the electronic health record used by the healthcare agency. Then, clinical outcomes can be assessed in the context of behaviors, which enables targeted coaching to sustain results or improve outcomes. Similarly, for managing diabetes, devices that track, upload, and trend blood glucose readings with other lifestyle behaviors can decrease diabetes-related complications.

Aesthetic and Social Dimensions

As noted under performance expectancy, aesthetic dimensions, and usability, the twofold nature of usability includes function as covered above under effectiveness/efficiency but also the affective dimensions. Quality of life is a closely related concept. Too often its measurement is limited to social, mental, and physical aspects of living. The dimensions in the Dishman (2007) model may be the most powerful predictors of continued use. Measures of these aspects in terms of digital devices are not known to the author. However, intuitively, dimensions with an emotional, artistic component could be powerful. (See factors such as a perceived sense of the helpfulness of the device, its support for creativity, and other affective aspects displayed in Figure 5.3.)

Using the Health Habitat

Integration with health habitat—self-care, social network, agency practices, provider links—is another predictor often ignored. The health habitat

(Jordan-Marsh, 2008) is the constellation of environments, networks, and resources that support the individual in meeting goals of survival and intent to thrive. To the extent that a device or collection of devices facilitates the individual's expectations and hope for independence (self-care), continued use is likely. In some instances, as noted by Vanderheiden (2007), the external observer may make different assessments of the contribution to self-care. The user may opt for less independence and greater speed in routine life tasks so that time is freed up for more rewarding activities.

Social Network Norm Setting and Integration

If one's social network—including formal and informal connections—relies heavily on digital devices to communicate, accomplish goals, and organize life, then each member is more likely to persist in using a device that may not be perfect. The network of digital users creates value for persisting with a device and sets an expectation that the savvy member will be a compliant user. Agencies important to the user will need to adapt their practices to accept input from the devices that support health. Increasingly, this will be done through a personal health record interface. Similarly, as games with their devices become a more routine part of healthcare regimens (Brown, 2009), patience with gaming devices will increase. As companies like Intel and GE move forward with collaborations (Intel, 2009), agencies will adapt their practices to accommodate the active and passive monitoring made possible by new software and new devices.

Congruence with anticipated meaning may be a make-or-break factor that is difficult for someone else to resolve with a dissatisfied user. This makes it important to set realistic expectations from the start. Scherer, Sax, Vanbierbliet, Cushman, and Scherer (2005) have developed an assessment of the match between the person and technology. This team reports that the tool has been validated with disabled people, has good reliability and validity, and is used in the United States, Canada, and Europe. The structure of the underlying model is such that it need not be limited to use with persons with disabilities.

The Importance of Cognitive Load

To some extent, congruence with meaning might be affected strongly by the cognitive load, which can be instantaneous or cumulative. Instantaneous load refers to transparency or complexity in starting to use a device. Cumulative load relates to the additive demands of paying attention to a task even when the neuromuscular requirements are minimal. Interacting with some devices requires great skill in concentration and repeated, timed interactions that might be immediately required and exhausting. Other devices might simply be tiring over time. An example could be body-sensor technology that requires hand entry of many variables in multiple screens. The potential for outright fatigue is such that emerging systems are designed to collect as much data as possible passively and to upload it with minimal key strokes and attention. In some cases, it is the setup that is exhausting as the user must go through multiple screens to enter baseline data and preferences. Error detection systems that require multiple rule-outs and trials of potential solutions are equally burdensome and discouraging. As devices are reviewed for recommendations, understanding the extent to which the software is self-healing is critical.

Cognitive load is appreciably diminished if the user finds interacting with the device makes minimal physical demands and summarizes the experience as comfortable. A device that is awkward to hold or hard to reach to change settings or requires heavy keyboarding creates physical fatigue and may create safety hazards as well. Few adults are aware of the desirability of tailoring keyboard style to their body frame and that simply downsizing a keyboard may make a great difference in comfort. So-called ergonomic keyboards come in many different styles that can minimize fatigue. Consumers can also examine whether they are more comfortable on a laptop versus a desktop; for someone with a smaller frame, the smaller laptop keyboard may be a good match.

In selecting a new keyboard, it is important to arrange a sufficient trial period as there is a learning curve. The University of Wisconsin—Milwaukee Rehabilitation Research Design and Disability Center has many projects related to accessibility (Rehabilitation Research Design and Disability Center, 2009). Other centers are the Assistive Technology Resource Center at Colorado State University (Colorado State University, 2009) and the Adaptive Technology Resource Centre (ATRC) at the University of Toronto (Adaptive Technology Resource Centre, 2009). A starting point for those new to using digital devices is the Technical Glossary at the ATRC. The glossary explains terms and has links to photos and related websites. The site covers alternative keyboards, alternative mouse, PDAs, electronic appliance controllers, Braille embossing, and signing avatars.

Comfort Matters

Comfort relates to the extent to which using the device is perceived to extend one's capabilities or stretches them in an unpleasant or frustrating manner. Portability is also an issue, particularly for adults who spend large amounts of time in a variety of environments.

Closely related to comfort is the robustness of the device to noise. Noise can take the form of mental distractions that interfere with the ability to concentrate. Screens that continuously interrupt to offer new options are an example of mental noise that increases cognitive load. Technical noise refers to extra pulses that are not specific to the task signal in digital devices. This kind of noise can create interference with the operation of other devices in the vicinity. Similarly, existing devices can create noise that distorts reception and transmission of signals in new devices. Good design of digital devices can be defeated if protection from this potential is not addressed. Even if the technical noise is infrequent, the unpredictability and irritation factor may diminish intent to continue with a device. In some cases, careful subtraction of devices must be carried out to see which device is the offender. Auditory noise is an unfortunate side effect of many digital devices—from the click of keyboard use to a low-volume hum. Some users adapt readily to this auditory intrusion, but others in the environment object to the point where discontinuance becomes a peace-keeping option.

The obsolescence curve refers to the speed with which a manufacturer declares a device or software application unworthy of continued support. This has become a major issue in gaming where devices and software must be adapted for the physical limitations of the user. Purchasing the kit that allows adaptation might be $250,000. This pricing scheme is targeted to companies that expect to reap large profits from games made for the major commercial platforms. However, there are no resources at present that cover the costs of these essential kits and no interest in creating accessibility on the part of Sony, Microsoft, and other major game device manufacturers. Finding someone to adapt a painstakingly built work-around one more time may be a barrier that leads to discontinuation.

In fact, as indicated earlier, access to sociotechnical capital (technical assistance) is important to a wide range of users. Technical assistance may come from the social network of friends, family, or neighbors, or from volunteer organizations, or it may be part of the device purchase or subscription. Adults new to technology may need coaching on the meaning of 24/7 access as their informal supports may not be available at extremes of the day. Similarly, learning how and when to use e-mail avenues, live chat through an Internet link, and telephone support can be empowering, especially when a decision to discontinue is under consideration due to unresolved problems.

Consumers need to be alerted to the risks of allowing the remote technician to access files, the advantages of saving applets that facilitate connection, saving purchase records with key access data, tracking the name or identifier of the technician, and preserving case numbers assigned by the service.

The act of interfacing with a device and the related support needed when a problem arises relies heavily on language and costs of access. For individuals who use English as a second language, interfacing with technical support can be cumbersome. Often e-mail or live chat facilitates communication as unfamiliar accents can distort perception of a word; written communication allows the sender and receiver to do a quick lookup if a word seems out of context or is unknown. Further, e-mail allows the user to send off the problem and do something else while waiting for the reply, whereas live chat and telephone support require a willingness and ability to sit for long periods as problem solving occurs. The advantage, however, is a quick trial of solutions offered and feedback to the technician. The cost of access in this context is both the energy and stress involved in securing a technician and then presenting the problem and trying solutions. Other costs relate to whether there is a charge by incident, minutes of contact, or an open subscription for a defined period of time. Individuals naïve to digital devices may be tempted to delay seeking assistance and inadvertently let the free support elapse.

Social Networking

The importance of social network engagement is increasingly recognized in mental and physical health. The evidence for this factor is discussed in the Chapter 2 overview of online engagement with the Internet. For device users, an important dimension is whether the engagement is invited versus required. In this instance, the network is assumed to include friends, family, neighbors, and professionals. If another person is required to use the device or to read trends and interpret findings, this creates a stress on the user.

If assistance is not readily available or is very unresponsive once accessed, users may discontinue using the device. On the other hand, if the device simplifies social contact or presence, such as the "presence amp" described by Intel (Dishman, 2007) or the telephones and doorbell links that display photos, adoption and use will be sustained. In some instances, if another person is required, use might be sustained as the system is highly functional for that person. This could be the case with activity-monitoring software that is set up by the caregiver so he or she can nap or engage in personally distinct activities, confident he or she will be alerted to any problems.

Correspondingly, if a user finds he or she cannot start or engage with a device without intervention by someone else, levels of use may rapidly diminish. A mobile phone device, for example, that is too complex in its functions and not intuitive might require continual coaching and direction. Over time, both the coach and the user may become sufficiently frustrated to sacrifice new and enriching options for simpler management.

If an intervention by another person in the social network is required to start or sustain device use, this is likely to decrease probability of sustained interaction. In many instances, members of the social network of seniors and the chronically ill will find increased peace of mind and lessened burden in caregiving as new devices emerge. That is, if the device is reliable, it can be mastered, integrated into existing self-care and home care arrangements, and if external technical assistance is available. If any one of these variables does not materialize or breaks down, the technical assistance burden is increased. As one student put it, "Now my grandmother is after me by phone, e-mail, and fax all day long!"

On the other hand, Pape (2002) notes that if persistent problems occur with a device intended to sustain the social network, the resulting frustration may promote social withdrawal. The risk of a self-perpetuating cycle of isolation is great if the device has been the fulcrum or mechanic by which social connections occur. Specifically assessing for social network connectivity is a critical variable in the contemporary clinical repertoire.

Continued economic feasibility is a dynamic variable that may be related to the overall economy. If government resources for health-related items shrink, individuals and families may find they are no longer reimbursed for items previously acceptable. Alternatively, the reimbursement process may slow to creating an unacceptable cash flow burden. Payment processes themselves may compromise long-term use. The burden of making payments or seeking reimbursement will be an important factor in sustained adoption. For some consumers, being able to make one payment versus having to track accuracy of billing for subscriptions and maintenance may be a critical factor. The more automatic, the less the everyday burden, but the more important that a review process is in place. There is always the risk of double billing or continued billing for a device no longer in use.

SUMMARY AND CONCLUSIONS

This is a field in which advances are rapid, with dramatic announcements of pilot projects. For this reason, the complementary website to the book will be updated periodically. However, a major issue is bringing exciting projects to a market that has the resources to take advantage of new products. As indicated in this chapter, tremendous capital must be available to the consumer even after the venture capital has been spent. *Economic capital* is a major issue and requires attention to whether government or private insurance will cover outright dollar costs. Device costs usually include purchase, maintenance, and subscription expenditures. Sociotechnical capital is required such that the device and user connect with social network and healthcare providers as required for optimal outcomes. Human capital is often a challenge as multiple forms of literacy are required to engage with digital devices and to take advantage of the events that devices can trigger and of the data that devices can supply. Finally, social capital is required to survive installation and early use and the frustrations of inevitable breakdowns and confusions.

The whole device picture is complicated by a pattern noted by the World Health Organization (cited in Martin et al., 2008) where adoption of digital technology usually happens without structure evaluations. Following their review, Martin et al. noted that this seems to be a global pattern in the race to fuse policy, investment, and changes in services. Progress in this area, they note, is slowed by a lack of national (US) and international terminology and standards. However, developments in digital devices for health technology targeted to consumers may be the most promising development in the emerging recognition that healthcare systems around the world are largely broken. The challenge will be to meld the creativity of the designers with the point-of-care wisdom of users, the clinical priorities of the professional healthcare providers, and the agendas of the policy makers at all levels. Attention to the complex of *influences* and array of *capital* available to consumers and their social network is equally critical in times of *transition* and stability where innovations have become routine.

REFERENCES

Aarsand, P. A. (2007). Computer and video games in family life: The digital divide as a resource in intergenerational interactions. *Childhood, 14*(2), 235–256.

Adaptive Technology Resource Centre. (2009). *Technical glossary*. Retrieved November 10, 2009, from http://atrc.utoronto.ca/index.php?option=com_content&task=blogsection&id=4&Itemid=9

Aldrich, F. K. (2003). Smart homes: Past, present and future. In R. Harper (Ed.), *Inside the Smart Home* (pp. 17–40). London: Springer-Verlag.

Altizer, R. (2010, April 30). Richard Marks and the PlayStation move to keynote the Games for Health Conference. Retrieved June 30, 2010, from http://playstation.about.com/b/2010/04/30/richard-marks-and-the-playstation-move-to-keynote-the-games-for-health-conference.htm

Alwan, M., & Nobel, J. (2008). *State of technology in aging services: Summary* (Summary Report for Blue Shield of California Foundation). Washington DC: American Association of Homes and Services for the Aging.

Alwan, M., Wiley, D., & Nobel, J. (2007). *State of technology in aging services*. Washington, DC: Center for Aging Services Technologies. Retrieved June 15, 2009, from http://www.agingtech.org/documents/bscf_state_technoloy_phase1.pdf

Associated Press. (2009). *Crystal Cruises has a new concierge for the gadget challenged*. Retrieved June 24, 2009, from http://www.baltimoresun.com/travel/bal-cruise-gadgets,0,339255.story

Au, A. (2009). *Game related illnesses and injuries: A review of articles, rhetoric, and realities*. Retrieved August 10, 2009, from http://www.slideshare.net/alanau/games-for-health-2009-game-related-illness-and-injuries-1578209

Barrett, L. (2009). *Health @ home*. Washington DC: AARP Knowledge Management.

Baur, C., & Kanaan, S. B. (2006). *Expanding the reach and impact of consumer e-health tools: Executive summary, a vision of e-health benefits for all* (Electronic No. 2006). Department of Disease Prevention and Health Promotion. Retrieved June 18, 2010, from http://www.health.gov/communication/ehealth/ehealthTools/summary.htm

Berk, L. E. (2004). *Development through the lifespan* (3rd ed.). Boston: Allyn and Bacon.

Brown, J. (2009). Game-care revolution: A health care game changer? *Center for Connected Health*. Retrieved June 22, 2009, from http://www.connected-health.org/about-us/get-connected-discussion/discussion/game-care-revolution-a-healthcare-game-changer.aspx

Brown, N. P. (2008). *At home with old age: Reimagining nursing homes.* Retrieved June 24, 2009, from http://harvardmagazine.com/2008/11/at-home-with-old-age.html

Brue, V., Hahn, J., Olmstead, R., Grimes, R. M., Zielinski, W. L. & Simoni, J. M. (2007). *A novel technology to promote HAART adherence.* Paper presented as part of innovations in adherence assessments and interventions symposium at the 2nd International Conference on HIV Treatment Adherence. Retrieved June 6, 2009, from https://www.medsignals.com/study01.aspx

Burg, B. (2009). *Medication dispenser respecting the physiological clock of patients.* Retrieved June 6, 2009, from http://www.freepatentsonline.com/y2009/0050645.html

Cella, G. (2010, June 23). *Wireless medication adherence study conducted at the Partners Center for Connected Health shows promising initial findings.* Retrieved June 29, 2010, from http://www.connected-health.org/media/288561/vitality%20interim%20data%20release%206.23.10.pdf

Chan, M., Esteve, D., Escriba, C., & Campo, E. (2008). A review of smart homes: Present state and future challenges. *Computer Methods and Programs in Biomedicine, 91*(1), 55–81.

Charness, N., & Schaie, K. W. (Eds.). (2003). *Impact of technology on successful aging.* New York: Springer.

Colorado State University. (2009). *Assistive technology resource center.* Retrieved November 10, 2009, from http://www.atrc.colostate.edu

Cress, C. J. (2009). *Care managers: Working with the aging family.* Sudbury, MA: Jones and Bartlett.

Curone, D., Dudnik, G., Loriga, G., Luprano, J., Magenes, G., Paradiso, R., et al. (2007). Smart garments for safety improvements of emergency/disaster operators. *Proceedings of the Annual International Conference of the IEEE Engineering in Medicine and Biology Society, 2007,* 3962–3965.

Czaja, S. J., Charness, N., Fisk, A. D., Hertzog, C., Nair, S. N., Rogers, W. A., et al. (2006). Factors predicting the use of technology: Findings from the Center for Research and Education on Aging and Technology Enhancement (CREATE). *Psychology & Aging, 21*(2), 333–352.

Davidoff, S., Lee, M. K., Zimmerman, J., & Dey, A. K. (2006). *Socially-aware requirements for a smart home for families.* Proceedings of International Symposium on Intelligent Environments. Retrieved June 24, 2009, from http://www.cs.cmu.edu/~sdavidof/pubs/davidoff-socially-aware-requirements-msr.pdf

Demiris, G., & Hensel, B. K. (2008). Technologies for an aging society: A systematic review of "smart home" applications. *Yearbook of Medical Informatics,* 33–40.

Demiris, G., Oliver, D. P., Dickey, G., Skubic, M., & Rantz, M. (2008). Findings from a participatory evaluation of a smart home application for older adults. *Technology & Health Care, 16*(2), 111–118.

Dishman, E. (2007). *Health technology and innovation at Intel.* Retrieved June 24, 2009, from http://hitanalyst.files.wordpress.com/2008/07/day1_1100_dishman21.pdf

Dishman, E., Matthews, J. T., & Dunbar-Jacob, J. (2004). Everyday health: Technology for adaptive aging. In R. Pew & S. Van Hemel (Eds.), *Technology for adaptive aging: Workshop report and papers* (pp. 179–208). National Research Council Steering Committee for the Workshop on Adaptive Aging. Washington, DC: National Academies Press.

Dunbar-Jacob, J., Schlenk, E. A., & Caruthers, D. (2002). Adherence in the management of chronic disorders. In A. J. Christensen & M. H. Antoni (Eds.), *Chronic Physical Disorders* (pp. 69–82). Oxford, UK: Blackwell.

e-Pill Medication Reminders. (2009). *e-Pill automatic pill dispensers.* Retrieved October 26, 2009, from http://www.epill.com/dispenser.html

European eHealth News. (2008). *Smart clothes: Textiles that track your health.* Retrieved June 6, 2009, from http://www.ehealthnews.eu/content/view/1063/27

Felong, A. (2008, January 7). *A fashion statement that merges man with machine.* [Web log post]. Retrieved November 10, 2009, from http://www.redwoodhouse.com/wearable

Fox, S. (2008). Recruit doctors. Let e-patients lead. Go mobile. *Pew Internet & American Life Project.* Retrieved on November 9, 2009, from http://www.pewinternet.org/Reports/2008/Recruit-doctors-Let-epatients-lead-Go-mobile.aspx

Frost & Sullivan. (2006, June 6). *European social alarms markets.* Retrieved June 29, 2010, from http://www.researchandmarkets.com/reportinfo.asp?report_id=358500

Fuoco, L. W. (2006). *Popularity of wireless ear pieces lessening the stigma of hearing aids.* Retrieved June 22, 2009, from http://www.post-gazette.com/pg/06025/643565-114.stm#ixzz0jC7LKeld&D

Hickman, J. M., Rogers, W. A., & Fisk, A. D. (2007). Training older adults to use new technology. *Journals of Gerontology Series B: Psychological Sciences and Social Sciences, 62*(Suppl. Special Issue 1), 77–84. Retrieved October 26, 2009, from http://psychsoc.gerontologyjournals.org/cgi/citmgr?gca=jgerob;62/suppl_Special_Issue_1/77

Horrigan, J. B. (2007). *Don't blame me: It's the phone's fault. Cell phone users find devices and applications too complicated or hardly worth the trouble.* Retrieved June 24, 2009, from http://pewresearch.org/pubs/517/dont-blame-me-its-the-phones-fault!

Intel. (2007). *Intel's proactive health lab.* Retrieved October 26, 2009, from http://www.intel.com/healthcare/hri/pdf/proactive_health.pdf

Intel. (2009, April 2). GE and Intel to form healthcare alliance. *Intel News Release.* Retrieved November 10, 2009, from http://www.intel.com/pressroom/archive/releases/2009/20090402corp.htm

Jordan-Marsh, M. (2008). Health habitat aspects of software as a service (SAAS/WEB2.0) reinforcing diabetic self-confidence: The PHRddBRASIL case. *DESAFIO International Symposium: Diabetes, Health Education and Guided Physical Activities,* 39–42.

Kvedar, J. C. (2009). *The connected health evidence base.* Retrieved June 24, 2009, from http://www.healthcareitnews.com/blog/connected-health-evidence-base

Lalley, H. (2006, September 18). Better health through PlayStation? *Health Beat.* Retrieved June 30, 2010, from http://www.spokesmanreview.com/blogs/healthbeat/archive.asp?postID=4032

Lauer, A., Rust, K. L., & Smith, R. O. (2006). *ATOMS project technical report—Factors in assistive technology device abandonment: Replacing "abandonment" with "discontinuance."* Retrieved June 24, 2009, from http://www.r2d2.uwm.edu/atoms/archive/technicalreports/tr discontinuance.html

Lundberg, S. (2007). Elite care brings elder-friendly technology to Oregon. *Aging Today.* Retrieved October 26, 2009, from http://www.elitecare.com/elite_care_brings_elder_friendly_technology_oregon

Marrero, D. G. (2009). Managing diabetes with mobile technology. *Forefront, 6*(1), 3–6. Retrieved July 5, 2010, from http://www.diabetes.org/assets/pdfs/forefront/forefront-winter-spring-09.pdf

Martin, S., Kelly, G., Kernohan, W. G., McCreight, B., & Nugent, C. (2008). Smart home technologies for health and social care support. *Cochrane Database of Systematic Reviews, 4,* CD006412. Retrieved November 10, 2009, from http://www.cochrane.org/reviews/en/ab006412.html

Matthews, J. T., LoPresti, E. F., Simpson, R. C., Kulyukin, V. A., Wang, J., & Nalitz, N. (2007, June). Preferences for interface design for a navigation assistant on a wheeled walker. *Proceedings of the 2nd International Conference on Technology and Aging,* Toronto, Canada.

Metros, S. (2008). *Visual literacy in the age of the big picture. Fighting the digital divide through education.* The Open University of Catalonia's UNESCO Chair in E-Learning Fifth International Seminar, Barcelona, Spain.

Meyer, J. (2004). Technology for adaptive aging: Workshop report and papers (pp. 253–282). *National Research Council Steering Committee for the Workshop on Adaptive Aging.* Washington, DC:

National Academies Press. Retrieved June 29, 2010, from http://www.nap.edu/openbook.php? record_id=10857

Morales Rodriguez, M., Casper, G., & Brennan, P. F. (2007). Patient-centered design. The potential of user-centered design in personal health records. *Journal of AHIMA, 78*(4), 44–46.

Morris, M. E., Lundell, J., Dishongh, T., & Needham, B. (2009). Fostering social engagement and self efficacy in later life: Studies with ubiquitous computing. In P. Markopoulos, B. De Ruyter, & W. Mackay (Eds.), *Awareness systems: Advances in theory, methodology, and design* (pp. 335–349). London: Springer London.

Musselwhite, C., & Haddad, H. (2008). Prolonging safe driver behaviour through technology: Attitudes of older drivers. *Strategic Promotion of Ageing Research Capacity.* Retrieved June 30, 2010, from http://www.sparc.ac.uk/media/downloads/executivesummaries/exec_summary_musselwhite.pdf

National Center for Chronic Disease Prevention and Health Promotion. (2009). *Chronic disease overview.* Retrieved November 10, 2009, from http:/www.cdc.gov/NCCdphp/overview.htm

National Highway Traffic Safety Administration (NHTSA). (n.d.). *Drowsy driving and automobile crashes.* Retrieved June 29, 2010, from http://www.nhtsa.gov/people/injury/drowsy_driving1/ Drowsy.html

Nielson, J. (2005). *Usability: Empiricism or ideology?* Retrieved November 9, 2009, from http://www.useit.com/alertbox/20050627.html

Pangher, N. (2008). Domotics in the counter-ageing society. *European Papers on the New Welfare 9,* 41–46.

Pape, T. L. B., Kim, J., & Weiner, B. (2002). The shaping of individual meanings assigned to assistive technology: A review of personal factors. *Disability and Rehabilitation, 24*(1/2/3), 5–20.

Professor says much of new technology should be known as nana-technology: Creates term to define technology to improve life for senior citizens. (2006, August 16). *Senior Journal.* Retrieved November 13, 2009, from http://seniorjournal.com/NEWS/Features/6-08-16-ProfessorSays.htm

Rehabilitation Research Design and Disability Center at University of Wisconsin–Milwaukee. (2009). *Current projects.* Retrieved November 10, 2009, from http://www.r2d2.uwm.edu/projects

Rialle, V., Duchene, F., Noury, N., Bajolle, L., & Demongeot, J. (2002). Health "smart" home: Information technology for patients at home. *Telemedicine Journal & E-Health, 8*(4), 395.

Ricciardi, L. (2009). *In-body sensors to monitor health.* Retrieved June 24, 2009, from http://projecthealthdesign.typepad.com/project_health_design/2009/02/inbody-sensors-to-monitor-health.html

Rogers, W. A., Mykityshyn, A. L., Campbell, R. H., & Fisk, A., D. (2001). Analysis of a "simple" medical device. *Ergonomics in Design, 1,* 6–14.

Ross, D. A. (2001). Implementing assistive technology on wearable computers. *IEEE Intelligent Systems, 16*(3), 47–53. Retrieved November 10, 2009, from http://www.computer.org/ portal/web/csdl/doi/10.1109/5254.940026

Roy, N., & Pineau, J. (2007). Robotics and independence for the elderly. In G. Lesnoff-Caravaglia (Ed.), *Growing old in a technological society* (pp. 209–242). Springfield, IL: Charles C. Thomas.

Ryder, P. T., & Brue, V. (2008, April). *Pills and patient behavior: Smarter experience tracking.* Paper presented at the American Geriatric Society Annual Meeting, Washington, DC. Retrieved October 26, 2009, from https://www.medsignals.com/study02.aspx

Scherer, M. J., Sax, C., Vanbierbliet, A., Cushman, L. A., & Scherer, J. V. (2005). Predictors of assistive technology use: The importance of personal and psychosocial factors. *Disability & Rehabilitation, 27*(21), 1321–1331.

SNOW Chat and Learn. (2008). *Alternative input devices.* Retrieved June 24, 2009, from http://inclusiveworkshop.ca/index.php?page=course-shell-2

Tapscott, D., & Williams, A. (2006). *Wikinomics: How mass collaboration changes everything.* New York: Penguin Group.

Tellzan, R. (2008). *Devices to get dressed with.* Retrieved June 28, 2009, from http://www. australianit.news.com.au/story/0,24897,23272622-5013037,00.html

Tonet, O., Marinelli, M., Citi, L., Rossini, P. M., Rossini, L., Megali, G., et al. (2008). Defining brain-machine interface applications by matching interface performance with device requirements. *Journal of Neuroscience Methods, 167,* 91–104.

Tyrer, H. W., Aud, M. A., Alexander, G., Skubic, M., & Rantz, M. (2007). Early detection of health changes in older adults. *Proceedings of the 29th Annual International Conference of the IEEE EMBS* (pp. 4045–4048). Lyon, France.

Vanderheiden, G. C. (2007). Redefining assistive technology, accessibility and disability based on recent technical advances. *Journal of Technology in Human Services, 25*(1/2), 147–148, 158.

Venkatesh, V., Morris, M. G., Davis, G. B., & Davis, F. D. (2003). User acceptance of information technology: Toward a unified view. *MIS Quarterly, 27*(3), 425–478.

Verza, R., Carvalho, M. L., Battaglia, M. A., & Uccelli, M. (2006). An interdisciplinary approach to evaluating the need for assistive technology reduces equipment abandonment. *Multiple Sclerosis, 12*(1), 88–93.

Vilamovska, A., Hatziandreu, E., Schindler, R., Oranje, C. V., Vries, H. D., & Krapels, J. (2009). *Study on the requirements and options for RFID application in healthcare: Identifying areas for radio frequency identification deployment in healthcare delivery: A review of relevant literature* (No. TR-608-EC). Cambridge, UK: RAND Europe.

Wielawski, I. M. (2006). Improving chronic illness care. In S. Issacs & J. Knickman (Eds.), *The Robert Wood Johnson Foundation anthology: To improve health and health care* (Vol. X, pp. 1–17). Retrieved June 28, 2009, from http://www.rwjf.org/pr/search.jsp?author=Wielawski%20IM

Appendix 5-A   Technical Capabilities and Potential Value for the Technology-Enabled Care Paradigm for Seniors and Caregivers in Their Network

Seniors	Informal Caregivers	Professional Caregivers		Payers
		Service Providers	Healthcare Professionals	
Capability				
Objective, up-to-date assessment of health, functional abilities, and care needs	Objective, up-to-date assessment of health, functional abilities, and care needs of their loved ones	Objective, up-to-date assessment of health, functional abilities, and care needs of seniors	Objective, up-to-date assessment of health, functional abilities, and care needs of seniors	Objective, up-to-date assessment of health and care needs of seniors
Values				
Health self-management Sense of security Prolonged or enhanced independence	Opportunity to participate in the management of the health and care needs of their loved ones Peace of mind	Identification of services needed Coordination of services Dispatching appropriate timely services as needed	Chronic disease management Detection of early disease onset Early and preventive interventions	Enhanced quality of care Reduced care costs Improved customer satisfaction

Seniors	Informal Caregivers	Professional Caregivers		Payers
		Service Providers	**Healthcare Professionals**	
		Values		
Improved quality of life	Reduced care burdens and strains	Improved caregiver efficiency	Monitoring efficacy of interventions	
	Improved quality of life	Reduced caregiver workloads	Improved efficiency	
		Improved customer satisfaction	Potential revenue opportunities	
		Revenue opportunity	Improved customer satisfaction	

Appendix 5-A *(continued)*

State of Technology Barriers/Benefits Matrix—Safety Technologies

Technology Description	Requirements, Advantages, Disadvantages	Value to Senior	Value to Care Provider	Value to Professional Caregiver	Value to Informal Caregiver	Value to Payer
Fall Detection/ Prevention	Reliability is a requirement; false negatives carry a higher weight than false positives. Reliability information is scarce. Effectiveness depends on the setting in which the technology is used and response protocols. Prevention is limited by the availability of the caregiver.	Sense of security Improved quality of life Improved health outcome in case of a fall	Reduced liability Improved professional caregiver efficiency Increased resident or family satisfaction	Reduced care burdens	Peace of mind Reduced caregiver strains	Reduced cost of care

State of Technology Barriers/Benefits Matrix—Safety Technologies

Technology Description	Requirements, Advantages, Disadvantages	Value to Senior	Value to Care Provider	Value to Professional Caregiver	Value to Informal Caregiver	Value to Payer
Wearable Mostly push-button and/or accelerometer and inclinometer based. Examples include LifeAlert, FallSaver, Stanley TABS, Tunstall	Limited by user's compliance Some could work outdoors, as well as indoors.	Sense of security Improved quality of life Improved health outcome in case of a fall	Reduced liability Improved professional caregiver efficiency Increased resident or family satisfaction	Reduced care burdens	Peace of mind Reduced caregiver strains	Reduced cost of care
Environmental Mostly motion-sensor based, sometimes in combination with other sensors. Examples include QuietCare, HealthSense, GrandCare, UVa's	Pet immunity of motion detectors is important. User's compliance is not required.	Improved sense of security Improved quality of life	Reduced liability Improved professional caregiver efficiency	Reduced care burdens	Peace of mind Reduced caregiver strains	Reduced cost of care

(continues)

Appendix 5-A   (continued)

State of Technology Barriers/Benefits Matrix—Safety Technologies

Technology Description	Requirements, Advantages, Disadvantages	Value to Senior	Value to Care Provider	Value to Professional Caregiver	Value to Informal Caregiver	Value to Payer
floor-vibrations fall detector; University of Missouri's imaging-based fall detector. Prevention systems include Samarion's imaging-based system in addition to bed and chair alarms.	Indoors only Effectiveness depends on the setting in which the technology is used and response protocols. Prevention is limited by availability of caregivers.	Improved health outcome in case of a fall	Increased resident or family satisfaction			
Mobility Aids Wheelchairs and walkers are being technologically enhanced to enable seniors to navigate safely in their environments.	User's compliance is required. Many still in research phase Cost is likely to be prohibitive	Added independence and freedom Improved quality of life	Increased resident or family satisfaction	Reduced care burdens	Peace of mind Reduced caregiver burdens	Reduced cost of care

State of Technology Barriers/Benefits Matrix—Safety Technologies

Technology Description	Requirements, Advantages, Disadvantages	Value to Senior	Value to Care Provider	Value to Professional Caregiver	Value to Informal Caregiver	Value to Payer
University of Virginia's, CMU's, and University of Michigan's walkers are examples.	without reimbursement. Liability is a potential barrier.	Improved health outcome				
Stove-Use Detectors Purely environmental; these technologies monitor stove use to automatically turn off the stove after a period of time or inferring a forgotten stove. Examples include University of Virginia's system, and commercially available StoveGuard and Tunstall gas shut-off valves.	Some devices are limited to electric stoves, others are limited to gas ranges (no manufacturer provides both types).	Improved sense of security Improved quality of life Reduced risk of fire damage, and possible reduced insurance premiums	Reduced liability Improved professional caregiver efficiency Reduced risk of fire damage, and possible reduced insurance premiums Increased resident or family satisfaction	Reduced care burdens	Peace of mind Reduced caregiver strains Reduced risk of fire damage, and possible reduced insurance premiums	Reduced cost of care

(continues)

Appendix 5-A *(continued)*

State of Technology Barriers/Benefits Matrix—Safety Technologies

Technology Description	Requirements, Advantages, Disadvantages	Value to Senior	Value to Care Provider	Value to Professional Caregiver	Value to Informal Caregiver	Value to Payer
Smoke and Temperature Monitors Purely environmental; Stanley, Honeywell, and GE have these products.	Wired (not easy to retrofit), wireless (easier to retrofit) Battery life may become an issue with some units.	Improved sense of security Improved quality of life Reduced risk of fire damage, and possible reduced insurance premiums	Reduced liability Improved professional caregiver efficiency Reduced risk of fire damage, and possible reduced insurance premiums Increased resident or family satisfaction	Reduced care burdens	Peace of mind Reduced caregiver strains Reduced risk of fire damage, and possible reduced insurance premiums	Reduced cost of care

	State of Technology Barriers/Benefits Matrix—Safety Technologies					
Technology Description	**Requirements, Advantages, Disadvantages**	**Value to Senior**	**Value to Care Provider**	**Value to Professional Caregiver**	**Value to Informal Caregiver**	**Value to Payer**
Door Locks Based on access control technology, currently targeted mainly to institutional settings. Some of these technologies do not entail wearing or carrying an ID badge, pendant, or wrist band, and rely on numeric keypads or biometrics (fingerprint) or a combination of the two. Vigil, Stanley, etc. offer these products.	Currently meant for institutional settings Badge-based systems require the compliance of the user. Systems that use the wearable badges rely on the user's compliance.	Improved sense of security Smart deterrents (like the ones employed by EliteCare) may enhance sense of independence and quality of life.	Reduced liability Improved professional caregiver efficiency Increased resident or family satisfaction	Reduced care burdens	Peace of mind Reduced caregiver strains	Reduced cost of care

(continues)

Appendix 5-A *(continued)*

State of Technology Barriers/Benefits Matrix—Safety Technologies

Technology Description	Requirements, Advantages, Disadvantages	Value to Senior	Value to Care Provider	Value to Professional Caregiver	Value to Informal Caregiver	Value to Payer
Wander Management Systems Requires a wearable ID badge, pendant, or wristband, and hence the user's compliance. HomeFree and Vigil have these products for institutional settings. Oatfield Estates also implemented this functionality in its system.	Currently meant for institutional settings. Systems that use wearable badges rely on the user's compliance.	Improved sense of security. Smart deterrents like the ones (employed by EliteCare) may enhance sense of independence and quality of life.	Reduced liability. Improved professional caregiver efficiency. Ability to locate wanderers quickly. Accurate record of wandering events may lead to better coordinated care. Increased resident or family satisfaction	Reduced care burdens. Ability to locate wanderers quickly. Accurate record of wandering events may lead to better coordinated care.	Peace of mind. Ability to locate wanderers quickly. Reduced caregiver strains	Reduced cost of care

	State of Technology Barriers/Benefits Matrix—Health and Wellness Technologies						
Technology Description	Requirements, Advantages, Disadvantages	Value to Senior	Value to Care Provider	Value to Professional Caregiver	Value to Informal Caregiver	Value to Payer
Wellness Monitoring Technologies— Wearable Gross activity monitoring based on accelerometers as well as other sensors; examples include simple pedometers and actigraphs to more sophisticated devices that incorporate physiological measurements, such as skin temperature. Mainly for self-managing fitness and wellness.	Rely on the user's compliance They work indoors as well as outdoors. Visual, auditory, and speech-disabled elderly will not be able to control some devices. Other physical or cognitive impairments may limit the use of the technology in the elderly.	Improved health outcomes Improved quality of life Empowerment and self-directed health (e.g., weight-loss management)	Potential added revenue opportunities if a service provider is in the loop Opportunity for prevention, early detection, and intervention	(If involved) More longitudinal health information available/better diagnosis and treament Opportunity for prevention, early detection, and intervention	More informed about senior's health Improved communication regarding health with senior and professional caregiver Opportunity for prevention, early detection, and intervention	Reduced cost of care through prevention, early detection, and intervention

(continues)

Appendix 5-A *(continued)*

State of Technology Barriers/Benefits Matrix—Health and Wellness Technologies

Technology Description	Requirements, Advantages, Disadvantages	Value to Senior	Value to Care Provider	Value to Professional Caregiver	Value to Informal Caregiver	Value to Payer
Examples include Minimitter Actiwatch and Bodymedia.	Some payers are encouraging their use and starting to consider reimbursement					
Nonwearable Embedding sensors in the environment to monitor daily life activities, behavior, ADLs, and sleep quality Mainly targeted at the professional and informal caregiver for coordinating care and early detection of decline in function or health issues	Do not require user's compliance Work indoors only, mostly on a person living alone Pet immunity feature of the motion detectors is important.	Prolonged independence Improved health outcome Improved quality of life	Potential for capturing lost revenue/added revenue opportunities Coordination of care Improved care provider efficiency	Coordination of care Improved data regarding the senior's health Improved diagnosis or better health outcomes	More informed about senior's health Improved communication with senior and professional caregiver Reduced burdens and strains of care	Reduced cost of care

State of Technology Barriers/Benefits Matrix—Health and Wellness Technologies

Technology Description	Requirements, Advantages, Disadvantages	Value to Senior	Value to Care Provider	Value to Professional Caregiver	Value to Informal Caregiver	Value to Payer
Examples include QuietCare, HealthSense, Grand Care, Elite Care, and University of Virginia	Technology could be viewed as an invasion of privacy.		Reduced caregiver turnover			
Hybrid Hybrid wearable and environmental wellness-monitoring systems require a wearable RFID and tagging objects in the environment with RFIDs, and they monitor ADLs. Still in research phase, e.g., at Intel and University of Washington	Require compliance, and may not be scalable/practicable (reliability and battery life of the reader)	Prolonged independence; Improved health outcome; Improved quality of life	Potential for capturing lost revenue/added revenue opportunities; Coordination of care; Improved care provider efficiency	Coordination of care; Improved data regarding the senior's health; Improved diagnosis or better health outcomes	More informed about senior's health; Improved communication with senior and professional caregiver; Reduced burdens and strains of care	Reduced cost of care

(continues)

Appendix 5-A *(continued)*

State of Technology Barriers/Benefits Matrix—Health and Wellness Technologies

Technology Description	Requirements, Advantages, Disadvantages	Value to Senior	Value to Care Provider	Value to Professional Caregiver	Value to Informal Caregiver	Value to Payer
			Reduced caregiver turnover			
Telemedicine and Telehealth **Traditional Telemedicine Stations** Targeted at the professional caregiver and used primarily by home health providers, physicians, and hospitals mainly in chronic disease management and for short-term follow-up after discharge from hospital	Require compliance of the user Limited by capacity of call center/ processing limitation Technology could be viewed as an invasion of privacy. Some equipment	Prolonged independence Improved health outcome Improved quality of life	Potential for capturing lost revenue/added revenue opportunities Coordination of care Improved care provider efficiency	Coordination of care Improved data regarding the senior's health Improved diagnosis or better health outcomes	More informed about senior's health Improved communication with senior and professional caregiver Reduced burdens and strains of care	Reduced cost of care

State of Technology Barriers/Benefits Matrix—Health and Wellness Technologies						
Technology Description	**Requirements, Advantages, Disadvantages**	**Value to Senior**	**Value to Care Provider**	**Value to Professional Caregiver**	**Value to Informal Caregiver**	**Value to Payer**
Examples created by Honeywell HomMed, Viterion, Phillips, Health Buddy, and numerous universities.	can be relatively expensive.					
Ambulatory and Wearable Monitors They connect via wire or wirelessly to a recording device that sends the data. These include cardiac event monitors. An example of these systems is LifeWatch's cardiac monitors that use a Bluetooth-enabled cell phone as a data recorder and for connectivity.	Require compliance of the user Limited by capacity of call center/ processing limitations Technology could be viewed as an invasion of privacy.	Prolonged independence Improved health outcome Improved quality of life	Potential for capturing lost revenue/added revenue opportunities Coordination of care Improved care provider efficiency	Coordination of care Improved data regarding the senior's health Improved diagnosis or better health outcomes	More informed about senior's health Improved communication with senior and profes- sional caregiver Reduced burdens and strains of care	Reduced cost of care

(*continues*)

Appendix 5-A   (continued)

		State of Technology Barriers/Benefits Matrix—Health and Wellness Technologies				
Technology Description	Requirements, Advantages, Disadvantages	Value to Senior	Value to Care Provider	Value to Professional Caregiver	Value to Informal Caregiver	Value to Payer
	Some equipment can be relatively expensive.					
Purely Interactive Q&A Systems These systems do not have dedicated peripheral measurement devices. An example of these technologies is ZumeLife Gateway. These devices rely on the compliance of the user as well; these technologies are generally not reimbursable, except possibly under	Require compliance of the user Limited by capacity of call center/ processing limitations Technology could be an invasion of privacy.	Prolonged independence Improved health outcome Improved quality of life	Potential for capturing lost revenue/added revenue opportunities Coordination of care Improved care provider efficiency	Coordination of care Improved data regarding the senior's health Improved diagnosis or better health outcomes	More informed about senior's health Improved communication with senior and professional caregiver Reduced burdens and strains of care	Reduced cost of care

State of Technology Barriers/Benefits Matrix—Health and Wellness Technologies						
Technology Description	**Requirements, Advantages, Disadvantages**	**Value to Senior**	**Value to Care Provider**	**Value to Professional Caregiver**	**Value to Informal Caregiver**	**Value to Payer**
PACE and MA-SNPs.	Some equipment can be relatively expensive.					
Video Phones and Two-Way Video Stations These devices are used to connect with a healthcare professional for telemedicine, televisits, and teleconsults; interventions with these technologies are generally reimbursable with limitations. An example of a simple system is KMEA's videophone.	Require compliance of the user Limited by capacity of call center/processing limitations Technology could be viewed as an invasion of privacy.	Prolonged independence Improved health outcome Improved quality of life	Potential for capturing lost revenue/added revenue opportunities Coordination of care Improved care provider efficiency	Coordination of care Improved data regarding the senior's health Improved diagnosis or better health outcomes	More informed about senior's health Improved communication with senior and professional caregiver Reduced burdens and strains of care	Reduced cost of care

(*continues*)

Appendix 5-A   *(continued)*

State of Technology Barriers/Benefits Matrix—Health and Wellness Technologies

Technology Description	Requirements, Advantages, Disadvantages	Value to Senior	Value to Care Provider	Value to Professional Caregiver	Value to Informal Caregiver	Value to Payer
	Some equipment can be relatively expensive.					
Passive/ Environmental/ Nonwearable University of Virginia's bed monitor for vitals and clinical sleep assessment (under validation) and instrumented walker for gait and balance assessment are two examples of this category of telemedicine/ telehealth technologies that are under research. Such	Does not require the compliance of the user Technology could be viewed as an invasion of privacy. Some equipment can be relatively expensive.	Prolonged independence Improved health outcome Improved quality of life	Potential for capturing lost revenue/added revenue opportunities Coordination of care Improved care provider efficiency	Coordination of care Improved data regarding the senior's health Improved diagnosis or better health outcomes	More informed about senior's health Improved communication with senior and professional caregiver Reduced burdens and strains of care	Reduced cost of care

State of Technology Barriers/Benefits Matrix—Health and Wellness Technologies						
Technology Description	**Requirements, Advantages, Disadvantages**	**Value to Senior**	**Value to Care Provider**	**Value to Professional Caregiver**	**Value to Informal Caregiver**	**Value to Payer**
technologies are generally not reimbursable, except possibly under PACE and MA-SNPs.						
Medication Compliance Technologies Most technologies stand alone and are targeted at the senior or the caregiver. Simple monitoring is offered by QuietCare. Intel and OHSU have prototypes of monitoring/reminding systems, and HomMed has a med monitoring and reminding system as part of their telemedicine suite.	Most products have usability/ user-interface issues. Some seniors have complicated medication regimens that some technologies are unable to accommodate.	Improved compliance Better health outcomes	Improved quality of care	Improved compliance Better treatment plans made on compliance outcomes	Reduced caregiver strains	Reduced cost of care

(*continues*)

Appendix 5-A *(continued)*

State of Technology Barriers/Benefits Matrix—Health and Wellness Technologies

Technology Description	Requirements, Advantages, Disadvantages	Value to Senior	Value to Care Provider	Value to Professional Caregiver	Value to Informal Caregiver	Value to Payer
MD2 has the dispensing functionality.	Dispensing systems require a professional caregiver to load and program them.					
Cognition Simulation and Entertainment Systems Computer-based cognitive stimulation with embedded assessment. Examples include Dakim, OHSU's research. Cognitive stimulation could be effective and may have positive impact on cognitive	Mostly research phase technology Little evidence of outcomes	Improved quality of life Improved cognition and/or function Prolonged independence	Improved resident and family satisfaction Competitive edge	Possible improved health outcomes	Improved satisfaction Reduced caregiver burdens	Reduced cost of care

State of Technology Barriers/Benefits Matrix—Health and Wellness Technologies

Technology Description	Requirements, Advantages, Disadvantages	Value to Senior	Value to Care Provider	Value to Professional Caregiver	Value to Informal Caregiver	Value to Payer
health outcomes in the short term. Entertainment systems for both physical and mental stimulation: Nintendo Wii and It's Never 2 Late.		Opportunity for social interaction in congregate settings				
Assessment Systems The embedded is generally based on measuring response time, and response is attention dependent and hence may require broader environment monitoring and complex context understanding. Response time may also depend on dexterity (flaring arthritis), vision, and hearing abilities, hence the assessment may not be reliable.	Mostly research phase technology May be subject to variability due to extraneous factors including dexterity, visual acuity, distractions, and familiarity with the input device Requires validation	Potential for early detection and intervention to improve health outcomes	Potential for standardized longitudinal assessment Opportunity for early detection and intervention Improved care provider efficiency	Potential for standardized longitudinal assessment Reduced caregiver workloads	Opportunity for early detection and intervention	Reduced cost of care

(continues)

Appendix 5-A   (continued)

State of Technology Barriers/Benefits Matrix—Health and Wellness Technologies

Technology Description	Requirements, Advantages, Disadvantages	Value to Senior	Value to Care Provider	Value to Professional Caregiver	Value to Informal Caregiver	Value to Payer
Reminder and Orthotics Systems Reminding systems: University of Toronto, University of Rochester, University of Michigan, University of Dundee, Intel research, and Accenture. Rely on environmental monitoring including video monitoring and complex context understanding, or hybrid monitoring.	May not be scalable, due to high computational complexity Unsure how effective they are, as they are not yet evaluated in the field	Prolonged independence	Reduced care demands	Reduced caregiver burdens or workloads	Peace of mind Reduced caregiver strains	Reduced cost of care

	State of Technology Barriers/Benefits Matrix—Social Connectedness Technologies						
Technology Description	Requirements, Advantages, Disadvantages	Value to Senior	Value to Care Provider	Value to Professional Caregiver	Value to Informal Caregiver	Value to Payer
Phones Adapted land line phones for senior use include amplified sound, big-button phones, caller ID with pictures	Most of these products are aesthetically unappealing.	Improved quality of life through increased social interaction Reduced isolation Improved quality of life	Improved client satisfaction	Improved communications	Improved communications	Most technologies and programs are self-elected and out-of-pocket.
Cell Phones Cellular phones intended for seniors' use JitterBug cell phone is an example of a cell phone designed for senior users.	Most have usability issues. Have the potential to deliver additional value-added services	Improved quality of life through increased social interaction Reduced isolation	Improved client satisfaction Potential to generate revenue streams from value-added services	Improved communications	Improved communications	Most technologies and programs are self-elected and out-of-pocket. Has potential to reduce cost of care

(continues)

Appendix 5-A (*continued*)

State of Technology Barriers/Benefits Matrix—Social Connectedness Technologies

Technology Description	Requirements, Advantages, Disadvantages	Value to Senior	Value to Care Provider	Value to Professional Caregiver	Value to Informal Caregiver	Value to Payer
		Potential for improved health outcome				
Social Monitoring Tracking an individual's reactions with others; research is mainly led by Intel. Research projects include a presence lamp to notify senior a friend or family member is available and a Web-based measure of social interaction.	Still in research phase Most effective method of promoting social interaction is unclear.	Improved quality of life through increased social interaction Reduced isolation Potential for improved health outcome	Improved client satisfaction Potential to generate revenue streams from value added services	Improved communications	Improved communications	Reduced healthcare cost

State of Technology Barriers/Benefits Matrix—Social Connectedness Technologies

Technology Description	Requirements, Advantages, Disadvantages	Value to Senior	Value to Care Provider	Value to Professional Caregiver	Value to Informal Caregiver	Value to Payer
Senior-Friendly E-Mail and Web Portal Efforts have been made to make the Internet and its services more available to seniors It's Never 2 Late, GrandCare, Celery (paper to e-mail scanner), etc.	Usability and awareness of product limit adaptation	Improved quality of life through increased social interaction Reduced isolation Potential for improved health outcome	Improved client satisfaction Potential to generate revenue streams from value-added services	Improved communications	Improved communications	Most technologies and programs are self-elected and out-of-pocket. Has potential for reduced cost of care

(continues)

Appendix 5-A   (continued)

	State of Technology Barriers/Benefits Matrix—Social Connectedness Technologies						
Technology Description	Requirements, Advantages, Disadvantages	Value to Senior	Value to Care Provider	Value to Professional Caregiver	Value to Informal Caregiver	Value to Payer
Video Phones and Two-Way Conferencing Phones offering both voice and video to improve social interaction	Cost prohibitive Require broadband connectivity	Improved quality of life through increased social interaction	Improved client satisfaction Potential to generate revenue streams from value-added services	Improved communications	Improved communications	Most technologies and programs are self-elected and out-of-pocket.
Motorola's Ojo Video Phone	Usability and awareness limit adoption	Reduced isolation Potential for improved health outcome				Has potential for reduced cost of care

Source: Alwan, Wiley, & Nobel, 2007. Used with permission.

CHAPTER 6

Digital Games: Consumer Resources for Health Capital

Maryalice Jordan-Marsh and Jae Eun Chung

The social ecology of health includes a new focus on games as part of the everyday experience of many adults across the globe. The Robert Wood Johnson Foundation (RWJF) Games for Health Initiative defines games as "rule-based activities that involve some degree of challenge to reach a goal and provide performance feedback to the player" (RWJF, 2009, p. 4). As of August 2008, the market for serious health games represented about 16% ($6.6 billion) of the worldwide video gaming industry (Goldstein, Loughran, & Donner, 2008). There are some surprises in data on who is playing games: Unlike the common stereotype, older adults play digital games as often as younger counterparts (Lenhart, Jones, & Macgill, 2008), and women like playing as much as men (Jackson & Keitt, 2008).

Games are "the latest tool in the medical care arsenal" (Hawn, 2009, p. 842). Games, Hawn notes, are expected to bridge fragmented public health and primary care resources. For example, games can extend the reach of specialists by being a new form of telemedicine. Hawn observes that games are powerful ways to engage consumers in their care and are part of new approaches that "are proliferating like viral spores in a virtual pond" (p. 842).

With age, adults are mentally and physically challenged by developmental changes, shifts in social interaction patterns, and requirements of managing chronic illnesses and environmental risks. For some adults, there is a reservoir of strengths in their knowledge, attitudes, behaviors, and health status— a pool of health capital. However, for others, sustaining health and health capital is a challenge. Changes in abilities and social circumstances, coupled with developmental changes in priorities, call for new strategies. Digital games may provide a powerful motivational platform for acquiring new knowledge, attitudes, and skills with respect to health and health behaviors.

Games can also create opportunities for social connectivity, adventure, and development of self-worth (Wang & Singhal, 2009), which can contribute to

303

engaged healthy aging. Features of digital gaming, including interactivity, narrative, and experiential learning, may offer advantages over more traditional methods of persuading adults to acquire health knowledge and change health habits. Both adult men and women are currently playing computer games with enthusiasm, providing validation for exploring game-based health applications. Particularly with the increasing popularity of casual computer games and Wii games among the baby boomers, we see the great potential of games for adult health.

Theories and research are presented in this chapter that suggest there may be cognitive, emotional, social, and physical benefits to engaging in games. New games specific to older adults are rapidly emerging as this market becomes better known. This chapter explores these new games and maps them onto four different categories depending on their intended goals: prevention, assessment and diagnosis, therapy, and education.

The platform for engagement in games may vary by user preference or developer design. Platforms include stand-alone game consoles, cell phones, computers, the Internet, handheld devices, CD-ROMS, arcades, and combinations of these. There are potential barriers and side effects to engaging older adults in games. These can include computer availability, economics, skill deficits, competition for limited resources, and physical side effects related to vision, physical strains, and effects specific to three-dimensional (3D) applications. Access to games can occur through purchases and gifts, freeware online, and may be available in community settings such as libraries or senior centers. Healthcare plans or programs may provide access to games to clients as well. Games can be played alone, with a partner in the same room or online across the globe in massively multiplayer online games (MMOGs), or asynchronously with partners online through a dedicated website or social networking site. The opportunities and challenges presented to consumers by digital games are the focus of this chapter.

Health games linked to provider–patient interactions represent a special case that is also explored in this chapter. Health professionals do need to be prepared to engage in game design and adaptation, to assist in creating guidelines for recommending games, and in developing ways for incorporating feedback and documentation into provider–patient interactions. These topics specific to providers will be discussed in a subsequent section.

GAME-RELEVANT AND AGE-LINKED ASPECTS OF HEALTH LEARNING

Healthy lifestyles can lower mortality risks and delay deterioration in health status (Ford, Spallek, & Dobson, 2007; Haveman-Nies, de Groot, & van Staveren,

2003). For many adults, this requires dramatic changes in daily habits and includes dropping some habits such as smoking and taking up other habits such as exercise. A great deal of information must be acquired in order to make the decision to change and then to select actions that will effect the change. Is such learning a priority for older adults? Some experts have raised concerns that developmental shifts may compromise willingness and ability to acquire the new knowledge and attitudes positive changes require.

For older adults, emotional goals may take priority over knowledge and information goals. Altruism and social engagement may become more important than learning. This shift to prioritizing emotions and altruism (Carstensen, Isaacowitz, & Charles, 1999) may create some problems in coping with chronic illnesses and rehabilitation requirements. Carstensen and colleagues (1999) argue there is the risk that older adults will take shortcuts in gaining health-related knowledge. Games may be an ideal platform for reinforcing beneficial health behaviors and attitudinal changes. The experience of play provides an emotional outlet in the context of gaining health knowledge and skill. In addition, the immersive nature of games creates situations where altruism and social engagement opportunities can occur.

Huizinga (1970) characterized games as a contest that is played with rules that restrict what players can and cannot do. In a summary of the state of the science (RWJF, 2009), experts concluded that not only are interactive games "engaging and fun," they have the potential to "provide powerful firsthand experiences that can motivate learning, skill rehearsal, and behavior change" (p. 3). A number of researchers have pointed out advantages of using games for health behavior change and have developed games using feedback mechanisms and vicarious learning experiences (Baranowski, Buday, Thompson, & Baranowski, 2008). There is great potential for developing health games for the older population as an increasing number of the boomer generation are recreational digital game players (Entertainment Software Association, 2010). A major caution is that games "must first be fun" (M. Gotsis, personal communication, November 29, 2009).

Gender and Age as Factors in Game Playing

Health, or serious games, should be targeted to both men and women, as despite common beliefs, both are heavy users of computer games (Jackson & Keitt, 2008). A survey by Digital Marketing Services reports that, among those who play online games, women over 40 years old play more often and for a longer period of time compared to male counterparts and even teenagers (Vance, 2004, as cited in Pearce, 2008). The Entertainment Software Association (2010) reported a 10% increase since 1999 in the number of adults over 50 who play video and computer games, bringing the rate to 26%. According to the Pew Internet and American Life Project (Lenhart et al., 2008), two in five adults between 50 and 64 years old (40%) and one in four adults 65 years and older (23%) are gamers. Older adult gamers in particular tend to play games more frequently than younger game players. Over a third of gamers 65 and older (36%) play games at least once a day compared with about a fifth of gamers younger than 65. According to a survey of massively multiplayer online gamers, older adults also tend to spend longer hours in game compared to younger adults (Dmitri, Yee, & Scott, 2008). According to the survey by the International Council on Active Aging (2008, as cited in Gerencher, 2008), older adults are also interested in purchasing gaming products: about 60% of seniors said that they intended to buy electronic games in the next 2 years. These numbers mean that in the future, older adults will reach their 60s and 70s with a history of game playing. Adults with a college education are likely to have work-related computer experience, which increases their comfort with trying games (Hargittai, 2002).

Recent research on a massively multiplayer online game (MMOG) purports to overturn previous assumptions about game play and gender. Sony Online Entertainment and a team at the University of Southern California collaborated in tracking game play by gender (Williams, Consalvo, Caplan, & Yee, 2009). The unobtrusive monitoring was complemented by a survey. The key features of MMOGs are summarized as built around characters that are part of an online social community that develops in a persistent world. Players select avatars (more than one is possible) who attain abilities and characteristics based on game play. Williams et al. (2009) cite figures from White (2008) of over 47 million active subscriptions to MMOGs worldwide. No MMOGs for health purposes were found. However, their study provides some new insights into gender aspects of game playing.

Williams et al. (2009) found patterns of play that validate gender role theory propositions about differences between men and women. Women (mean age of 33.49) played for longer periods than men (mean age of 32.82) but under-reported their time by three times the male rate of underreporting. Williams et al. speculate this low estimation may be due to prevailing cultural norms about gender and games. There were fascinating gender differences in motivation for playing, play patterns with romantic partners, and self-reported health (BMI and fitness).

Games promoting healthy lifestyles generally result in positive outcomes for children, such as an increase in health knowledge and positive changes in health behaviors and attitudes (Baranowski et al., 2008). Games may have similar benefits for adults. There is an extensive list of game features that make games an ideal platform for changing health behaviors and attitudes for all ages. However, so far, games for healthy lifestyles are mostly targeted at young audiences such as children and adolescents.

Older adults are often neglected as game players and treated as unlikely gamers. Most age-specific research on games is targeted to children and adolescents (Pearce, 2008). Furthermore, games developed for older adults often use limited features of games and not their full potentials. For example, in a review of video games, Baranowski and colleagues (2008) found no health-related behavior-change games with stories for adults. Storytelling is a core feature of many successful games (Jenkins, 2004) and of successful aging. Other features of games are that the player is the "star," failure is part of success, and "there's always a solution—you just have to find it" (Maney, 2004, para. 16). Bringing these norms to gerontologists may revolutionize health and other interactions with older adults.

Older adults with limited or no game experience may need to become familiar with gaming features and unstated customs. Many games do not come with the set of instructions and rules of traditional commercial games. Younger generations who grow up with digital interactive games may not even be aware that these expectations are learned. The risk is that not getting the game right on their first few tries could be frustrating to naïve players. If the younger clinician who recommends games to older adults has grown up playing digital games, it may not be obvious that inexperienced players will require coaching on many features of digital games. Games also have an allure for adults as a way to connect to younger generations. In fact, there is some speculation that game-related injuries may be caused by adults trying to compete at the same level as younger, more fit family members (M. Apostolos, personal communication, May 20, 2009).

Older adults may experience changes generally attributed to aging that may affect game play. These are highlighted in Table 6.1 and linked to design guidelines. Changes in vision, audition, movement, and cognition are normal aspects of aging. While these changes may be initial barriers to successful game play, a knowledgeable coach can assist adults with impairments. Across age groups, Folmer (2009) notes that 25.9 million individuals with disabilities are unable to fully experience many digital games. Research issues in game accessibility are reviewed in a SlideShare presentation by Folmer (2009).

Some attempts have been made to adapt games for such individuals and for older adults. However, any adaptations to hardware are complex and software adaptations often require an expensive development kit. The kits are sufficiently expensive that they are not cost effective. A superior approach would be accommodations built in by the designers of games.

Table 6.1   Age-Related Sensory and Cognitive Changes and Guidelines for Game Designs for Older Adults

	Age-Related Changes	Guidelines
Vision	• Decreased sensitivity to low-contrast displays • Increased susceptibility to glare • Decreased ability to resolve small details • Decreased motion sensibility • Difficulty in selecting relevant information among cluttered displays • Difficulty in discriminating certain wavelengths, particularly blue-greens	• Using high-contrast colors for texts and images • Deploying illuminating strategies to minimize glare effects • Adapting font and image sizes to optimize legibility • Adapting the speed of moving targets • Placing target objects within central vision field and minimizing the need to use peripheral vision • Using long wavelength colors
Audition	• Decreased ability to separate speech from background noise • Decline in sensitivity to high frequencies • Decreased ability to discriminate similar sounds and distinguish among tones • Decreased speech perception	• Reducing background noise and avoiding long-term exposure to high levels of noise • Minimizing the use of high-frequency acoustic information • Provide proper training for auditory information processing and adjusting audio systems based on feedback from users • Using semantically well-structured speech materials and adapting the pace of words
Movement	• Decreased ability to manipulate very small controls • Decline in accuracy of rapid movements	• Removing tasks requiring manual dexterity • Increasing sensitivity of game devices to detect slow motion

	• Decline in sensitivity to pressure and vibration • Reduced grip strength and range of motion	• Reducing vibrotactile detection thresholds • Removing, the need to carry out complex actions using mouse or handheld devices
Cognition	• Decreased ability to filter out irrelevant information and increased distraction • Slow acquisition of new knowledge • Poorer explicit memory for specific events and their contexts • Reduced capacity to maintain information in active memory • Reduced ability to hold and operate on spatial representations in working memory • Difficulty in processing multiple tasks simultaneously and switching from one task to another	• Using simple symbolic icons to reduce ambiguity and misunderstanding • Providing enough evidence to link stimuli and learned responses • Providing consistent interfaces and feedback about errors • Easy access to help system for game-playing instructions and strategies • Avoiding complex visual displays and using simple visual cues to reduce the search • Presenting tasks in small chunks and minimizing the number of steps and controls needed to complete a task

Source: Adapted from Gamberini et al., 2006, and Schieber, 2003.

Later in the chapter, we explore how these age-related changes shape the ways that games could assist in their health-related purposes. We also explore how the guidelines can assist in the design of games and in their value for older adults.

EMERGENCE OF SERIOUS AND HEALTH GAMES

In the literature on digital gaming, a distinction between casual, recreational games and serious games is emerging. Casual games are described by the Casual Games Association (2007) as based on concepts today's adults experienced as children with games played in arcades or on the Atari gaming system. Casual games require no special skills or long time commitments to play. The association summarizes that they are fun and played by over 200 million people each month in short time increments. However, some people will not admit to their predilection for casual online games, feeling embarrassed. Prensky (2003) notes the prevalence of media story labels that encourage dismissing games as "frivolous at best and harmful at worst" (p. 4).

Labeling some games as being serious conveys added value that may attract different audiences. The new label of *serious* is an attempt to overcome the social expectation that games are strictly frivolous and without benefit. Developers of games that go beyond entertainment searched for key words to signal added value, and eventually they named the games with goals beyond fun and entertainment as "serious games" (Prensky, 2003; Whatley, 2005). This label has become popular with the launch of the Serious Games Initiative by the Woodrow Wilson International Center for Scholars in 2002. Games for Health is a special division that the Serious Games Initiative founded to develop a community and a platform to gather best practices of games being built for healthcare applications. These health games are expected to foster patients' engagement in health care and adoption of healthy behaviors while delivering fun (Hawn, 2009).

Serious game developers are increasing their endeavors to embrace entertainment aspects and use various complicated game features to attract game players and sustain participation, and thus the boundary of serious and casual games has become blurred (Sawyer, 2007). Games such as Nintendo's Wii Fit and Electronic Arts' EA Sports Active are examples of the reverse—a game with entertainment priorities that offers new versions with health, or serious, features. This game system is discussed in the section on examples of the physical benefits of "exergames."

BENEFITS OF GAMES

Shifting Goals for Existing Games

There are applications, such as Wii Sports, where the initial intent was entertainment, but serendipitous side effects of body movements indeed provide exercise. A strategy video game was also shown to have an unintentional effect, a slowdown of cognitive declines among older adult gamers (Basak, Boot, Voss, & Kramer, 2008). Now, *serious* or *health* may be an appropriate label. Some game applications are specifically designed to increase the participant's willingness to engage in desired behaviors. For example, Glucoboy is a game designed for children to measure and monitor blood glucose levels (Guidance Interactive Healthcare, n.d.). Wellness Partners (Gotsis, Valente, Jordan-Marsh, Spruijt-Metz, 2008), funded by the Robert Wood Johnson Foundation's games initiative, encourages increasing physical activity across generations. Players are encouraged to engage their social network as cheerleaders if not partners. Points are earned for activities in the real world. Points are used to buy minigame access. The game format has also been used by nurses to inform people of the dangers of malaria and to improve adherence to malaria prevention (Bauman & Hartjes, 2008). There are some applications that are simply intended to distract the participant while he or she is engaged in an otherwise tedious practice, such as stationary cycling for exercise (Warburton et al., 2007). In an exercise cycling study (Warburton et al., 2007), one group that exercised along with playing a video game, compared to a group that exercised without, had better health outcomes at the end, such as improved blood pressure and increased attendance in exercise programs. Similarly, physical therapists utilize Wii as a tool to sustain interests and engagement in otherwise boring repetitive behaviors (Baertlein, 2007; Fagan, 2008; Tanner, 2008). Other examples are Wii Sports for Parkinson's disease patients (Medical College of Georgia, 2008) and the Guitar Hero game for rehabilitation after hand surgery (Ballenger, 2009; Shachtman, 2008).

Future studies might explore whether there is a unique aspect to the gaming experience that goes beyond attendance to intensity of engagement. There is almost no research on adult outcomes specific to health measures, such as blood pressure, weight management, blood glucose, reduced incidence of complications, or prevention of onset of chronic illnesses or reduction in age-related risks for falls or other accidents. Physiological measures during the exercise period or during game playing without exercise would be very useful in understanding the causative mechanisms that create benefits and risks.

Some recreational applications may provide useful assessment or monitoring data. An area where games can be of particular use is early detection of dementia symptoms or assessment of cognitive impairment (Jimison, Pavel, McKanna, & Pavel, 2004; Liu, Chen, Xie, & Gao, 2006). Though cost of game development can be high, benefits from early detection of symptoms can outweigh costs for both individuals and the entire healthcare system. Games can be also useful at measuring disease progress or the effects of different treatment approaches. As the elderly population living independently at home is increasing, an unobtrusive monitoring of changes in cognitive functions can be valuable (see section on cognitive benefits). There are some promising applications for moderating or treating symptoms related to dementia and stroke. Use of video games in senior centers has been frequently reported in the news as a strategy for passing time and motivating social encounters (Schiesel, 2007; Yam, 2007).

In considering serious games for health, it is important to distinguish whether the health benefits are directly caused by playing the game, or if participation in the game serves as a reward or an incentive for adhering to healthy behaviors. With interests in health games rising, the recent conference on health games garnered attention from a diverse set of players, including game developers, medical practitioners, and researchers, and acknowledged the need for continued efforts to develop health games and promote their benefits (Gaudiosi, 2009). Theory and preliminary studies do suggest potential benefits of games, some of which have been validated by empirical studies. These benefits include cognitive, emotional, social, and physical activity outcomes and are described separately in the following sections.

Cognitive Benefits

With a global increase in the older population, public attention to the topic of cognitive impairment, its consequences, and potentially effective interventions is rising. Continued exercise and stimulation of brain function are thought to slow the decline of mental functions and even improve cognitive performances in the elderly (Rosenzweig & Bennett, 1996). In writing about recent brain health interventions, Morrison-Bogorad, Cahan, and Wagster (2007) noted such rising attention to cognitive health and gave a list of relevant campaigns and books from highly respected sources and best-seller publishers. The list includes campaigns, such as:

- The Cognitive and Emotional Health project launched by the National Institutes of Health (NIH) in 2001
- The Staying Sharp project led by AARP
- The Maintain Your Brain program sponsored by the Alzheimer's Association

Such rising attention to cognitive health is also seen in many books, for example:

- *Keep Your Brain Young* (McKhann & Albert, 2002)
- *The Memory Cure: How to Protect Your Brain Against Memory Loss and Alzheimer's Disease* (Fotuhi, 2003)
- *Age-Proof Your Mind: Detect, Delay, and Prevent Memory Loss—Before It's Too Late* (Tan, 2005)

The apparent success of some cognitive interventions gives strength to advertisements for digital games promising to improve cognitive functioning. Therefore, video and computer game developers have started targeting older generations in advertising. Well-known games include Nintendo's Brain Age, Posit Science's Brain Fitness Program, and CogniFit's MindFit (see Table 6.2 for details). Risks and unintended consequences are discussed separately.

These game-based cognitive intervention programs are based on the evidence that cognitive training interventions are helping people think faster, focus better, and memorize more. One early success was demonstrated in the Advanced Cognitive Training for Independent and Vital Elderly (ACTIVE) study (Jobe et al., 2001), sponsored by the National Institutes for Health, specifically, the National Institute on Aging and the National Institute for Nursing Research. The investigators randomly assigned 2832 healthy adults with an average age of 74 years to one of four groups—memory training, reasoning training, speed training, or a control group. Each of the training programs was effective at improving the targeted cognitive functions. Five years later, researchers revisited those who participated in one of three cognitive training sessions and found persistent positive long-term effects of those training sessions (Willis et al., 2006). Participants in cognitive training sessions showed persistent advantages compared to those who were not trained. Those advantages, however, were limited to the specific functions for which participants were previously trained.

Barnes et al. (2006) conducted a randomized controlled trial of computer-based cognitive therapy in older adults with mild cognitive impairment. Participants in this study were patients with cognitive impairment, and the results were similar to the above study that used healthy older adults. Barnes and colleagues asked intervention group participants to perform a series of computer-based, progressive listening exercises that were designed to enhance learning and memory. The exercises lasted 100 minutes a day, and were performed 5 days a week for about 6 weeks. The control group participants were asked to read online newspapers, listen to audio books, and play rudimentary computer games for comparable amounts of time. Findings showed that verbal memory and the primary outcome consistently favored the intervention group.

Posit Science and CogniFit collaborated with investigators at research institutes and universities and published studies to demonstrate their games' effectiveness in improving cognitive health. For example, Zelinski and her colleagues (Zelinski, Yaffe, Ruff, Kennison, & Smith, 2007) recruited 468 adults 65 years or older and randomized them to one of two groups. One group used the game-based Posit Science's Brain Fitness Program and the other group used a DVD-based educational training program on computer skills. Results suggest significantly greater improvement in memory scores and perception of cognitive performance in everyday life for those who used the game-based program compared to those who used the DVD-based program.

A similar study that used another kind of cognitive training game, CogniFit's MindFit, demonstrated the effectiveness of game-based cognitive training programs (Korczyn, Peretz, Aharonson, & Giladi, 2007). In this study, 121 healthy adults ages 50 years old or older were asked to play specific games for 20 minutes every 2 or 3 days for 24 sessions. Compared to those in a control group who played classic popular computer games downloaded from a CD, those who played MindFit games scored significantly higher for spatial short-term memory tests, visual–spatial learning measures, and simple reaction-time measures.

However, less is known about the long-term effects of these games. These video games are at a very early stage, and their evaluation is limited to short-term effects. Vigorous research is needed to show whether effects of mental exercise games are persistent over time (Salthouse, 2006). Also, a cautionary warning should be made against claims about generalized cognitive efficiency. Improvement in a specific cognitive skill practiced does not translate to improvement in other cognitive skills (Jobe et al., 2001). Different games focus on different sets of cognitive skills, such as short-term memory, reaction time, or spatial learning, and consumers need to compare them and make a choice based on their needs (Greene, 2007). This choice presumes a very knowledgeable consumer. The publishing of a guidebook on the topic of brain training and its related products (Fernandez & Goldberg, 2009) attests to the difficulty in navigating through various claims made on cognitive training products. Cost is also a consideration discussed in the section on clinical implications.

Emotional Benefits

Games, in any format, offer a way to discharge surplus energy, provide relaxation that permits recovery from stress, and grant pleasure from the experience of *play* (Hoppes, Hally, & Sewell, 2000). Wang and Singhal (2009) argue that the experiential aspect of play in digital games is what distinguishes them the most from other forms of entertainment. This play dimension, they argue, goes beyond arousal and diversion and creates the emotional engagement that sustains participation and facilitates outcomes. The emotional engagement of *play* is "crucial to achieve any outcome, whether enjoyment and relaxation, or knowledge gains and skill building, or other attitudinal and behavioral change" (Wang & Singhal, 2009, p. 274). Emotional benefits may be tied to the ability of games to fill time, diminish loneliness, and create a sense of self-worth. To some extent, social dimensions of games may be critical to achieving emotional benefits. Earlier studies suggested that digital games can satisfy older adults' needs for entertainment and relaxation (Weisman, 1983), enhance their self-esteem by giving the feeling of success and achievement (Goldstein et al., 1997; Hollander & Plummer, 1986; McGuire, 1984), and improve their sense of well-being (Goldstein et al., 1997). In a more recent study on single-player games from PopCap (http://popcap.com), Russoniello and Park (2008) found dramatic decreases in depression and anger and improvement in mood after game play. For one game, stress as measured by heart rate variability was reduced by half with no gender differences. Though the sample was small, subjects were randomly assigned, and outcomes of this study show the positive role that these games play in terms of mood improvement and stress management. Along with positive outcomes, negative effects of game playing on older adults' emotions also need to be considered. In some cases frustration with game playing can result in negative outcomes (Riddick, Drogin, & Spector, 1987).

Social Benefits

In our increasingly global and digital world, we have fewer face-to-face encounters and more virtual interactions. There is also some evidence that older adults trim their social networks with time use and strength of emotional connection as priorities (Charles & Carstensen, 2010). Developmental stages shape choices. For older adults who are parents, interactions with the larger social world on behalf of their child diminish as the child gains autonomy, independence, and geographical distance from the family. Another way that familiar, in-person contacts diminish is on retirement when an older adult leaves the workplace with its emotional, social, cognitive, and physical demands. At that time, the spouse or partner of the older adult who was engaged in the workplace also loses interrelated social contacts. These may be as simple as social chitchat when the partner received phone calls at home, when delivering forgotten lunches or reports, transporting a partner to the work site, or attending recurring work-related social events such as parties or award ceremonies.

Parenting, working, and supporting a working partner provide opportunities not only for social networking, but for doing good for others that meets altruism needs. Altruism provides a sense of being useful in caring for others. This web of mutual or reciprocal obligations and trust creates a resource often labeled as "social capital" (see Chapter 1). Social capital losses can create emotional stress that leads to depression. Many older adults may require opportunities to develop social capital in new arenas. Games can be an important new resource for social contact. Providing for satisfaction of altruism and social needs within a game may draw older adults into games where an equally important goal is delivery of health knowledge and reinforcement of healthy lifestyles. The potential for promoting altruism within games is being explored by Nowak and Roch (2007). Games can have other useful social consequences that increase social capital. Some benefits of gaming include development and maintenance of new relationships, diminishment of isolation and loneliness, and social leveling that enhances the life of disabled adults.

Relationship Support

Participating in an interactive game provides multiple opportunities for the development and maintenance of social relationships. As Mangrum and Mangrum (1995) note, many games are social activities. Schott and his colleagues (Schott & Hodgetts, 2006; Schott & Horrell, 2000) assert that digital gaming enhances social interaction and that gaming is not a solitary act. Game play often requires collective action and provides shared spaces where a sense of belonging can be fostered. This sense of belonging can become compromised with aging. Today, social motivations are often found to be the primary driver for video game play among the elderly (Figure 6.1). Learning a game from the younger generation can provide rewarding interactions and new topics of conversation and reasons to connect. Vanden Abeele and Van Rompaey (2006) reported that one of the core themes that the elderly want to see in digital games was "connection with others." Their interviewees raised a need for games that specifically connect them with significant others, such as their children,

Figure 6.1   Older Adults Enjoy Social and Physical Aspects of Digital Games

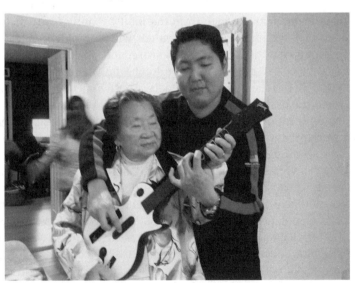

Source: Enrile, 2009. Used with permission.

grandchildren, and friends. The older adults rejected designs that isolated game players. Games can assist older adults to "keep up" with younger family members. Games can allow older adults to reconnect with friends in a new way.

In that regard, multiplayer games were found to be preferred to solo games among the elderly. Also, according to self-determination theory (Ryan, Rigby, & Przybylski, 2006), a desire for relatedness is one important game motivation regardless of game players' ages. This psychological need for relatedness, or a feeling of connectedness with others (Ryan & Deci, 2001), is one critical motivation behind video game play. Games satisfying such a need generate greater enjoyment, enhance self-esteem, and lead to positive affect.

Intergenerational Relationship Potential

Intergenerational relationships can become strained with age and changing needs. Games offer a new potential for relating to others as individuals or in groups, as players and onlookers can feel socially engaged (Figure 6.2). In the real world, game players may have roles that are power-based by nature. Examples where the inherent power base is age include parent, grandparent, and uncle or aunt relationships with a younger person. However, in games, "age" or seniority can come from experience in the game or the skills of gaming. A child can be the expert or senior partner. When one player is "older" in the game by length of time playing and development of core skills, the balance of power shifts

Figure 6.2   Digital Games Provide Intergenerational Opportunities for Play and Cheerleading

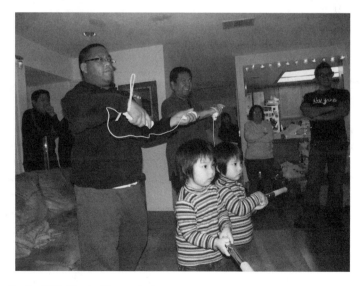

Source: Enrile, 2009. Used with permission.

(Aarsand, 2007). New opportunities for negotiation evolve that may be very engaging for all of the players and increase interaction across the generations.

A story about a local library setting up video games as an effort to bridge generations shows us how playing games can easily become an intergenerational activity (Kurutz, 2008). This public library in Pittsburgh launched a weekly program of social video game playing and reported having drawn not only children but also parents and grandparents. Games can be encouraged as a comfortable venue for intergenerational connections. In the future, games may be developed or marketed specifically to create opportunities for dialogue between the generations. Validation of experience and shared practical solutions to challenges of living with an illness can occur as a direct goal of a game or in incidental conversations.

In an effort to maximize intergenerational benefits of games, a research group in Singapore invented a game called Age Invaders that is specifically designed to connect two different generations such as grandparents and grandchildren (Cheok, Lee, Kodagoda, Tat, & Thang, 2005; Khoo, Merritt, & Cheok, 2009). This game is designed to be enjoyed by both older and younger generations because its parameters are adjustable to the ages of the game players. For example, older players can be given more time to react to rockets fired by younger players; whereas younger players have to react faster to the ones launched by their older counterparts. This game attempted to bridge the generational gap by balancing out differences in physical abilities across generations. A demonstration video on YouTube helps elucidate how the game works (http://www.youtube.com/watch?v=kkA9iFrHq_0), and its companion website also provides detailed information about the game (http://www.mixedreality.nus.edu.sg/index.php/projects/all-projects/age-invaders).

As part of efforts to attract the elderly and publicize video game playing as an activity for everyone in the household, one of the largest video game makers, Nintendo, recently hosted an event for grandparents (Nintendo, 2006). The same company also took their products to an annual convention sponsored by AARP and courted the older gamer (Taub, 2006). With the rising popularity of easy, casual games among all age groups, the gaming industry expects to find a move toward intergenerational video game play (Macgill, 2007). No health games designed specifically for intergenerational play were found at the time of this writing. However, there is great potential for intergenerational learning and play around any health condition with genetic links or environmental influences on diet, exercise, and stress management. The generations can learn from each other and act in ways that support rather than sabotage each other's intentions to engage in more healthy behaviors. Intergenerational games can take advantage of existing social capital and, over time, increase social ties and build trust and willingness to assist each other. The Wellness Partners Game developed under the RWJF initiative is an example where exercise can be encouraged (Gotsis, Valente, Jordan-Marsh, & Spruiijt-Metz, 2008).

Social Leveling Potential for Stigmatized Groups

In the past, most gaming experiences required a physical presence, such as participating in bowling, a board game, or poker night. The use of digital games for socialization is especially useful for stigmatized groups in promoting social interaction. Absent face-to-face contact, stereotypes about disability or other overt physical differences are not evoked (Cassidy, 2008; Deeley, 2007; Stein, 2007). Online, globe-spanning tournaments of well-known games such as Scrabble are increasingly popular. According to a survey by Information Solutions Group (2008), those with mental or physical disabilities play games more often and for a longer time, compared to those without disabilities. About two-thirds of respondents with disabilities also cited distraction from disability as a core reason to play computer or video games.

Gaming in virtual worlds in particular can be a venue for social interaction for those who are disadvantaged in a face-to-face interaction, freeing the disabled from restrictions of their real life (Schlender, 2008). Cole and Griffiths (2007) characterize virtual world gaming as a space where players can express themselves in "ways they may not feel comfortable doing in real life because of their appearance, gender, sexuality, and/or age" (p. 575). With digital technology, the use of an avatar in the virtual world affords an opportunity to mingle with people at each individual's preferred geographic location. Physical characteristics such as a disability or skin color or gender can be masked, changed, or hidden. The potential of virtual reality has not been fully explored as a tool in minimizing health disparities.

Social Presence Aspects

The experience of social presence inherent in games can be a major attractor for older adults when social contact is limited by geography or disability. Social presence is "the degree of salience of the other person in interaction and the consequent salience of the interpersonal relationships" (Short, Williams, & Christie, 1976, p. 65). This feeling of being with others is especially strong in massively multiplayer online role-playing games (MMORPGs) where game players develop and control game characters and interact with others online who also have those embodied characters (Tamborini & Skalski, 2006). Unlike the long-held stereotype that game players are socially inactive, a survey of MMORPG players showed that the most salient motivation to play a MMORPG is social companionship and connectedness (Cole & Griffiths, 2007; Griffiths, Davies, & Chappell, 2004). In a survey of MMORPG players (Cole & Griffiths, 2007), about three-quarters of all respondents said that they had made good friends within the game. Of all respondents, 40% also answered that they would discuss sensitive issues with friends they had met through MMORPGs before they would discuss them with their real-life friends. These survey numbers suggest that well-designed online games can be an attractive venue for older adults whose social network and physical boundary have become diminished by mobility issues. Game play may promote incidental socialization. Participant comments indicate that MMORPGs brought game experiences to a new, social dimension where players interacted to form networks of communities while playing games.

However, at present, the number of adults over 65 playing such games is unknown. A recent census reported that the oldest respondents were 50–65 and represented only 4% of the players (Williams, Yee, & Caplan, 2008). Williams et al. did note that older players and women were spending more time playing than young males. Game developers in this genre were encouraged to rethink audiences who might be new players.

Networking through games may be valuable as one's network shrinks because of mortality in one's peer group and when family members are a long distance away. In addition, many social interchange games are played around the clock, which can be an advantage for older adults with shorter sleep cycles. Games can be an important counterbalance to isolation and loneliness triggered by changes experienced by older adults.

Physical Benefits

Recent development of games that incorporate exercising has also spurred interest among the elderly. These applications are called "exergames" and are promoted as a way to improve physical performance while having fun. According to a report by the Centers for Disease Control and Prevention (CDC; 1999), older adults can obtain significant health benefits with only a moderate amount of physical activity, such as walking or stair climbing. Playing exergames can replace time spent sitting in a couch and watching television and bring positive health benefits to older adults. Exergaming may not help much to fulfill the daily amount of exercise recommended to adolescents. However, for older adults with sedentary lifestyles and slow metabolism, even gentle and light body movements stimulated by exergames can prevent muscles and joints from becoming stiff from inactivity.

Digital games' physical benefits are not limited to exergames. One early study showed that even nonexergame video games can slow down deterioration of perceptual–motor functions and improve hand–eye coordination (Drew & Waters, 1986). Similarly a Japanese game company in its collaborative research efforts with Kyushu University found an increase in both alertness and physical balance among female elderly video game players, lowering the risk of falling (Hug, 2004).

Exergames can maximize games' potentials to realize physical benefits. An experiment that compared calorie consumption levels between a sedentary game (Project Gotham Racing 3 on Xbox360) and an activity-promoting exergame (Wii Sports) found a significantly higher level of energy consumption among exergame players compared to sedentary game players (Graves, Stratton, Ridgers, & Cable, 2007). Another team of researchers compared physical activity levels across different types of games and found that children playing exergames had significantly higher levels of heart rates and energy expenditure than children playing seated games (Mellecker & McManus, 2008). More studies on exergames can be found in a review article by Daley (2009). Though participants of these studies were not older adults but children, the same results are expected to be true for older adults. Altered stamina and cardiovascular conditions may result in greater energy expenditures. This will be an important topic for research as exergames are more widely used in rehabilitation (Baertlein, 2007) and game companies expand their efforts to partner with the health industry (Lewis, 2009).

A cautionary note is appropriate as current versions of exergames have a relatively low activity level compared to traditional exercise (Daley, 2009). As some exergames require as little activity as a swing of the wrist, virtual gaming cannot be a replacement for real exercise. However, new versions of exergames require full body movement and use a full-vision lens or weight pressure to provide feedback. One example is the EyeToy: Kinetic (Lieberman, 2006). An exergame can also involve the active use of certain body parts, such as upper body, that a person is less likely to move during his or her everyday activity (Graf, Pratt, Hester, & Short, 2009). Future versions would ideally include heart rate monitoring or sway assessment for balance interventions. Even games with a lower physical demand can be a useful transition from a totally sedentary lifestyle. This transition seems promising as it was for those with the more sedentary lifestyles who expressed greater interests and more positive attitudes toward exergames (Klein & Simmers, 2009).

Virtual reality applications for rehabilitation are emerging as a new field as well. This technology has great potential for observing and coaching human motor behaviors (Broeren, Rydmark, Bjorkdahl, & Sunnerhagen, 2007). A game called 3DBricks is an example of combining virtual reality and haptics[1]. The player strikes a virtual ball to topple bricks. The advantage is that speed and level of difficulty can be varied.

---

[1]Haptics is "the sensation of shape and texture a computer user feels when virtually 'touching' a digital object with a force-feedback device" (McLaughlin, Jung, Peng, Jin, & Zhu, 2008, p. 158).

STRUCTURE OF GAMES AS MECHANISM FOR BENEFITS

Properties of games, such as interactivity, storytelling (narrative), nonlinearity, simulation, and role playing, make gaming an ideal platform for changing health-related behaviors and attitudes (Baranowski et al., 2008) and enhancing health knowledge (Lieberman & Brown, 1995). Other key features of games include multimodality, options for social (multiplayer) use, and the game's frame of experience (Klimmt, 2009). Games are often based on stories, featuring back stories and narrative introductions (Jenkins, 2004).

Taking control of game characters in a story, game players perceive themselves as the center of events or a driver of change and progress and become an active participant in a narrative, rather than a passive observer (Kelso, Weyhrauch, & Bates, 1993). They feel as if they were being transported into, or absorbed in, a story, and they become emotionally involved with game characters. This phenomenon is called narrative or dramatic transportation (Green, 2004; Green & Brock, 2000). Such transportation translates into deep engagement and, as a result, increases the likelihood of being persuaded by messages embedded in game designs. This engagement can be an advantage when health professionals are designing or recommending games to change health attitudes, or behaviors. However, it is equally a caution in that older adults may be susceptible to embedded messages that promote unhealthy behaviors in commercially available or freeware games.

Interactivity

An essential feature of games is interactivity. Games that are interactive respond to game players; such feedback influences the course of events occurring in the game world (Klimmt & Vorderer, 2007; Lee, Park, & Jin, 2006). This interactive feature of games allows a player to choose the unfolding of a story. Games can progress in a nonlinear fashion, presenting unique story lines for each individual game player. Depending on game players' feedback, game designers can deliver customized messages to their players. Such increased customization leads players to build direct, self-related connections with the game world and pay more attention to messages conveyed within a game (Fogg, 2003). The interaction feature creates a sense of presence that adds to the social dimension of a game and may be a key aspect of the potential for emotional engagement. This ability to respond to individual players creates conditions that facilitate changes in health behaviors and attitudes specific to the individual. A well-designed game would adjust to the differing needs of players with chronic conditions across their illness journey. Similarly, a game's infrastructure can accommodate changes in attitudes and acquisition of skills and deliver a different experience.

Stories as Developmental Tasks

Reflecting on one's history is considered a major task of aging successfully, and games are known to facilitate story sharing. Mangrum and Mangrum (1995) found that domino games provided the elderly an opportunity to exchange their life stories with others. In analyzing games, it is important to distinguish story as a back structure provided by the developer or a feature built with participant input. Back stories are recognized as a critical aspect of games for children and act to sustain engagement (Baranowski et al., 2008).

Role-playing games are one aspect of using stories. They are common in the recreational game area and are recently emerging in the health game category. Life and Death in the Age of Malaria is one example of a health game where players take on the role of advisor to other travelers (Bauman & Hartjes, 2008). Creating and playing with an avatar in Second Life is a kind of participant storytelling. However, relatively little is known about the role of structured narratives or sharing of participant stories in digital games for adults.

Research on how health games might facilitate conversation with other players could provide valuable insights into developmental task achievements and illness coping processes. Games often provide a context for discussion during and after games. Conversations taking place inside and outside of the gaming arena can facilitate learning by story sharing. Such story sharing also helps to spread the word to those who do not play games (Shaffer, Squire, Halverson, & Gee, 2005). According to Jenkins and colleagues (2009), benefits of in-game learning can be maximized when game players articulate what they have learned. Thus they emphasized the importance of peer-to-peer conversation among game players and proposed building an environment (such as a discussion forum or online conversation board) where game players can exchange ideas and insights. Especially among those with illnesses, sharing experiences and emotional disclosure can affect therapeutic outcomes (Pennebaker, 1997). The gaming environment can offer opportunities for emotional disclosure to peers, information sharing, and empathic connections.

Potential Outcome Mechanisms

In sum, properties of games, such as storytelling and interactivity, when fully used, lead to deep engagement, feeling of empowerment, and delivery of personalized and tailored messages. Using such features of games, game developers designed games that promote healthy lifestyles and educate about disease conditions and management. Examples include games that teach adolescents and children about diabetes and the relationships between diet, insulin, and blood sugar levels (Brown et al., 1997); obesity prevention

(Thompson et al., 2008); asthma management for children (Lieberman, 2001); and cancer treatment (Kato, Cole, Bradlyn, & Pollock, 2008).

However, little is known about the outcomes of the currently available health games for adults. Often commercial games do not offer any data that researchers can easily access. Though game sites often record and post highest scores, these numbers and ranking data are too coarse to be useful for clinical purposes. The work of Russoniello and Park (2008) is groundbreaking in its inclusion of physical parameters such as heart rate variability and electroencephalography (EEG) readings. The study was funded by Popcap, a major commercial game supplier. More stratified sampling across age groups and longitudinal findings are urgently needed. The Robert Wood Johnson Foundation's games initiatives are expected to deliver quality research as that was a condition of awards. As with drugs, determining the mechanism of action is important to making sound recommendations with minimal side effects. Monitoring eyestrain and carpel tunnel and other musculoskeletal impacts is as important as understanding benefits. As therapists and healthcare providers adopt games as part of their clinical routines and researchers respond to funding initiatives, more will be known.

SKILL AS A VARIABLE IN PARTICIPATION

For all players, but especially older adults, it is important to consider the level of skill required to play. For some adults, loading a CD and starting a file are already familiar. Others will need a walk-through. The health professional can increase the likelihood of playing by not assuming computer capabilities. For Internet-based games, entering URLs spontaneously or clicking on a URL in an e-mail may be required and problematic. In one study, for example, investigators observed Internet use by older adults and reported a frequent tendency to click on irrelevant text and difficulties in scrolling and using tabbed navigation (Chadwick-Dias, McNulty, & Tullis, 2003). Difficulty in navigating early steps in computer use can interfere with game play experience and lower the degree of confidence and diminish feelings of spatial presence (Schaik, Turnbull, Wersch, & Drummond, 2004). A perception of incompetence in game playing can lead to negative affects and low self-esteem (Ryan et al., 2006). Healthcare providers will want to provide access to games that fit the skill levels of older players. For some older adults, special eyeglass prescriptions are needed for computer tasks at work. No information was found on whether this adaptation was required for playing online games.

Fisk and colleagues (2004) conducted focus group interviews with older adults and found the most often reported issue with the use of new technology is usability. This could be solved by better design and proper training and early engagement of potential players in the design process (Morales-Rodriguez,

Casper, & Brennan, 2007). To enhance usability especially among the elderly, they suggest making it learn to use devices and memorize their functions. They also suggest making devices that are less prone to induce errors. A paper from Eldergames project, a project funded by the European Union (EU), also acknowledges a variety of sensory, cognitive, and physical impairments that occur with aging and have put forward specific design guidelines for games targeting older adults (Gamberini et al., 2006). Table 6.1 lists changes in cognitive and sensory functions among the elderly and specific guidelines to cater to elderly gamer players' needs. Natural interfaces as well as simplified game commands are important because they will determine whether games will become popular among older adults (Gamberini et al., 2008).

Games that must be accessed from consoles also require special skills. One of Japan's largest game developers, Namco, runs adult day care facilities where the elderly as well as people with disabilities can learn how to operate consoles and play games (Andersen, 2006; "Video game company, Namco," 2006). At these facilities, the elderly learn how to turn on gaming consoles, how to insert a game CD into the machine, and which button to press on the handheld game devices. The development of a game-learning center for the elderly demonstrates the fact that skills needed for video game playing do not come naturally for older adults who are less familiar with the operation of new technology. Another category of games that needs special consideration for older adults are exergames. Exergames are based on motion-sensing technology, and motion sensors might not be sensitive enough to catch the narrow angle and slow speed of older adults' movements. For example, older adults with weak muscles or severe arthritis might not be able to operate exergames without proper adjustment of sensor devices. Some issues that gamers with limited body movements experience are well addressed in an open letter sent to Nintendo by a muscular dystrophy gamer (Crecente, 2006).

Children and Teens as Coaches

Engaging a younger person as coach may also increase both parties' investment in having the older adult participate enthusiastically in the game. Highlighting the potential to give a younger person an opportunity to be the teacher may diminish the embarrassment of asking for help. This role reversal can be significant if there is competition in the household for using the computer. It is important that provider, client, and coach appreciate that beginning to use a health game can be frustrating. Some problems will arise related to skill level and some will be related to equipment failures and Internet connection disruptions, which are well known to experienced users. A younger person who expresses interest, declares these problems are normal, and checks on progress can provide the social support that increases the likelihood of continued participation.

SELECTING GAMES FOR CLINICAL OBJECTIVES

Sawyer and Smith (2008) introduced a taxonomy for serious games that covered a wide range of areas, such as health, education, and military defense. Following their categories for health games, we present examples of health games that are specifically relevant to the older adult population in Table 6.2. This table is not created to introduce all available games. Rather the intent is to show current uses and future potential of games for a wide range of health issues for older adults. As Table 6.2 shows, games are not only developed for therapeutic purposes but also for prevention, assessment, and education goals. When available, studies or ongoing research relevant to specific games are also cited.

Games as Prevention

As older adults suffer from natural declines in physical and cognitive functions, such as decreasing manual dexterity and hand–eye coordination, impaired balancing ability, and slowdown of processing speed, video games can be one powerful solution to slow, stall, or reverse the natural consequences of aging.

Entrepreneurial companies and university-affiliated research labs, such as Posit Science, CogniFit, HAPPYneuron, and Lumos Labs, are marketing their brain-training products for their effectiveness in reversing or slowing cognitive impairment among older adults. Games are also freely available with registration on a few websites, such as eons.com (http://fun.eons.com/brain_games) and AARP sites (http://games.aarp.org).

Exergaming is another area that is booming with the rising popularity of motion-sensitive games, such as Wii. Though the concept of exergames has been around since the 1980s, it is only recently that exergames have been marketed on a massive scale. Examples of exergames include Nintendo's Wii Sports, Konami's Dance Dance Revolution (DDR), Sony PlayStation's EyeToy Cycle, Gamercize's GZ Sport, and Fisher-Price's Smart Cycle. These games require skills that are relatively less complex and easy to learn because they resemble real-world movements. Instead of learning a series of complex buttons on a control pad, exergamers can move their bodies in a natural way because motion sensors can monitor and reflect the movement of bodies into the game screen.

Unlike the stereotype that only children enjoy games, one study found no significant difference between young adults (21–30) and older adults (59–80) in the degree of enjoyment earned from Sony's EyeToy exergames (Rand, Kizony, & Weiss, 2004). All participants, regardless of age, found the game enjoyable and easy to operate. Some game companies are also prioritizing games specifically targeting older adults. For example, DanceTown is designed for older adults, using simple high-contrast graphics and background music

Table 6.2   Health Games for Older Adults: Examples by Types

Purpose	Types	Game Title	Maker	Platform	References
Preventive	Exergame	Dance Dance Revolution	Konami	Dance pad and monitor	White, Lehmann, & Trent, 2007
	Exergame	Wii Sports	Nintendo	Video game console	
	Exergame	Wii Fit	Nintendo	Video game console	
	Exergame	DanceTown	TouchTown	Dance pad and monitor	
	Cognitive training	Brain Age	Nintendo	Handheld video game device	
	Cognitive training	Brain Fitness Program	PositScience	Computer CD and Internet	Zelinski, Yaffe, Ruff, Kennison, & Smith, 2007
	Cognitive training	MindFit	CogniFit	Computer CD and Internet	Korczyn, Peretz, Aharonson, & Giladi, 2007
	Cognitive training	[m]Power	Dakim	Touch screen	

(continues)

Table 6.2   Health Games for Older Adults: Examples by Types (*continued*)

Purpose	Types	Game Title	Maker	Platform	References
Assessment	Unobtrusive monitoring –Dementia detection	Computer game for the detection of dementia		Computer	Jimison et al., 2004
	Self-assessment –Dementia detection	Gesture-based game		Computer and camera	Liu, Chen, Xie, & Gao, 2006
Therapeutic	Pain distraction/ Rehabilitainment –Poststroke patients	Virtual reality (VR) simulation Exercises on Xbox	Microsoft	Video game console	Morrow et al., 2006
	Pain distraction/ Rehabilitainment –Poststroke elderly patients	EyeToy on PlayStation	Sony	Video game console	Rand, Kizony, & Weiss, 2004
	Disease management –Alzheimer's patients	VR simulation game		Computer	Hofmann et al., 2003
	Pain distraction/ Rehabilitainment –Poststroke patients	Spatial rotation and space tube games		Computer and haptic device	McLaughlin et al., 2005

Rehabilitainment	Taiko Drum Master RT-Japanese Mind, Wani Wani Panic RT, Sweet Land 4RT, GateBall Club RT	Namco	Arcade game machine	Namco and Kyushu University research team (Hug, 2004)
Pain distraction/ Rehabilitainment –Poststroke patients	Wii Sport	Nintendo	Video game console	Stacy Fritz at the University of South Carolina is exploring the Wii Sport in motivating stroke patients.
Rehabilitainment –Parkinson's disease patients	Wii Sport	Nintendo	Video game console	Funded by NIH, Glenna Dowling at the University of California at San Francisco, in collaboration with Red Hill Studio, is studying Wii for Parkinson's disease patients

familiar to the older generation. To prevent falls, this gaming device also provides safety bars that older adults can hold while playing. To the extent that a game is intended to provide aerobic exercise, a heart rate monitor is essential (Ijsselsteijn, de Kort, Westerink, Jager, & Bonants, 2006). Ideally, the monitor would be linked to a component of the visual display.

Games as Therapy

Games are also used as distractions and therapeutic tools. The immersive nature of games helps hold the attention of a game player for a prolonged time and alleviate boredom resulting from repetition of similar tasks. A Japanese company, Namco, joined two terms, *rehabilitation* and *entertainment*, and coined a word, *rehabilitainment*, to describe the use of entertainment for recovery of functions (Baindai Namco Group, 2007). As mistakes in games do not have real-life consequences and learning is often by trial and error, simulation games are also developed to let patients make errors and learn from simulated game environments. For example, Hofmann and colleagues (2003) asked 10 patients suffering from Alzheimer's disease to move their avatars through a virtual environment that simulated each patient's typical surroundings, home or usual shopping route, and photographs of the patient at an earlier age. Results indicated that after 3 weeks of training, patients could perform the task more quickly and, equally important, needed less help navigating the environment in their real lives.

Another game with stress management applications is the Cloud game developed at the University of Southern California. Chen (2007) developed this game as a meditative experience using flow theory developed by Csikszentmihalyi (1975; 1997), which is captured by the phrase "being in the zone." No research data for outcomes is available, although the game has won several prizes and has been downloaded by thousands of users across the world. The Cloud game is available free at http://www.jenovachen.com/flowingames/cloud.htm. SilverFit is an exergame developed by a Dutch company that enhances physical therapy and rehabilitation of older adults (SilverFit, n.d.). Unlike other commercially available games, such as Wii Fit, this game allows customization of game course and plan based on game play data collected during previous sessions. Keeping in mind that the targeted players of SilverFit may not have good mobility skills and may become easily fatigued, its developers designed this game in a way that it can be played with no handheld controllers in a sitting position with stretching of the arms and legs, or in a standing position with the support of a walking stick.

Researchers who are interested in using games for therapeutic purposes not only develop new games (Hofmann et al., 2003; McLaughlin et al., 2005), but they also adapt commercial games for rehabilitation purposes (Morrow, Docan, Burdea, & Merians, 2006; Rand et al., 2004). Especially with the development and popularity of motion-sensitive gaming devices, such as Wii, rehabilitation and therapy centers are increasing their uses of commercial gaming platforms. Examples include use of games for rehabilitation of Parkinson's disease patients, post-stroke individuals (Medical College of Georgia, 2008; Tanner, 2008), and brain-injured patients (Goldberg et al., 2008). Occupational therapists are finding Wii to be an excellent tool to increase engagement in therapy as well as to enhance the amount of physical activities. The National Institutes of Health and Robert Wood Johnson Foundation are also funding studies that test effectiveness of commercial games, such as Wii Sport, in rehabilitation. A Google keyword search for *Guitar Hero* shows informal reports of use to regain hand and shoulder function after burns and other health applications. As more health professionals have the opportunity to play with and study games involving movement, more applications will emerge.

Games as Assessment Tool

Games as an assessment adjunct is perhaps the least developed area. Engaged aging at home as independently as possible is a clear preference of older adults. Digital game playing among baby boomer generations is potentially an everyday activity. Data from game play, if analyzed correctly, can provide useful predictive information about changes in cognitive and physical functions. This data can help track changes in an unobtrusive way and detect symptoms of certain diseases, such as dementia, at their beginning stages.

For example, Liu and colleagues (2006) used a camera to capture motions of a player doing a traditional game, rock–paper–scissors, against a computer character, and developed an algorithm to analyze motion data from a player's gestures. This game helps a player make an initial judgment regarding any changes in his or her mental status. Another team of researchers at the Oregon Center for Aging and Technology (Jimison & Pavel, 2006; Jimison et al., 2004) wrote cognitive performance assessment algorithms for a card game called FreeCell, which is a popular casual game installed as a default on the Microsoft Windows system. The researchers' objective was to facilitate early detection of dementia among older adults. Other applications are bound to emerge as body-sensor technology advances.

Games as Education

There has been a rapid increase in applications to educate and inform consumers about a wide range of health and public health issues (Wang & Singhal, 2009). These are often labeled as "edutainment" or entertainment–education (E-E) applications. Wang and Singhal (2009) have defined entertainment–education as "a theory-based communication strategy for purposefully embedding educational and social issues in the creation, production, processing, and dissemination process of an entertainment program, in order to achieve desired individual, community, institutional, and societal changes among the intended media user populations" (p. 272). One famous education game is Re-Mission, a shooting game developed to teach young cancer patients what happens inside the bodies of cancer patients and how they can most effectively cope with their ailments. Education, or the increase in cancer knowledge, was not the sole outcome from this game. As a result of game playing, children also showed greater adherence to treatment (Kato et al., 2008).

Unlike prevalence of health education games developed for children and adolescents, older adults have been largely neglected as potential beneficiaries of health and physical education games. Papasterigiou (2009) reviewed papers on computer and video games developed for health and physical education during the last 10 years. The topics covered in these games include nutrition, disease management and prevention, first-aid education, and symptom awareness. Although some of these topics are equally relevant and important to an aging population, no education games have been developed for or tested on older adults. Games have been developed as instructional tools to improve health knowledge not only for children and adolescents but also for health professionals and medical students (Akl et al., 2008). For example, a game was developed that teaches medical school students to locate risk factors for fall during home visit (Duque, Fung, Mallet, Posel, & Fleiszer, 2008). A similar game may be developed and used to teach the elderly about healthy lifestyles, disease management, and prevention techniques. Educational games were found to be effective for the younger population in the majority of cases (Papasterigiou, 2009) and are expected to be of great use for the older generation as well. One risk in this field is being too pedantic and boring and losing the audience engagement built by play.

Games as Informatics

Health games for informatics are the least developed among the five types of games. Although incomplete and still under development, a game-based personal health record (PHR) system is an example of games as informatics. Sawyer ("Eye on innovation," 2007) in an interview introduced his team's efforts to develop a game-based PHR system where an in-game avatar embodies and visually represents a patient's health information. A patient's health record can be fed into a game character, and the appearance and traits of the game character can change accordingly. The graphical display of health information can help players understand their own health status. Also, people often develop an emotional attachment to their in-game characters, and this can result in more accurate and honest reporting of their health information and deeper engagement in health care. Video gaming consoles that come with advanced graphics processing power can also be used as an affordable viewer of medical images, such as a CT scan and MRI images ("Video gaming graphics," 2008). Microsoft runs both video game and PHR platform units, Xbox and HealthVault (Brown, 2009), and we may expect to see the synergies of these two units in the development of a game-based PHR system.

PLATFORMS FOR GAMES

Some games use a computer as the platform and use a CD, but more often games require an Internet connection. Some games are also played on a video game console, such as Xbox and Wii. Other games are on handheld devices, such as a PDA or a cell phone.

According to a recent survey on video game players in the United States (Jackson & Keitt, 2008), the most often used game platform among older adults is a tethered or desktop computer. As more than two-thirds of adults age 43 or older have computers at home, a computer is the most easily accessible gaming device (Golvin, 2008). According to the same report, the frequency of downloading free or paid online games is almost equal or greater for older adults as it is for younger adults. Older adult gamers are often categorized as PC casual gamers who do not have video game consoles but who frequently play online or computer games (Nielsen Entertainment, 2006).

Ownership of video game consoles is relatively less common in the older adult-dominated house compared to that of computers. However, a recent survey predicts shifts will emerge as a high percentage of younger boomers between ages 42 and 51 own video game consoles, such as Xbox, PlayStation, or Wii, in comparison to older boomers (Golvin, 2008). Compared to 22% of adults ages 52 to 62, 43% of adults between 42 and 51 years of age said they own video game consoles and play video games. Numbers also show that baby boomers will continue or resume buying video games (IBISWorld, 2008). Princess Cruises and Holland America have recently announced not only the availability of digital exergames but plans to project them on giant poolside screens. The social component is a primary motivator as well as updating the cruise ship image (Princess Cruises, 2008).

As the major game platforms are computers and video game consoles, health games on mobile devices are still rare. However, with the increase in sales of advanced phones, such as smartphones, and advancement in location-tracking and motion-sensing technologies, development of health applications based on these phones is well underway (Lovelock, 2009; Suhonen, Väätäjä, Virtanen, & Raisamo, 2008). The potential for an innovative use of mobile phones has started receiving attention from researchers and health professionals. For example, a research team at the University of Houston (Fujiki et al., 2007) developed a mobile phone-based game called NEAT-o (Non-Exercise Activity Thermogenesis). Using a sensor that detects movement such as running and walking, this game wirelessly transmits the movement data of each game player from a sensor to a server and moves avatars in a game world according to real-world movement data for each player. A team at the University of Southern California is developing a casual game to encourage healthy lifestyle behaviors in a social network. Wellness Partners, funded by the Robert Wood Johnson Foundation's games initiative can be played on a cell phone or on the Web (Gotsis et al., 2008). The team is exploring the potential of "wearable" sensors to detect movement and whether gaming with points increases healthy lifestyle behaviors. Also under development in Europe is Health Defender, a motion-based mobile phone game incorporating cardiovascular feedback (Wylie & Coulton, 2009). This game rewards players for successfully increasing their heart rate exertion to the goal set by the game system based on real-time cardiovascular data. New serious or health games are constantly emerging, as the evidence of benefits accumulates and new partnerships form.

RISKS OF GAME ENGAGEMENT

Some experts have been concerned that children who engage in computer games are at risk for social isolation from peers (Colwell & Payne, 2000), as well as diminished physical activity and interaction with the external environment, including exposure to sunlight (Subrahmanyam, Kraut, Greenfield, & Gross, 2000). These concerns are equally appropriate for older adults. Exergames are often based on motions used in real exercises and the issues resulting from physical exertion such as aching backs and sore shoulders need to be addressed. Hand injuries are the most often reported issue among Wii players (Sparks, Chase, & Coughlin, 2009). Even with growing media coverage on game-related injuries (Das, 2009; "Doctors warn," 2008; Raby, 2008; Warren, 2006), safety and fall risk issues have been minimally addressed with respect to the Wii Fit or other exergames (Au, 2009).

The vulnerability of the older adult to advertising pitches for games that promise extravagant results for high costs must be considered. Some games simply have no evidence for stated or implied outcomes. In other cases, older adults may not be clear that they are purchasing a subscription to use the game that will expire. Some games require a subscription such as Happy Neuron, and others require a console and later purchase of new modules.

There is some risk that involving one's adult children or grandchildren in selection and purchase could lead to credit card abuse. Similarly, equipment purchased for the older adult may be taken over by younger members of the family. Many older adults would be unwilling to assert their rights. A comprehensive assessment of the individual and the family circumstances and history would be critical to setting up targets for monitoring aspects of game play.

The brain game market is rapidly expanding, and marketers are creating an expectation that playing digital games forestalls dementia and other cognitive problems attributed to aging. Serious game researchers place part of the blame on game companies for "shoveling" out health or brain games without research (Orland, 2008). Kawashima, the neuroscientist behind the smash-hit Brain Age, also warns against liability problems in the serious games market and raises the need for game companies to collaborate with researchers in designing serious games for health. This echoes with Coyle and his colleagues' (2007) call for more collaborative efforts between health professionals and game software and hardware engineers.

Video and computer games can be costly. It is unknown whether traditional methods of more inexpensive play would lead to similarly effective results. For example, can playing with paper-and-pencil puzzles or card games be as effective in managing some cognitive deficits? However, no studies were found comparing digital or video games to traditional games. Most studies use a control group that does not engage in games (Jobe et al., 2001; Zelinski et al., 2007). Testing whether the play or gaming aspect is the core mechanism might be done with games that are not digital.

CLINICAL PRACTICE IMPLICATIONS

When games are introduced, the clinician has responsibility to consider the evidence base, costs, skill level required, available training, and potential documentation in electronic health records (EHRs) and personal health records

(PHRs), as well as monitor outcomes, track side effects, and participate in interdisciplinary collaboration efforts to meet emerging opportunities and demands. Some implications for practice are summarized in Table 6.3.

Table 6.3   Games in Care Plan: Practice Implications

- Costs: one time, ongoing subscription, freeware, library access
- Coverage: eligibility for reimbursement by healthcare plan
- Skill level of patient: comfort with and availability of CD player, Web access, console use, mobile phone
- Training available through agency: hands-on return demonstration, coaching, technical assistance after introduction
- Outcome monitoring: interim results, clinical goal achievement
- Side effects tracking: carpal tunnel, addiction, social isolation
- Interdisciplinary collaboration: communicating expectations and outcomes
- EHR and PHR documentation: capacity for monitoring
- Social network impact: expansion, narrowing, diversification
- Interdisciplinary communication and feedback: motivation, reinforcement

---

Evidence Base

Adding games to a care plan for adults has the potential to lead to improved outcomes that may be specific to the game and its mechanisms. Equally likely is that, much like online support groups, playing a game is empowering but may not lead to specific clinical outcomes (Barak, Boniel-Nissim, & Suler, 2008). Although the clinician is seeking increased knowledge, positive change in health habits, improved weight management and blood pressure, or compliance with regimens, it may be that games simply achieve more global outcomes. For online groups, the most consistent outcomes are well-being, a sense of control, self-confidence, feelings of independence, social interactions, and improved feelings (Barak et al., 2008).

It may be that health games are similarly limited in their impact. These achievements are worthy in themselves and may be a platform for subsequent interventions. To date, for games, as presented earlier, the most rigorous evidence for older adult applications has been for cognitive outcomes. As Ijsselsteijn, Nap, de kort, and Poels (2007) argue, further well-controlled empirical studies are needed to establish literature on games' effects on older adults. This literature then can be used to persuade older adults to engage in the potentially rewarding and beneficial digital game activities. Many other serious or health games for older adults are in the developmental stage. Research on the relative value of digital games compared to other therapies will continue. Multiple studies are underway based on funding from such groups as the Robert Wood Johnson Foundation (2009).

Humana is another primary agency and sponsor of health games. In a recent press release, it explicitly states its goal as making people healthier and motivating healthy lifestyle choices through video games (Humana, 2007). Humana recently reported adding its new dance game platform designed for seniors to its Guidance Centers (Thomas-Ross, 2009). This placement in a health insurance service facility increases exposure to games for an audience focused on health. The Dance Dance Revolution pad was adapted for seniors for use as a supported standup or hand-controlled lap option. A dashboard tracks calories burned, skill level, and experience. Pilot research on Dancetown conducted by Humana's Health Services Research Center found that the game had positive results; for example, feelings about general health and perceived ability to perform specific activities such as ability to climb stairs, walk more than a mile, and a reduction in overall bodily pain, as well as lower levels of depression (Keller et al., 2009). A few game studios, such as Archimage, are also closely working with research teams at universities and health institutions to develop health games. Archimage's partnership with a research team at the University of Texas to develop casual health games is also funded by a major health insurance company, Aetna. Nonprofit organizations are also contributing to the development of health games. For example, HopeLab has collaborated with the insurance company Cigna and developed a game for cancer patients. Major universities are developing products with promises of rigorous evaluations. They collaborate with game developers and often receive financial support from various health agencies and foundations. Sony, in a groundbreaking collaboration, partnered with researchers to provide real-time data on game play (Williams et al., 2009).

As a part of the Serious Games Initiative, funded by the Woodrow Wilson Center, Games for Health (www.gamesforhealth.org) is another project dedicated to health games with annual conferences. The Games for Health and Health Games Research initiatives will be contributing to the evidence base in the years to come. The Woodrow Wilson International Center for Scholars supports the Games for Health website led by Sawyer and Smith. Interested healthcare providers can access this site to stay abreast of developments in the health game field. There are also archives back to 2004 (http://www.gamesforhealth.org/index3.html).

Trends to watch in health gaming are summarized in Table 6.4. New developments have been spurred not only by technology but the commercial success of games and evidence of their effectiveness as tools in healthcare arsenal.

Table 6.4   Trends in Health Games

- Well-designed games have improved players' behavioral and/or clinical outcomes
  - "Intensified anti-smoking attitudes, improved prevention behaviors, influenced dietary habits, increased physical activity, enhanced self-care, strengthened adherence to one's medical treatment plan and improved chronic disease self-management" (RWJF, 2009, p. 3)
  - Rehabilitainment uses games for occupational and physical therapy goals
- Expanding range of platforms and interfaces
  - Traditional video games on game consoles, handheld game players, arcade machines, computers, websites and multiplayer online worlds, social networking sites
- New kinds of delivery for games
  - "Mobile networked computing, exertion interfaces (e.g., dance pads, cameras pointed at players, motion-detecting remote controllers), robots, interactive television, virtual environments, electronic toys, context-sensitive programs (e.g., using sensors, physiological and health monitors, global positioning systems)" (RWJF, 2009, p. 4)
  - Social networking sites, such as Facebook
- New data potentials: body-sensor technology and self-report of play
  - Real-time data on body sway for falls, accelerometer for activity
  - Real-time data on physiological responses, HR, EEGs
  - Real-time data on observations of daily life related to games
- New access and data collection/reporting platforms
  - Online PHRs through mobile phone
  - Commercial and nonprofit web-based applications; see Zyked.com
  - Gyms, cruise ships, community centers, waiting rooms
  - Social networking applications
  - Health insurance claims facilities (e.g., Humana Guidance Centers)
- Healthcare providers, foundations, and game companies partnering with university researchers
  - Humana-sponsored Games for Health Conference 2008
  - Robert Wood Johnson Foundation's Health Games Research Initiative (2009)
  - Sony collaboration for gender play analysis (Williams et al., 2009)
  - Cognitive improvement systems developed or tested by universities
  - Collaborations with university experts on developing games

Source: Adapted from RWJF, 2009.

Costs

Games can come from many sources. The clinical practice group may have partnerships with game developers for specific clinical conditions. The stroke rehabilitation games are one example (McLaughlin et al., 2005; Morrow et al., 2006). At present, the rehabilitation games are the focus of research projects and are made available without cost to participants. Occupational therapists are increasingly using Wii for a variety of clinical goals (Fagan, 2008; Tanner, 2008). The *rehabilitainment* developments in Japan by Namco are clearly for commercial purposes (Bandai Namco Group, 2007).

Nurse-directed designs for comprehensive clinical centers are incorporating leisure activities (Penprase, 2006). Such centers, senior housing sites, and the existing multipurpose senior centers are targets for aggressive campaigns by groups such as Dakim. This company, affiliated with the University of California, Los Angeles, makes a stand-alone console with a touch screen that requires a subscription. Although individuals could purchase the system, it is marketed to centers for multiple users. Posit Science's Brain Fitness Program is marketed to individual users, but has application in group settings as well. In 2009, the price of programs ranged from $395 for a single user to $495 for a shared use between two users. It is clear in the advertising that ideally one buys multiple versions to have truly excellent results. Although other options from Nintendo's Brain Age are less expensive, at the time of this writing, $19.95 per game, one can quickly rack up a large bill. Health professionals who recommend health games will have to be very specific about what they are endorsing. The risk is that clients may overspend for dubious results. Clients may also be tempted to "save money" by purchasing cheaper versions of well-known and well-researched games.

Skill Level

Clinicians who decide to include games will want to become familiar with the demands of the media platform as well as the game itself. Dakim's Brain Fitness games, for example, are explicitly designed with a turnkey approach. A caregiver or aid can turn on the system, explain the purpose, and briefly coach on the mechanics of a touch screen and leave. The game system is self-directed to minimize staff or caregiver burden. Some games simply require knowing how to insert a CD and select an application. Others require Internet search skills and understanding the use of a URL that might come in an e-mail or be on a health agency website. Some, like Wii, are more complex in requiring psychomotor coordination as well as linking up peripherals, such as the Fitness Pad. The availability of technical assistance from the manufacturer can be a major consideration. In some cases, the older adult can make sense of user forums provided on related websites. In other cases, the usual failures of any computer-based application can cause great frustration and anxiety. Planning ahead for these glitches is important to launching games as a therapeutic option.

Planning for Training and Technical Assistance

As with any other computer application, finding a way to provide initial training and coaching to maximize results is critical. If the manufacturer offers no assistance, building a user group is one option. Some strategies currently in use, such as frequently asked questions (FAQs) and user group forums, actually require a fair amount of sophistication to find even the relevant topic. Health-care settings may make good use of adolescent volunteers who can be available by phone or at onsite computer centers. YouTube videos are emerging that can provide a friendly chat style and motivate use. Videos that walk the new user through the steps using actual screen choices to start a game and to play more effectively can be useful. For many older adults, these resources will be totally unfamiliar. For older adults who use dial-up connections, Internet-accessed videos are impractical. The least desirable option is creating a situation where the health professional is the technical coach. This quickly compromises the professional's capacity for assessing the impact of the game on clinical goals and for monitoring any undesirable side effects.

Creative Subscription Options

It is possible that subscription services for software will emerge to match Dell and Microsoft customer service applications. For a fee, subscribers would get access to e-mail, live chat, and phone support that is specific to questions and problems the user is experiencing. As these applications are designed, a fee schedule similar to that for term life insurance would be a creative option. New users would pay a higher monthly fee and have unlimited support. As they progressed over the next few months, support would be more limited until the user decides he or she has mastered the game and discontinue or suspend the subscription. This option may be more attractive than pay-by-request plans. This diminishing cost and decreased access manner of accounting would help users who are reluctant to engage in the intense byplay of games to get started and engaged in a new application.

Potential Documentation in EHRs and PHRs

There is emerging interest in measuring outcomes. At present, game data is fed back to the individual. Linking this data to electronic health records, insurance, and benefits seems a logical step (Donner, Goldstein, & Loughran, 2008, as cited in Hawn, 2009), but it may be that consumers will be the ones to insist on this link (Brown, 2009).

Case for Integrating Games in Patient Care Assessment

In doing an intake assessment or follow-up visit, there is sufficient data and experience to support learning whether patients are engaging in any digital games and what the patient goal is for their engagement. The clinician can learn a great deal about the individual's personal and social priorities and networks through a gaming history.

In some cases, a clinician may have recommended a game to teach or motivate, as noted above as part of a telemedicine therapy. It is important to document the clinician's recommendation to incorporate games in a case management plan. At health checkups, the care provider then follows up on recommended game play and other digital applications in use. This can result in early detection of any problems. The location of the notes will vary by the medical record format. If patient education activities are documented separately, then games intended to increase knowledge and change attitudes would be documented there. When games are recommended as part of a plan to improve health habits, such as exercise, the note would be attached to discussion of specific habits or to a general discussion of health promotion. It is important for the clinician to document the specific game, the purpose for the recommendation, the "dose"—frequency of play, expectation of weeks or months of adherence, outcomes to be measured, and methods for assessing results. Clients and clinicians would negotiate outcomes and method of data collection (see Table 6.5). Clients with PHRs would be encouraged to do real-time monitoring with pedometer, pulsometer, and so on as appropriate. Nintendo announced a plan to ease the transition to real-time monitoring and coaching on game workouts. According to its plan, a new Wii channel will be set up connecting patients and health professionals, and patients will be able to send their Wii Fit and Wii Balance workout data to, and receive health instructions from, health professionals ("Nintendo creates," 2009).

Table 6.5   Elements of Documentation for Game in Care Plan

Name of game: _____

Platform: ☐ Wii ☐ Xbox ☐ PlayStation ☐ Computer with Internet ☐ Mobile phone

Supplier: ☐ Commercial (name): _____ ☐ Agency-developed (name): _____

Access: ☐ One-time purchase ☐ Free ☐ Subscription

Dose: Number of times to play [ ] Number of minutes [ ] Times per day [ ]

Days per week [ ]

Task achievement (specify): _____

Extent of time: ☐ Until next visit ☐ Level of proficiency (specify) _____

Reminders supplied to client: ☐ Flash drive ☐ CD ☐ iPod ☐ Calendar

☐ E-mail ☐ Other

Outcomes to assess (circle or bold):

- Changes in physiological parameters: BP, pulse, weight, BMI, lab values, etc.
- Changes in endurance: Will vary with outcome (e.g., minutes of exercise, distance, range of motion)
- Changes in mood: Self-report on standardized tool, anecdotal
- Changes in social parameters: Engagement, network size, strength, variety
- Changes in ADL: Anecdotal, standardized measure (name):_____

Data collection:

- Self-report: ☐ Oral at visit ☐ E-mail ☐ Online survey ☐ Diary ☐ Health Buddy or other peripheral ☐ Monitoring through personal health record
- Clinician observation: Live/Virtual: using ☐ Weight scale ☐ BP check ☐ Lab values ☐ Specialized assessment (specify: RN, OT, PT)

Reporting to interdisciplinary team: Oral and written communications

- ☐ Summaries in electronic health records of agency ☐ Personal health records of clients ☐ Kardex or other agency quick summary devices

Outcome Monitoring

Clinician discussion with clients and documentation should be specific as to whether the game play is intended to increase knowledge, change attitudes, or promote adherence to a plan of treatment. Increasing social support for health changes may be an equally important goal of health gaming. In a useful record, a time frame is specified as well as the dose as described above. PHRs would provide the opportunity to cross-check medication adherence and improvement in symptoms.

Limited Research on Gaming Contributions to Health Outcomes

A major dilemma in recommending or using games in a healthcare plan is the lack of outcome data on the efficacy of games (Hawn, 2009). This is a surmountable problem. Donner et al. (2008, as cited in Hawn, 2009) note that digital games produce a great deal of data. Researchers can harness this data on proxy measures (steps per day, minutes of exercise, weight, calories, blood pressure, heart rate) to track relationships to long-term outcomes. A well-designed electronic record with a PHR component will go a long way in documenting the additive effects of games in a therapeutic or rehabilitation program.

Lieberman and Donner (2008, as cited in Hawn, 2009) suggest that self-efficacy may be a very important outcome of health gaming. She explains that the game provides a rehearsal opportunity with feedback and mistakes that are not dangerous, and this may be a precursor to behavior change.

Side Effect Tracking

It will be very important to include inquiries about game playing and Internet/computer interactions that are client initiated—both before and after recommending game play. It will be useful to encourage clients to report any changes in their symptoms or emergence of new symptoms. There is the potential for development of symptoms specific to excessive digital interactions ("Doctors warn," 2008; Raby, 2008; Sparks et al., 2009; Warren, 2006). For some clients, eye strain, hand and wrist pain, and headaches may occur related to poor visual acuity or eye corrections (glasses, contact lenses) not adapted to computer screen use and poor light or ergonomics. Client coaching on screen distance, chair position, stretch breaks, and paying attention to pain and cramps is as important for game play as for any other extended computer experience.

Addiction to gaming is a frequent topic in lay and scientific literature (Griffiths, 2008). No reports of cases for older adults were found. However, older adult game play is relatively new. Games can become an "easy day care device" for children. Similarly, older adults may be abandoned and encouraged to play games as a substitute for interaction. There is a risk that older adults may choose to engage in game play to the exclusion of other activities. There is also a risk that others in a social network will be discouraged from usual interactions because the game player looks so immersed in his or her gaming. Monitoring social interaction status is as important as tracking desired clinical outcomes and potential physical side effects.

Playing some games requires creating an avatar that is a virtual representation of the person. This allows for creativity and, to some extent, anonymity. However, the avatar is visible in the virtual world and data related to the individual linked to their IP address might be available to unforeseen groups. However, "there is an astounding silence in the peer-reviewed literature regarding what rights a person ought to expect to retain when being represented by an avatar rather than a biological body" (Graber, 2010, p. e28). As games become more widely played across groups, there will be more opportunity, and pressure, to determine rights relating to avatars, including the role of informed consent for research or marketing.

At some point, health professionals and others will want to turn their attention to the massive data being collected when individuals and groups play online games. Who owns this data? Can it be mined more often in the manner of Williams et al. (2008, 2009)? In what ways are game companies using data they collect? All of the issues related to privacy and research discussed under Personal Health Records in Chapter 4 may have relevance to online game playing. Relevant issues related to morality in telehealth and data mining are discussed in Chapter 7.

Interdisciplinary Collaboration

Health games are a unique example of the potential for powerful collaboration across disciplines. Becoming aware of trends in health gaming opens new possibilities for changing healthcare management (see Table 6.4). Consumers are clearly the experts on themselves and their experience. However, colleagues in patient education and health communication can provide valuable information and insight for choosing games for achieving and measuring health goals.

Physicians, nurse practitioners, and social workers can provide assessment of needs and work with patient education colleagues to match available games with clients. Taking advantage of PHRs to record daily experiences will provide a means for clients to be active in managing their care. Team members who validate the contribution of game playing to the plan of care increase the potential impact of this intervention. Care management team members can help build research evidence by coaching clients on the value of granting consent to record health information from game play. In the final chapter, areas for interdisciplinary collaboration from the provider and game developer perspective will be discussed.

SUMMARY

Games are just emerging as a tool for providers and consumers seeking to sustain or improve health. There is a distinct lack of rigorous clinical trials and minimal follow-up. The fact that older adults form a new market for the very lucrative digital game business makes it likely that games will proliferate. Labeling such games as "health" games provides a mantle of respectability. Claims of preventing disability will make them very appealing to older adults who are feeling vulnerable as they experience changes associated with aging. Providers in all disciplines need to be aware of the potential uses of games. In time, games may form a regular part of the repertoire of health promotion and rehabilitation providers. It will be important to pay attention to the ecology of gaming experience for consumers who make personal choices about what to play; clients who are guided or prescribed games for independent learning or rehabilitation; and situations where through telemedicine, the specialist engages patients in gaming under supervision. Equally important will be appreciating the extent to which an organization sets policies on use of games, documents the role of games in care plans for individuals, and engages in setting a climate for valuing games and arranging necessary training for healthcare providers and patients.

REFERENCES

Aarsand, P. A. (2007). Computer and video games in family life: The digital divide as a resource in intergenerational interactions. *Childhood, 14*(2), 235–256.

Akl, E. A., Sackett, K., Pretorius, R., Erdley, S., Bhoopathi, P. S., Mustafa, R., et al. (2008). Educational games for health professionals. *Cochrane Database of Systematic Reviews, 1*.

Andersen, J. (2006). *The state of serious games in Japan.* Retrieved December 22, 2009, from http://seriousgamessource.com/features/feature_041806_sg_japan.php

Au, A. (2009, June 11–12). *Game related illness and injuries: A review of articles, rhetoric, and realities.* Paper presented at Game for Health 2009, Boston, MA. Retrieved August 10, 2009, from http://www.slideshare.net/alanau/games-for-health-2009-game-related-illness-and-injuries-1578209

Baertlein, L. (2007, December 6). Physical therapists prescribe Wii time. *Reuters.* Retrieved August 4, 2009, from http://www.reuters.com/article/technologyNews/idUSLAU65942220071206

Ballenger, T. (2009, June 15). Video games boost patient rehabilitation. *Boston Globe.* Retrieved August 7, 2009, from http://www.boston.com/news/local/massachusetts/articles/2009/06/15/video_games_boost_patient_rehabilitation

Bandai Namco Group. (2007). *Providing entertainment to everyone, including children, adults, and the elderly* (CSR Report). Tokyo: Bandai Namco Group. Retrieved December 21, 2009, from http://www.bandainamco.co.jp/en/social/pdf/csr_en2007.pdf

Barak, A., Boniel-Nissim, M., & Suler, J. (2008). Fostering empowerment in online support groups. *Computers in Human Behavior, 24*, 1867–1883.

Baranowski, T., Buday, R., Thompson, D. I., & Baranowski, J. (2008). Playing for real: Video games and stories for health-related behavior change. *American Journal of Preventive Medicine, 34*(1), 74–82.

Barnes, D. E., Yaffe, K., Belfor, N., Reed, B., Jagust, W., DeCarli, C., et al. (2006). Computer-based cognitive therapy for mild cognitive impairment: Results of a pilot randomized, controlled trial. *Alzheimer's & Dementia: The Journal of the Alzheimer's Association, 2*(3S), 508–509.

Basak, C., Boot, W. R., Voss, M. W., & Kramer, A. F. (2008). Can training in a real-time strategy video game attenuate cognitive decline in older adults? *Psychology and Aging, 23*(4), 765–777.

Bauman, L., & Hartjes, L. (2008). *Life and death in the age of malaria*. Retrieved December 20, 2009, from https://wiki.doit.wisc.edu/confluence/display/MALSIM/Life+and+Death+in+the+Age+of+Malaria

Broeren, J., Rydmark, M., Bjorkdahl, A., & Sunnerhagen, K. S. (2007). Assessment and training in a 3-dimensional virtual environment with haptics: A report on 5 cases of motor rehabilitation in the chronic stage after stroke. *Neurorehabilitation and Neural Repair, 21*(2), 180–189.

Brown, J. (2009, May 15). *Game-care revolution: A healthcare game changer?* Center for Connected Health. Retrieved August 10, 2009, from http://www.connected-health.org/about-us/get-connected-discussion/discussion/game-care-revolution-a-healthcare-game-changer.aspx

Brown, S. J., Lieberman, D. A., Gemeny, B. A., Fan, Y. C., Wilson, D. M., & Pasta, D. J. (1997). Educational video game for juvenile diabetes: Results of a controlled trial. *Informatics for Health and Social Care, 22*(1), 77–89.

Carstensen, L. L., Isaacowitz, D. M., & Charles, S. T. (1999). Taking time seriously: A theory of socioemotional selectivity. *American Psychologist, 54*(3), 165–181.

Cassidy, M. (2008). Flying with disability in Second Life. *Eureka Street, 18*(10), 22–24.

Casual Games Association. (2007). *Market report 2007: Industry summary*. Retrieved December 20, 2009, from http://www.casualconnect.org/newscontent/11-2007/CasualGamesMarketReport2007_Summary.pdf

Centers for Disease Control and Prevention (CDC). (1999). *A report of the Surgeon General: Physical activity and health—Older adults*. Retrieved December 20, 2009, from http://www.cdc.gov/nccdphp/sgr/pdf/olderad.pdf

Chadwick-Dias, A., McNulty, M., & Tullis, T. (2003). Web usability and age: How design changes can improve performance. *Proceedings of the 2003 Conference on Universal Usability*, 30–37.

Charles, S. T., & Carstensen, L. L. (2010). Social and emotional aging. *Annual Review of Psychology, 61*, 383–409.

Chen, J. (2007). Flow in games (and everything else). *Communications of the ACM, 50*(4), 31–34.

Cheok, A. D., Lee, S., Kodagoda, S., Tat, K. E., & Thang, L. N. (2005). A social and physical intergenerational computer game for the elderly and children: Age invaders. *Proceedings of the 2005 Ninth IEEE International Symposium on Wearable Computers (ISWC'05)*, 202–203.

Cole, H., & Griffiths, M. D. (2007). Social interactions in massively multiplayer online role-playing gamers. *CyberPsychology & Behavior, 10*(4), 575–583.

Colwell, J., & Payne, J. (2000). Negative correlates of computer game play in adolescents. *British Journal of Psychology, 91*, 295–310.

Coyle, D., Doherty, G., Matthews, M., & Sharry, J. (2007). Computers in talk-based mental health interventions. *Interacting with Computers, 19*(4), 545–562.

Crecente, B. (2006, November 22). *The disabled and the Wii: An open letter to Nintendo*. Retrieved August 11, 2009, from http://kotaku.com/gaming/wii/the-disabled-and-the-wii-an-open-letter-to-nintendo-216826.php

Csikszentmihalyi, M. (1975). *Beyond boredom and anxiety*. San Francisco: Jossey-Bass.

Csikszentmihalyi, M. (1997). *Creativity: Flow and the psychology of discovery and invention*. New York: Harper Collins.

Daley, A. J. (2009). Can exergaming contribute to improving physical activity levels and health outcomes in children? *Pediatrics, 124*(2), 763–771.

Das, A. (2009, April 20). More Wii warriors are playing hurt. *New York Times*. Retrieved December 21, 2009, from http://www.nytimes.com/2009/04/21/health/21wii.html

Deeley, L. (2007, March 24). Is this a real life, is this just fantasy?: Second Life is the online world where disabled people can reinvent themselves and enjoy a better life. *Times*. Retrieved December 22, 2009, from http://women.timesonline.co.uk/tol/life_and_style/women/body_ and_soul/article1557980.ece

Dmitri, W., Yee, N., & Scott, E. C. (2008). Who plays, how much, and why? Debunking the stereotypical gamer profile. *Journal of Computer-Mediated Communication, 13*(4), 993–1018.

Doctors warn: Wii puts 10 in hospital a week. (2008, December 23). *Foxnews.com*. Retrieved August 11, 2009, from http://www.foxnews.com/story/0,2933,471364,00.html

Donner, A., Goldstein, D., & Loughran, J. (2008). *e-Health games market report, status and opportunities*. San Francisco: Physic Ventures.

Drew, B., & Waters, J. (1986). Video games: Utilization of a novel strategy to improve perceptual motor skills and cognitive functioning in the non-institutionalized elderly. *Cognitive Rehabilitation, 4*(2), 26–34.

Duque, G., Fung, S., Mallet, L. P. D., Posel, N., & Fleiszer, D. (2008). Learning while having fun: The use of video gaming to teach geriatric house calls to medical students. *Journal of the American Geriatrics Society, 56*(7), 1328–1332.

Entertainment Software Association. (2010). *2010 sales, demographics and usage data: Essential facts about the computer and video game industry*. Washington, DC: Entertainment Software Association. Retrieved July 21, 2010, from http://www.theesa.com/facts/pdfs/ esa_essential_facts_2010.pdf

Eye on innovation: Games-based personal health records. (2007, March 28). Retrieved August 4, 2009, from http://www.hcplive.com/mdnglive/webexclusives/phr-games

Fagan, A. (2008, May 30). Hidden health benefits of video games studied. *Washington Times*. Retrieved December 22, 2009, from http://www.washingtontimes.com/news/2008/may/30/hidden-health-benefits-of-video-games-studied

Fernandez, A., & Goldberg, E. (2009). *The sharp brains guide to brain fitness: 18 interviews with scientists, practical advice, and product reviews, to keep your brain sharp*. San Francisco: SharpBrains.

Fisk, A. D., Rogers, W. A., Charness, N., Czaja, S. J., & Sharit, J. (2004). *Designing for older adults: Principles and creative human factors approaches*. London: CRC Press.

Fogg, B. J. (2003). *Persuasive technology—Using computers to change what we think and do*. San Francisco: Morgan Kaufmann.

Folmer, E. (2009). Game accessibility research. Presentation at Games 4 Health Conference Boston. Game Accessiblity Workshop [PowerPoint]. Available at http://www.slideshare.net/eelkefolmer/ game-accessibility-research-at-the-university-of-nevada

Ford, J., Spallek, M., & Dobson, A. (2007). Self-rated health and a healthy lifestyle are the most important predictors of survival in elderly women. *Age and Ageing, 37*(2), 194–200.

Fotuhi, M. (2003). *The memory cure: How to protect your brain against memory loss and Alzheimer's disease*. New York: McGraw-Hill.

Fujiki, Y., Kazakos, K., Puri, C., Pavlidis, I., Starren, J., & Levine, J. (2007). Neat-o-games: Ubiquitous activity-based gaming [Abstract]. *CHI '07 Extended Abstracts on Human Factors in Computing Systems*, 2369–2374.

Gamberini, L., Alcaniz, M., Barresi, G., Fabregat, M., Ibanez, F., & Prontu, L. (2006). Cognition, technology and games for the elderly: An introduction to Eldergames project. *PsychNology Journal, 4*(3), 285–308. Retrieved December 22, 2009, from http://www.psychnology.org/File/PNJ4(3)/ PSYCHNOLOGY_JOURNAL_4_3_GAMBERINI.pdf

Gamberini, L., Alcaniz, M., Barresi, G., Fabregat, M., Prontu, L., & Ibanez, F. (2008). Playing for a real bonus: Video games to empower elderly people. *Journal of CyberTherapy & Rehabilitation, 1*(1), 37–48.

Gaudiosi, J. (2009, June 25). Health games become serious business. *Reuters.* Retrieved August 9, 2009, from http://www.reuters.com/article/technologyNews/idUSTRE5502LQ20090625

Gerencher, K. (2008, December 11). Gaming your way to better health: Interactive games seek to get people moving, help them manage disease. *MarketWatch.* Retrieved September 1, 2009, from http://www.marketwatch.com/story/e-games-catch-on-as-fun-way-to-improve-health-manage-disease?pagenumber=1

Goldberg, G., Rubinsky, H., Irvin, E., Linneman, E., Knapke, J., & Ryan, M. (2008). Doing Wiihab: Experience with the Wii video game system in acquired brain injury rehabilitation. *Journal of Head Trauma Rehabilitation, 23*(5), 350.

Goldstein, D., Loughran, J., & Donner, A. (2008). *Health egames market report: How video games, social media and virtual worlds will revolutionize health.* Alexandria, VA: iConecto.

Goldstein, J., Cajko, L., Oosterbroek, M., Michielsen, M., Houten, O., & Salverda, F. (1997). Video games and the elderly. *Social Behavior and Gerontology, 25,* 345–352.

Golvin, C. S. (2008). *Benchmark 2008: Gen X loves gadgets the most.* Cambridge, MA: Forrester Research.

Gotsis, M., Valente, T., Jordan-Marsh, M., & Spruijt-Metz, D. (2008). Effectiveness of social mobile networked games in promoting active lifestyles for wellness. Los Angeles: University of Southern California. Proposal submitted to the Robert Wood Johnson Foundation's Health Games Research Initiative.

Graber, M. A. (2010). Get your paws off of my pixels: Personal identity and avatars as self. *Journal of Medical Internet Research, 12*(3), e28. Retrieved July 23, 2010, from http://www.jmir.org/2010/3/e28

Graf, D. L., Pratt, L. V., Hester, C. N., & Short, K. R. (2009). Playing active video games increases energy expenditure in children. *Pediatrics, 124*(2), 534–540.

Graves, L., Stratton, G., Ridgers, N. D., & Cable, N. T. (2007). Comparison of energy expenditure in adolescents when playing new generation and sedentary computer games: Cross-sectional study. *British Medical Journal, 335*(7633), 1282–1284.

Green, M. C. (2004). Understanding media enjoyment: The role of transportation into narrative worlds. *Communication Theory, 14*(4), 311–327.

Green, M. C., & Brock, T. C. (2000). The role of transportation in the persuasiveness of public narratives. *Journal of Personality and Social Psychology, 79*(5), 701–721.

Greene, K. (2007, February 3). Putting brain exercises to the test. *Wall Street Journal,* p. R1.

Griffiths, M. D. (2008). Videogame addiction: Further thoughts and observations. *International Journal of Mental Health and Addiction, 6*(2), 182–185.

Griffiths, M. D., Davies, M. N. O., & Chappell, D. (2004). Online computer gaming: A comparison of adolescent and adult gamers. *Journal of Adolescence, 27*(1), 87–96.

Guidance Interactive Healthcare. (n.d.). *Glucoboy.* Retrieved December 22, 2009, from http://www.glucoboy.com

Hargittai, E. (2002). Second-level digital divide: Differences in people's online skills. *First Monday, 7*(4), 1–20.

Haveman-Nies, A., de Groot, L. C., & van Staveren, W. A. (2003). Dietary quality, lifestyle factors and healthy ageing in Europe: The Seneca Study. *Age and Ageing, 32*(4), 427–434.

Hawn, C. (2009). Games for health: The latest tool in the medical care arsenal. *Health Affairs, 28*(4), 842–848.

Hofmann, M., Rosler, A., Schwarz, W., Müller-Spahn, F., Kräuchi, K., Hock, C., et al. (2003). Interactive computer-training as a therapeutic tool in Alzheimer's disease. *Comprehensive Psychiatry, 44*(3), 213–219.

Hollander, E, K., & Plummer, H. R. (1986). An innovative therapy and enrichment program for senior adults utilizing the personal computer. *Activities, Adaptations & Aging, 8*, 59–68.

Hoppes, S., Hally, C., & Sewell, L. (2000). An interest inventory of games for older adults. *Physical and Occupational Therapy in Geriatrics, 18*(2), 71–84.

Hug, D. (2004, July 7). Playing arcade games yields positive effects on elderly rehabilitation: Namco and Kyushu University. *Japan's Corporate News (JCN) Network*. Retrieved December 22, 2009, from http://www.japancorp.net/Article.Asp?Art_ID=7764

Huizinga, J. (1970). *Homo Ludens: A study of the play element in culture*. New York: Harper & Row.

Humana. (2007, September 7). Humana launches initiative to reach consumers through games [Press release]. Retrieved December 20, 2009, from http://www.humanagames.com/assets/pdf/Humana %20Games%20for%20Health_News_G4H%20Conference_20080505.pdf

IBISWorld. (2008, August 18). The new American players: Baby boomers and women take on video gaming [Press release]. Los Angeles: IBISWorld. Retrieved December 22, 2009, from http://www.ibisworld.com/pressrelease/pressrelease.aspx?prid=133

Ijsselsteijn, W. A., de Kort, Y. A. W., Westerink, J., Jager, M., & Bonants, R. (2006). Virtual fitness: Stimulating exercise behavior through media technology. *Presence: Teleoperators and Virtual Environments, 15*(6), 688–698.

Ijsselsteijn, W., Nap, H. H., de Kort, Y., & Poels, K. (2007). Digital game design for elderly users. *Proceedings of the 2007 Conference on Future Play*, 17–22.

Information Solutions Group. (2008, June 11). "Disabled gamers" comprise 20% of casual video game audience [Press release]. Retrieved December 20, 2009, from http://www.infosolutionsgroup. com/pdfs/disabled_gamers.pdf

Jackson, P., & Keitt, T. J. (2008). *Understanding the US video game player*. Cambridge, MA: Forrester Research.

Jenkins, H. (2004). Game design as narrative architecture. In N. Wardrip-Fruin & P. Harrigan (Eds.), *First person: New media as story, performance, game*. Cambridge, MA: MIT Press. Retrieved August 5, 2009, from http://web.mit.edu/cms/People/henry3/games&narrative.html

Jenkins, H., Camper, B., Chisholm, A., Grigsby, N., Klopfer, E., Osterweil, S., et al. (2009). From serious games to serious gaming. In U. Ritterfeld, M. J. Cody, & P. Vorderer (Eds.), *Serious games: Mechanisms and effects* (pp. 446–466). New York: Routledge.

Jimison, H., & Pavel, M. (2006). Embedded assessment algorithms within home-based cognitive computer game exercises for elders. *Proceedings of the 28th IEEE EMBS Annual International Conference*, 6101–6104.

Jimison, H., Pavel, M., McKanna, J., & Pavel, J. (2004). Unobtrusive monitoring of computer interactions to detect cognitive status in elders. *IEEE Transactions on Information Technology in Biomedicine, 8*(3), 248–252.

Jobe, J. B., Smith, D. M., Ball, K., Tennstedt, S. L., Marsiske, M., Willis, S. L., et al. (2001). Active: A cognitive intervention trial to promote independence in older adults. *Controlled Clinical Trials, 22*(4), 453–479.

Kato, P. M., Cole, S. W., Bradlyn, A. S., & Pollock, B. H. (2008). A video game improves behavioral outcomes in adolescents and young adults with cancer: A randomized trial. *Pediatrics, 122*(2), e305–e317.

Keller, V. F., Spadola, J., Yang, Y., Hershorin, J., Garcia, J., & Studenski, S. (2009). Assessing the impact of an exer-game in a healthy elderly population. Miami, FL: Humana. Unpublished manuscript.

Kelso, M., Weyhrauch, P., & Bates, J. (1993). Dramatic presence. *Presence: The Journal of Teleoperators and Virtual Environments, 2*(1), 1–15.

Khoo, E. T., Merritt, T., & Cheok, A. D. (2009). Designing physical and social intergenerational family entertainment. *Interacting with Computers, 21*(1–2), 76–87.

Klein, M. J., & Simmers, C. S. (2009). Exergaming: Virtual inspiration, real perspiration. *Young Consumers: Insight and Ideas for Responsible Marketers, 10*(1), 35–45.

Klimmt, C. (2009). Serious games and social change: Why they (should) work. In U. Ritterfeld, M. J. Cody, & P. Vorderer (Eds.), *Serious games: Mechanisms and effects* (pp. 246–259). New York: Routledge.

Klimmt, C., & Vorderer, P. (2007). Interactive media. In J. J. Arnett (Ed.), *Encyclopedia of children, adolescents, and the media* (pp. 417–419). London: Sage.

Korczyn, A. D., Peretz, C., Aharonson, V., & Giladi, N. (2007). Computer-based cognitive training with MindFit improved cognitive performances above the effect of classic computer games: Prospective, randomized, double-blind intervention study in the elderly. *Neurodegenerative Diseases, 1*(Suppl. 1), 113.

Kurutz, D. R. (2008, August 28). Bellevue Library 's Wii program designed to bridge generations. *Pittsburgh Tribune-Review.* Retrieved December 22, 2009, from http://www.pittsburghlive. com/x/pittsburghtrib/search/s_584919.html

Lee, K. M., Park, N., & Jin, S. (2006). Narrative and interactivity in computer games. In P. Vorderer & J. Bryant (Eds.), *Playing video games: Motives, responses, and consequences* (pp. 259–274). Mahwah, NJ: Erlbaum.

Lenhart, A., Jones, S., & Macgill, A. R. (2008, December 7). Adults and video games. *Pew Internet & American Life Project.* Retrieved November 15, 2009, from http://www.pewinternet.org/ Reports/2008/Adults-and-Video-Games/1-Data-Memo.aspx?r=1

Lewis, L. (2009, January, 29). Tempus analysis: Wii Fit on prescription. *Times Online.* Retrieved August 11, 2009, from http://business.timesonline.co.uk/tol/business/industry_sectors/ technology/article5611223.ece

Lieberman, D. A. (2001). Management of chronic pediatric diseases with interactive health games: Theory and research findings. *Journal of Ambulatory Care Management, 24*(1), 26–38.

Lieberman, D. A. (2006, April). Dance games and other exergames: What the research says. Retrieved December 22, 2009, from http://www.comm.ucsb.edu/faculty/lieberman/exergames.htm

Lieberman, D. A., & Brown, S. J. (1995). Designing interactive video games for children's health education. In K. Morgan, R. M. Satava, H. B. Sieburg, R. Mattheus, & J. P. Christensen (Eds.), *Interactive technology and the new paradigm for healthcare* (pp. 201–210). Amsterdam, The Netherlands: IOS Press and Ohmsha.

Lieberman, D. A., & Donner, A. (2008). *Using electronic games to empower healthy lifestyles, prevention and self-care: Theory and research findings.* San Francisco: PhysicVentures.

Liu, J.-F., Chen, Y.-Q., Xie, C., & Gao, W. (2006). SSC: Gesture-based game for initial dementia examination. *Journal of Zhejian University—Science A, 7*(7), 1253–1258.

Lovelock, B. (2009, May 7). Healthy phones? Paper presented at Health Beyond: e-Heath Consumer Day, Melbourne, Australia. Retrieved August 7, 2009, from http://www.healthbeyond.org.au/files/u2/ hb_lovelock.pdf

Macgill, A. (2007, November 19). Is video gaming becoming the next family bonding activity? *Pew Internet*. Retrieved August 7, 2009, from http://www.pewinternet.org/Commentary/2007/November/Is-video-gaming-becoming-the-next-family-bonding-activity.aspx

Maney, K. (2004, November 17). "Halo 2" shows new generation gap: Boomers vs. gamers. *USA Today*. Retrieved December 22, 2009, from http://www.usatoday.com/money/industries/technology/maney/2004-11-16-halo2-generation-gap_x.htm

Mangrum, F. G., & Mangrum, C. W. (1995). An ethnomethodological study of concerted and biographical work performed by elderly persons during game playing. *Educational Gerontology, 21*(3), 231–246.

McGuire, F. A. (1984). Improving the quality of life for residents of long-term care facilities through video games. *Activities, Adaptation & Aging, 6*(1), 1–7.

McKhann, G. M., & Albert, M. (2002). *Keep your brain young*. New York: Wiley.

McLaughlin, M. L., Jung, Y., Peng, W., Jin, S. A., & Zhu, W. (2008). Touch in computer-mediated communication. In E. A. Konjin, S. Utz, M. Tanis, & S. B. Barnes (Eds.), *Mediated interpersonal communication* (pp. 158–176). New York: Routledge.

McLaughlin, M. L., Rizzo, A. A., Jung, Y., Peng, W., Yeh, S., & Zhu, W. (2005). Haptics-enhanced virtual environments for stroke rehabilitation. *Proceedings of IPSI 2005*. Cambridge, MA. Retrieved December 22, 2009, from http://imsc.usc.edu/haptics/paper/manuscript_ipsi2005usa.pdf

Medical College of Georgia. (2008, April 7). Occupational therapists use Wii for Parkinson's study. Retrieved December 22, 2009, from http://www.sciencedaily.com/releases/2008/04/080407074534.htm

Mellecker, R. R., & McManus, A. M. (2008). Energy expenditure and cardiovascular responses to seated and active gaming in children. *Archives of Pediatrics & Adolescent Medicine, 162*(9), 886–891.

Morales-Rodriguez, M., Casper, G., & Brennan, P. F. (2007). Patient-centered design: The potential of user-centered design in personal health records. *Journal of AHIMA, 78*(4), 44–46.

Morrison-Bogorad, M., Cahan, V., & Wagster, M. V. (2007). Brain health interventions: The need for further research. *Alzheimer's & Dementia: The Journal of the Alzheimer's Association, 3*(2S), 80–85.

Morrow, K., Docan, C., Burdea, G., & Merians, A. (2006, Aug 29–30). *Low-cost virtual rehabilitation of the hand for patients post-stroke*. Paper presented at the International Workshop on Virtual Rehabilitation, New York. Retrieved July 23, 2008, from http://ieeexplore.ieee.org/stamp/stamp.jsp?arnumber=1707518&isnumber=36031

Nielsen Entertainment. (2006). *Active gamer benchmark study*. New York: VNU Corporation.

Nintendo. (2006, August 29). Nintendo crowns "Coolest grandparent of the year" [Press release]. Retrieved December 22, 2009, from http://gonintendo.com/?p=5120

Nintendo creates Wii health advisory unit. (2009, January 28). *United Press International*. Retrieved August 12, 2009, from http://www.upi.com/Top_News/2009/01/28/Nintendo-creates-Wii-health-advisory-unit/UPI-58151233160361/

Nowak, M. A., & Roch, S. (2007). Upstream reciprocity and the evolution of gratitude. *Proceedings of the Royal Society B: Biological Sciences, 274*(1610), 605–609.

Orland, K. (2008, May 27). GFH: The "overheated" state of DS learning games in Japan. Retrieved December 22, 2009, from http://www.gamasutra.com/php-bin/news_index.php?story=18596

Papastergiou, M. (2009). Exploring the potential of computer and video games for health and physical education: A literature review. *Computers & Education, 53*, 603–622.

Pearce, C. (2008). The truth about baby boomer gamers: A study of over-forty computer game players. *Games and Culture, 3*(2), 142.

Pennebaker, J. W. (1997). Writing about emotional experiences as a therapeutic process. *Psychological Science, 8*(3), 162–166.

Penprase, B. (2006). Developing comprehensive health care for an underserved population. *Geriatric Nursing, 27*(1), 45–50.

Prensky, M. (2003). Digital game-based learning. *Computers in Entertainment (CIE), 1*(1), 1–4.

Princess Cruises. (2008, June 24). Retrieved July 24, 2020 from http://www.princess.com/news/article.jsp?newsArticleId=na958

Raby, M. (2008, January 24). Wii injuries make headlines. *TG Daily.* Retrieved August 10, 2009, from http://www.tgdaily.com/content/view/35770/118

Rand, D., Kizony, R., & Weiss, P. L. (2004, September 20–22). *Virtual reality rehabilitation for all: Vivid GX versus Sony PlayStation II EyeToy.* Paper presented at the 5th International Conference on Disability, Virtual Environments, and Associated Technologies, Oxford, UK. Retrieved December 22, 2009, from http://www.icdvrat.reading.ac.uk/2004/papers/S03_N2_Rand_ICDVRAT2004.pdf

Riddick, C. C., Drogin, E. B., & Spector, S. G. (1987). The impact of video game play on the emotional states of senior center participants. *Practice Concepts, 27*(4), 425–427.

Robert Wood Johnson Foundation (RWJF). (2009). Health games research: Advancing effectiveness of interactive games for health. Retrieved August 9, 2009, from http://www.rwjf.org/files/applications/cfp/cfp_HGR2009.pdf

Rosenzweig, M. R., & Bennett, E. L. (1996). Psychobiology of plasticity: Effects of training and experience on brain and behavior. *Behavioural Brain Research, 78*(1), 57–65.

Russoniello, C., & Park, J. (2008, May 8). *A randomized controlled study of the effects of PopCap games on mood and stress.* A paper presented at the Games for Health Conference, Baltimore, MD. Retrieved December 22, 2009 from http://core.ecu.edu/hhp/russoniello/PopCap_results.mht

Ryan, R. M., & Deci, E. L. (2001). On happiness and human potentials: A review of research on hedonic and eudaimonic well-being. *Annual Reviews in Psychology, 52*(1), 141–166.

Ryan, R. M., Rigby, C. S., & Przybylski, A. (2006). The motivational pull of video games: A self-determination theory approach. *Motivation and Emotion, 30*(4), 344–360.

Salthouse, T. A. (2006). Mental exercise and mental aging: Evaluating the validity of the "Use it or lose it" hypothesis. *Perspectives on Psychological Science, 1*(1), 68–87.

Sawyer, B., & Smith, P. (2008, February 18–22). *Serious games taxonomy.* Paper presented at the Game Developers Conference, San Francisco, CA. Retrieved December 22, 2009, from http://www.dmill.com/presentations/serious-games-taxonomy-2008.pdf

Sawyer, R. K. (2007). *Group genius: The creative power of collaboration.* New York: Basic Books.

Schaik, P. V., Turnbull, T., Wersch, A. V., & Drummond, S. (2004). Presence within a mixed reality environment. *CyberPsychology & Behavior, 7*(5), 540–552.

Schieber, F. (2003). Human factors and aging: Identifying and compensation for age-related deficits in sensory and cognitive function. In N. Charness & K. W. Schaie (Eds.), *Impact of technology on successful aging* (pp. 42–84). New York: Springer.

Schiesel, S. (2007, March 30). Video games conquer retirees. *New York Times.* Retrieved December 22, 2009, from http://www.nytimes.com/2007/03/30/arts/30seni.html

Schlender, S. (2008, September 17). Second Life frees disabled from restrictions of everyday life. *Voice of America.* Retrieved December 21, 2009, from http://www1.voanews.com/english/news/american-life/a-13-2008-09-17-voa24.html

Schott, G., & Hodgetts, D. (2006). Health and digital gaming: The benefits of a community of practice. *Journal of Health Psychology*, *11*(2), 309–316.

Schott, G. R., & Horrell, K. R. (2000). Girl gamers and their relationship with the gaming culture. *Convergence*, *6*(4), 36–53.

Shachtman, N. (2008, August 26). Wounded G.I.s' new rehab: Wii Sports, Guitar Hero. *Wired*. Retrieved August 2, 2009, from http://www.wired.com/dangerroom/2008/08/wounded-gis-new

Shaffer, D. W., Squire, K. D., Halverson, R., & Gee, J. P. (2005). Video games and the future of learning. *Phi Delta Kappan*, *87*(2), 104–111.

Short, J., Williams, E., & Christie, B. (1976). *The social psychology of telecommunications*. London: Wiley.

SilverFit (n.d.). *What is SilverFit?* Retrieved August 10, 2009, from http://www.silverfit.nl/en/index.htm

Sparks, D., Chase, D., & Coughlin, L. (2009). Wii have a problem: A review of self-reported Wii related injuries. *Informatics in Primary Care*, *17*(1), 55–57.

Stein, R. (2007, October 6). Real hope in a virtual world: Online identities leave limitations behind. *Washington Post*. Retrieved May 23, 2008, from http://www.washingtonpost.com/wp-dyn/content/article/2007/10/05/AR2007100502391.html

Subrahmanyam, K., Kraut, R. E., Greenfield, P., & Gross, E. (2000). The impact of home computer use on children's activities and development. *The Future of Children: Children and Computer Technology*, *10*(2), 123–144.

Suhonen, K., Väätäjä, H., Virtanen, T., & Raisamo, R. (2008). Seriously fun: Exploring how to combine promoting health awareness and engaging game play. In A. Lugmayr, F. Mäyrä, H. Franssila, & K. Lietsala (Eds.), *Proceedings of the 12th International Conference on Entertainment and Media in the Ubiquitous Era* (pp. 18–22). New York: ACM.

Tamborini, R., & Skalski, P. (2006). The role of presence in the experience of electronic games. In P. Vorderer & J. Bryant (Eds.), *Playing video games: Motives, responses, and consequences* (pp. 225–240). Mahwah, NJ: Erlbaum.

Tan, Z. S. (2005). *Age-proof your mind: Detect, delay, and prevent memory loss before it's too late*. New York: Warner Books.

Tanner, L. (2008, February 8). Doctors use Wii games for rehab therapy. *USA Today*. Retrieved December 22, 2009, from http://www.usatoday.com/tech/science/2008-02-08-wii-rehabilitation_N.htm

Taub, E. (2006, October 30). Nintendo at AARP event to court the grayer gamer. *New York Times*. Retrieved December 22, 2009, from http://www.nytimes.com/2006/10/30/technology/30aarp.html

Thomas-Ross, B. (2009, December 15). Humana Games for Health adds new dance pad video game to product line. *Forbes Business Wire*. Retrieved December 21, 2009, from http://www.forbes.com/feeds/businesswire/2009/12/15/businesswire132866169.html

Thompson, D., Baranowski, T., Buday, R., Baranowski, J., Thompson, V., Jago, R., et al. (2008). Serious video games for health: How behavioral science guided the design of a game on diabetes and obesity. *Simulation Gaming*. Retrieved August 7, 2009, from http://sag.sagepub.com/cgi/content/abstract/1046878108328087v1

Vance, M. (2004). *Casual online gamer study*. Lewisville, TX: Digital Marketing Services for AOL Games.

Vanden Abeele, A. V., & Van Rompaey, V. (2006, April 22–27). Introducing human-centered research to game design: Designing game concepts for and with senior citizens [Abstract]. *CHI '06 Extended Abstracts on Human Factors in Computing Systems*, 1469–1474.

Video game company, Namco makes games for elderly people. (2006, June 5). *Techshout.* Retrieved December 22, 2009, from http://www.techshout.com/gaming/2006/05/video-game-company-namco-makes-games-for-elderly-people

Video gaming graphics supercharge medical imaging. (2008, November 11). *HealthBlog.* Retrieved August 1, 2009, from http://blogs.msdn.com/healthblog/archive/2008/11/11/video-gaming-graphics-supercharge-medical-imaging.aspx

Wang, H., & Singhal, A. (2009). Entertainment–education through digital games. In U. Ritterfeld, M. J. Cody, & P. Vorderer (Eds.), *Serious games: Mechanisms and effects* (pp. 260–290). New York: Routledge.

Warburton, D. E. R., Bredin, S. S. D., Horita, L. T. L., Zbogar, D., Scott, J. M., Esch, B. T. A., et al. (2007). The health benefits of interactive video game exercise. *Applied Physiology, Nutrition, and Metabolism, 32*(4), 655–663.

Warren, J. (2006, November 25). A Wii workout: When video games hurt. *Wall Street Journal.* Retrieved August 5, 2009, from http://online.wsj.com/public/article/SB116441076273232312-IHR8Xf3YEG61QlW0e7hA_kHAA8w_20061224.html?mod=tff_main_tff_top

Weisman, S. (1983). Computer games for the frail elderly. *Gerontologist, 23,* 361–363.

Whatley, D. (2005, October 31). *What's so serious about game design?* Paper presented at the Serious Games Summit 2005, Washington, DC.

White, M., Lehmann, H., & Trent, M. (2007). Disco dance video game-based interventional study on childhood obesity. *Journal of Adolescent Health, 40*(2S), 32.

White, P. (2008). *MMOGData: Charts.* Tuxedo Park, NY: Voig.

Williams, D., Consalvo, M., Caplan, S., & Yee, N. (2009). Looking for gender: Gender roles and behaviors among online gamers. *Journal of Communication 59* ,700–725.

Williams, D., Yee, N., & Caplan, S. (2008). Who plays, how much, and why? A behavioral player census of virtual world. *Journal of Computer Mediated Communication, 13*(4), 993–1018.

Willis, S. L., Tennstedt, S. L., Marsiske, M., Ball, K., Elias, J., Koepke, K. M., et al. (2006). Long-term effects of cognitive training on everyday functional outcomes in older adults. *Journal of the American Medical Association, 296*(23), 2805–2814.

Wylie, C. G., & Coulton, P. (2009). Persuasive mobile health applications. In D. Weerasinghe (Ed.), *Electronic healthcare* (pp. 90–97). Berlin, Germany: Springer.

Yam, M. (2007, February 22). Wii invades retirement home. *Daily Tech.* Retrieved December 22, 2009, from http://www.dailytech.com/article.aspx?newsid=6191

Zelinski, E. M., Yaffe, K., Ruff, R. M., Kennison, R. K., & Smith, G. E. (2007, November 16–20). *The impact study: A randomized controlled trial of a brain plasticity-based training program for age-related cognitive decline.* Poster session presented at the Gerontological Society of America Meeting, San Francisco, CA. Retrieved December 22, 2009, from http://www.dcprovidersonline.com/pres_file.php?id=2011&file=PSC_GSASF_handout.pdf

Consumer-Centric Health Technology: Wicked Problems and Deliciously Disruptive Solutions

THE CHALLENGES AND OPPORTUNITIES OF THE NEXT ERA IN HEALTH CARE

Implementation of Telehealth: Messes and Wickedness

This chapter is written with the assumption that the reader is familiar with and accepting of the wide-ranging benefits of telehealth and its component parts (personal health records, online information, devices, games). This chapter contains three major topics: (1) the challenges and risks of telehealth implementation in a climate of *participatory health*, (2) the documentation of the return on investment (ROI) of telehealth implementation, and (3) new partnerships with issues specific to those stakeholders who are not the patient "consumers," but consumers of policy and implementers of practice. Challenges to the implementation of telehealth are examined in terms of larger socioecological contexts such as unexpected ethical or moral issues.

Telehealth is characterized as a messy, *wicked problem* (Rittel & Webber, 1973) in a social context. Some specific risks of implementing telehealth are outlined. The term *telecare* is used when the component of monitoring is central. The state of knowledge about return on investment—the research base and its limitations—is outlined. The chapter concludes with balancing these dilemmas with the potential benefits to a wide range of stakeholders. The prospect of overcoming current telehealth challenges is presented through highlighting some *delicious* disruptive opportunities on the horizon. *Delicious* was selected as a designation as it conveys a sense of excitement and possibilities to which all stakeholders might look forward with pleasure. The Delicious social bookmarking function of finding one's way back to remembered resources for sharing with others (see http://www.delicious.com) was also a factor. Equally important was the bookmarking strategy where tags are chosen by consumers—an apt feature for consumer-centric technology of any kind. *Disruptive* is used to connect to Christenson's theory of disruptive innovation (1997, as cited in Christensen, Bohmer, & Kenagy, 2001). He looked at the introduction of new ideas to consumer markets that "break" or "disrupt" established patterns so dramatically that old, secure companies or systems of service delivery become obsolete abruptly. Christensen et al. (2001) observed that disruptions at play in the healthcare system are likely to result in higher quality, lower cost, and more convenient health care. Part of this disruption is the new paradigm of *participatory health* that is centered on the patient. Understandings of patient-centered care, Disch argues, are fortuitously shifting (2009). In the new journal of *Participatory Medicine*, she draws on her career in nursing, the work of Virginia Henderson, and the Institute of Medicine to build a case for new partnerships in patient-centered care. Based on her paper, a definition is proposed that has transdisciplinary application.

Participatory health is a lens that begins with a holistic view of the strengths, will, and knowledge of the patient, the health professionals, and available social support in the context of their shared environment and daily experiences. It builds on patient values, needs and preferences given available capital as the guide to all clinical decisions with the patient or designee as the source of control and full partner at each transition in the health and illness journey.

The definition proposed here is novel in that it recognizes the influences of the environment and daily life, acknowledges the limitations that may be imposed by various forms of capital available to the team, and takes into account the powerful influence of characteristics of not only the patient, but the professionals and social support prospects. Partners in participatory health would empower each other at each clinical transition as they share data, information, knowledge, and wisdom in the context of available and potential capital and the range of influences in the environment. Telehealth facilitates this empowerment process by making new resources available at a time when the healthcare system is in chaos with the impact of healthcare reform in the United States a massive unknown.

Limitations of the Scientific Method Search for One Solution

Clearly, we have what Ackoff (1981) labeled a *mess*—an experience of external circumstances that cause dissatisfaction. The everyday experience of these messes and the struggle to sort out the systems is described by Schön (1987) as occurring in a "swampy lowland" of problems that "defy technical solution" (p. 28). Rittel and Webber (1973) note that in the 1950s, there was a consensus that a mass society would emerge with great homogeneity. The scientific method took over as the dominant paradigm for social problems. In the Western world, this led to a long tradition of conceptualizing public messes as systems or systems of systems—a mechanistic view (Rittel & Webber, 1973). However, Rittel and Webber argue that the "cognitive and occupational style" of the social professions that adopted the style of engineers and scientists "have just not worked on a wide array of social problems" (p. 160), particularly where equity is involved. The implication was that with good science, one powerful solution would evolve that would work for most cases.

Instead, across the globe, societies are becoming more heterogeneous. Rittel and Webber (1973) observed that the increased volume of information and knowledge and the expansion of options related to technology could create conditions where diversity would thrive. Rittel and Webber thought, in 1973, that affluence could increase the desire for a subcultural identity, promoting homogeneity. Lacking knowledge of the World Wide Web and related technological device and software developments, they underestimated the potential for heterogeneity. Today, social values and individual choice are in continual dynamic tension fueled by these conditions. A case might be made that in the face of the denouement of the "affluent forever" taken for granted by the wealthy countries, personal solutions and any personal advantages will be protected even more zealously. This guarding is playing out in the healthcare reform debates. People want the system to change but not for them.

Alternative to the Scientific Method: Re-Solving Social Problems

An alternative to the scientific method is to appreciate that social policy problems are *wicked problems* (Rittel & Webber, 1973). "Social problems are never solved. At best they are only *re-solved*—over and over again" (p. 160). These planning theorists emphasized that everything is connected and that *context* is critical in complex adaptive human-engaging systems (Table 7.1). Wicked problems emerge because stakeholders have divergent views, values, and preferences. A socioecological or ecosystems perspective that values disruptive innovation accommodates this diversity. A map of stakeholders engaged in medical home implementation is presented in Table 7.2 to illustrate the wide range of anticipated beneficiaries and actors in participatory health linked to technology. These are the stakeholders whose perspectives are key in any attempt to solve the social problem of quality health care for a diverse world.

It is the context of the diverse values, preferences, and experiences of the stakeholders that creates the wicked dimension of a *mess*—a generalized dissatisfaction with a social policy or resource. Therefore, policy makers should not be distracted by apparent similarities in messes. An ecological analysis often

Table 7.1   Characteristics of Wicked Problems: Diversity of Stakeholders Complex

Recognizing the problem: A whole that is greater than the sum of parts

- There is no definitive formulation of a wicked problem. The problem cannot be understood until solutions have been conceived.
- Every wicked problem is essentially unique. Applying the same solution to seemingly similar wicked problems may be problematic.
- Every wicked problem can be considered to be a symptom of another problem. Broad societal issues are connected to lesser societal problems.
- There are numerous explanations for wicked problems, and the choice of explanation determines the nature of the resolution. Stakeholders choose explanations that are most plausible to them and that affects the solution they implement or at least endorse.

Building and evaluating solutions: Optimizing trade-offs

- There is no way to know that all potential solutions to a wicked problem have been identified. Judgment must be used to determine which potential solutions should be pursued. Determining the stakeholder base becomes critical.
- Wicked problems have no "stopping rule." There is no single definitive solution.
- Solutions to wicked problems are not correct and incorrect, but better or worse. Assessments are often made based on the planner's values.
- There is no test of a solution to a wicked problem. Solutions to these problems will generate unforeseen consequences that continue indefinitely.
- Every solution to a wicked problem has consequences that will likely lead to new wicked problems. There is no opportunity to learn by trial and error.
- The goal of solving wicked problems is to improve people's lives. Thus planners are liable for the consequences of their implemented solutions.

Sources: Adapted from Rittel & Webber, 1973, and Conklin, 2005. See website resource: Building Shared Understanding of Wicked Problems, available at http://cognexus.org/id42.htm

Table 7.2   The Medical Home Offers Potential Benefits to Stakeholders Across the Healthcare Ecosystem

Stakeholder	Potential Benefits of the Medical Home
Patient/family	• Help from a trusted resource to navigate healthcare system • Empowered to make better-informed healthcare decisions • Receive safe, effective care with compassion • Achieve healthier outcomes collaboratively with extended care delivery team • Improved relationship with PCP, health plan

Table 7.2   The Medical Home Offers Potential Benefits to Stakeholders Across the Healthcare Ecosystem (*continued*)

Stakeholder	Potential Benefits of the Medical Home
Primary care provider	• Redefine patient relationship to deliver more comprehensive, coordinated care • Fair compensation for PCMH services, as well as rewards for improved clinical outcomes • Through a shift in incentives, able to more effectively provide wellness and preventative care • Better supported to deliver quality care to patients
Specialist	• Receive higher quality referrals, with more complete documentation • Improved focus on area of expertise without having to assume management of patient's primary care • Opportunity to offset income losses by participating in financial incentives for coordination and quality (for example, telephone consultations)
Nurse	• Develop better relationship with patients • More involvement with patient care and support (for example, patient education, behavioral change, preventive care, proactive care planning)
Pharmacist	• Participate fully in team-based care (for example, help determine medication and reasonable formularies)
Social worker	• More integrated role to address key patient needs (for example, Medicaid)
Hospital	• Serve PCMH patients whose conditions may not be as severe as non-PCMH patients • Potentially reduce admissions from patients who cannot pay • Potentially reduce number of readmissions, for which there may be no or reduced payment
Health plan	• Improved member and employer satisfaction • Expend healthcare resources with less waste and greater effectiveness though coordinated, evidence-based care

(*continues*)

Table 7.2   The Medical Home Offers Potential Benefits to Stakeholders Across the Healthcare Ecosystem (*continued*)

Stakeholder	Potential Benefits of the Medical Home
Employer	• Purchase health care based on value and potentially see medical cost savings • Maintaining more present and productive workforce, in part, through improved wellness and prevention
Pharmaceuticals and other life sciences	• Improved appropriateness of and compliance with therapeutics • Enhanced pharmacovigilance of products, post clinical trials
Government	• Potential to improve care quality, reduce wasteful health-care expenditures • Address frustration with the current uncoordinated and impersonal system
Communities and society	• Potential for a healthier, more productive citizenry • Potential to allocate dollars so that they have greater return

Notes: PCP = primary care provider; PCMH = patient-centered medical home.

Source: Adams, Grundy, Kohn, & Mounib, 2009. Used with permission.

reveals that the particulars of a problem under consideration may outweigh apparent similarities. For example, what works for the Veterans Health Administration (VHA) in saving costs by cutting visits (Darkins et al., 2008) may sharply decrease income for private healthcare providers. This heterogeneity creates multiple dilemmas for dissolving healthcare problems at high policy levels.

For wicked problems of society, working on one node in a network and "solving" that situation has consequences across the network. These consequences may be worse than the trigger problem itself. The danger is by reacting to a symptom, new structures or rules are created that cripple other interactions inadvertently. Disruptive innovations come from radically different approaches and create opportunities independent of existing systems.

Socioecological Solutions: Wisdom and Influence

In the traditional model, Rittel and Weber (1973) point out that reconciliation was entrusted to "wise and knowledgeable professional experts and politicians" (p. 169). As the World Wide Web emerged and related technology of devices and software connected, the opportunities for individuals and special interest groups to become "experts" and dispensers of wisdom exploded. New experts have been adopted as definitive resources independent of credentials or face-to-face encounters. Consumers are increasingly *expert* and operate in a social context (Bos, 2007).

Lewis (2006) reviewed the literature on the nature of health information on the Internet and studied patterns of access. She concluded that the information available and the patterns of use do represent "a significant challenge to the hegemony of the medical profession" (p. 536). This evolution of expertise has not meant that Internet users do not consult health professionals. Rather, Lewis argues that we are moving toward a more socially contextualized perspective on health. The Internet is a new and charismatic source of expertise—mostly a complement to health expert advice (Bos, 2007; Fox & Jones, 2009). Some individuals consider their Web-based interactions in the nature of a close friend who provides reliable advice (see Figure 7.1).

Figure 7.1   Reliance on the Internet for Information and Support

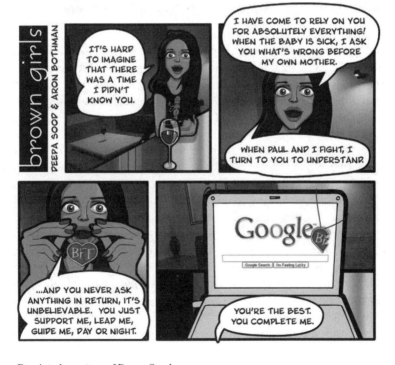

Source: Reprinted courtesy of Deepa Sood.

Each of the disciplines is called on in participatory telehealth to make the case for their specific intelligence. The intelligence called on in each social problem varies with the stakeholder perspective. In nursing intelligence (May, 2008, as cited in Jordan-Marsh & May, 2008), for example, there is an acumen related to nursing's unique interface with the social aspects of health in a persistently mind–body engagement with patients. Social work in turn has a unique intelligence specific to social justice as a primary value. This plays out in social workers' focused attention to the legal and ethical issues of health care (McCarty & Clancy, 2002).

Long-standing social contracts have become, if not null and void, certainly weakened and blurred. Charisma has become a more powerful influence than the obligations of traditional social ties and organizational hierarchies. Building and conserving capital by individuals and special interest groups is the engine of the consumer society.

Using a socioecological framework provides a context for appreciating the flow of events, dilemmas, and opportunities provided by telehealth implementation. There is certainly no going back to an era when politicians and professionals guarded access to social power and knowledge and expertise.

Sociotechnical Theory as Resource for Optimizing Choices

Westbrook et al. (2007) advocate looking at the deep structure of *wicked problems*. Their focus is the challenge of how to deliver safe and sustainable healthcare systems using information and communication technology (p. 747). They propose design and evaluation schemas using principles of sociotechnical theory and analysis. In health care, they note the social system includes coalitions or groups that deliberate and act to optimize the system. The system is nonlinear, erratic, and complex, and confronts unpredictable events and trends. In a wicked problems sociotechnical model, the dynamic tension of the interdependency between social and technical subsystems is predictive of the impact of the organization. Systems are analyzed independently and interdependently. The analysis requires attention to context, to technology in particular.

Westbrook and colleagues (2007) demonstrate how the social and technical framework informs evaluating a new electronic medication management system. In their project, a series of technical tasks were computerized to save valuable time for patient care. Unfortunately, the tasks themselves consumed very little time before the interactive computer conversion. This mismatch between technical priorities and social systems is typical of the rush to implement interactive communication technology undertaken in a vacuum. New attention is being given through the National Institutes of Health workshop mechanism to the perspective of the consumer, given the capital and influences in their specific environment (McFarland-Horne & Li, 2010).

Wicked problems are best resolved by examining perspectives, habits, and preferences of the stakeholder aggregate. Another example of change at one level with undesirable consequences is the loss of family face-to-face time with the advent of new online technologies. The abrupt nature of the drop was surprising to the director of the Center for the Digital Future, Michael Gilbert: "Families are the social building blocks of virtually every society, and this [loss of face time] can't be a good thing" (Gardner, 2009, para. 3). Gilbert pointed out that current Internet applications are demanding interactions, unlike TV or radio where family members might gather and share the experience. As telehealth becomes more integrated into multigenerational families, planning for face-to-face time may require formal scheduling. The risk is there will be diminished levels of social commitment to the family, which could have implications for instrumental and emotional support commitments essential to successful telehealth implementations.

Discussed less often is the lack of exposure to sunlight resulting from long sessions linked to a tethered computer (desktop). New developments in mHealth (mobile phone based telehealth) may have the serendipitous and *disruptive* effect of moving people outside of their home again. Health professionals and consumer advocates can work with individuals and families so that the geography of fixed devices does not limit choices. In this move toward zero geography or pan geography, location does not affect access, or access is everywhere.

Social Dimensions of the Mess: Aging and Chronic Illness Issues

Nearly two in three publicly insured adults under the age of 65 have one or more chronic conditions, based on a Medical Expenditures Panel survey (Machlin & Woodwell, 2009). An issue brief from the Center for Studying Health System Change reported that 75% ($1.7 trillion) of healthcare dollars were spent on managing chronic illness conditions (Carrier & Reschovsky, 2009). However, the report notes that few recognized care management tools are used by physicians, especially in small practices. Even the knowledgeable California Healthcare Foundation expert exclaimed that the expenditures for chronic care in the United States were "staggering" (Sarasohn-Kahn, 2009, p. 2). Unfortunately, the data on return on investment (ROI) for these expenditures in the care of the chronically ill was characterized with "pervasive problems" and as "disturbing" (Sarasohn-Kahn, p. 2). Few people are getting adequate care. However, telehealth applications were seen as offering the most promising avenues for changing the care of the chronically ill. Given that half of all the healthcare resources in the United States are used by 5% of the population, new approaches must be explored that take advantage of new technologies (McFarland-Horne & Li, 2010).

Chronic disease is most effectively managed through frequent, near continuous monitoring (Sarasohn-Kahn, 2009). Sarasohn-Kahn observes that many patients spend only a few minutes a year with their clinicians. According to the National Council on Aging, a third of all chronically ill people say they leave a doctor's office or hospital feeling confused about what they should do to manage their disease, and 57% report that their providers have not asked whether they have anyone to help implement a care plan at home. New technology tools are emerging to bridge these gaps. Some of these technologies fall under the utilization of personal motion technology, which can provide information in community context, in real time (McFarland-Horne & Li, 2010). A report from the California Health Foundation, *Participatory Health: Online and Mobile Tools Help Chronically Ill Manage Their Care* (Sarasohn-Kahn, 2009), describes some of the online and mobile platforms and applications that can assist patients in managing their health care—not only at home but almost anywhere outside their clinician's office. Sources include extensive interviews with stakeholders in the field whose experiences and views are presented throughout the report (Sarasohn-Kahn, 2009). (See also the monograph by Johnston & Solomon [2008] on telemedicine and other reports under *Health IT* at the California Health Foundation, available at http://www.chcf.org/topics/index.cfm?topic=CL108.) A review of the tools and their availability to specific healthcare agencies may prompt changes in budgets and policies as the advantages of telehealth suggest new priorities.

New Demographics of Health and Aging

Most consumers and health professionals are well aware of the high costs of caring for older adults and that their numbers are swelling. Less frequently discussed is the massive costs of caring for the "near elderly"—baby boomers ages 55–64. In 2007 alone, hospitals spent $56 billion on care for this group (Russo, Wier, & Elixhauser, 2009). The number of near-elderly individuals is expected to increase by 18% by 2020, which is a greater increase than any other group under age 65 due to the sizeable baby boom population (Russo et al., 2009). The hospital cost summary does not include costs related to outpatient or rehabilitation following surgery or accidents.

The near elderly have new expectations of lively and engaged aging. The healthcare-related costs of their new hobbies may be significant. As noted in the games chapter, even exergames such as Wii Sports and Wii Fit have led to age-specific injuries related to "keeping up" with the younger generation.

Statistics like this are important to understanding the scope of the need for new approaches to health care. There is the sheer size of the no longer young adult group (middle aged, near old, and old) with the attendant burden of multiple conditions and related financial implications. Nonetheless, it is important to keep a personal face on the complexity of what individuals and families face (Table 7.3).

Table 7.3   Context for Telehealth: A Scenario

Earlier today I had a terrifying experience when visiting my 80-something-year-old parents in their little house in Islip, Long Island. It's not much of a house, but we all love it, and, not surprising, my parents want to live there forever. I was in good spirits as I made the familiar sharp turn into the driveway, reflecting on my last telephone call with my dad just 2 days ago. He was upbeat—everything was just fine, and both Mom and Dad were looking forward to my visit from Portland, where I am a division head at Oregon Health & Science University.

After a seemingly cheerful hug from Dad, I knew instantly something was terribly wrong. Mom did not come to the door, and the house was unusually dark and messy—even for my parents. A pile of dishes in the sink, the stench of old garbage—this was not Mom's kitchen—a wonderful cook in her day. When I found Mom in her bed, she gave me a big smile, but it was hard for her to move as she attempted to cover up a bruise on her right arm. None of this had come up during my phone call!

Reluctantly, Dad told me that Mom's bruise was caused by a fall in her bedroom several days ago. The scary part was that he hadn't discovered her fall for several hours, even though she was wearing an alert pendant and says she was screaming—at the time, Dad was deeply into his favorite TV show. Mom did not press the pendant because she dreaded the havoc of an ambulance—as had happened with a false alarm a few years ago.

Dad also admitted that Mom was sometimes confused, but he did not make much of it because more often than not she was as sharp as ever, and after all, we all have our senior moments. While washing my hands, I discovered a full container of Lasix—medication my Mom swore she was taking religiously once a day. Obviously she was not.

Watching my Dad walk, I could not help noticing a hesitation and shuffle in his gait. It turned out that my parents had stopped taking walks in the nearby park— their main form of exercise—after an unexpected October snowstorm, and they had never resumed them.

I was uneasy. Did Mom have a serious cognitive decline—a mild cognitive impairment? Should I do something? Should I tell their doctor? Should I convince them to move to an elder care facility? I doubt if I could…and I live 3000 miles away.

The parents of Misha Pavel described above belong to the fastest growing, economically dangerous, "epidemic" threat to society—the aging population. . . . Fifty years ago, it was indeed a regular pyramid with straight sides. Today, however, there is a large bulge in the middle—a "tsunami" wave of baby boomers racing toward retirement age.

Source: Pavel et al., 2009. Reprinted with permission of the National Academy of Engineering, Washington, DC.

Social Dimensions of the Mess: Disparities and the Health Visit Experience

In the Chapter 1 introduction to telehealth, a case was made for how systems of telehealth could be arranged to support patient-centered, cost-effective care. The literature of persuasion is vast. However, issues of equity and the potential impact on health disparities are rarely discussed. One-third of residents in the United States are a minority (Center for Health Care Quality at the George Washington University & Robert Wood Johnson Foundation, 2009). Data keeps emerging that document disparities for minorities: they are sicker and have more environmental challenges of pollution, crowding, and physical hazards. Recent data from the National Health Interview Surveys and the Medical Expenditure Panel Surveys analyzed by Muennig, Fiscella, Tancredi, and Franks (2009) suggest that poverty itself is a more powerful variable in explaining disease burden than any behavioral variables. Responsive policies are difficult to formulate, the authors indicate. The care experience was not discussed, but beyond access there are issues of delivery that are relevant to telehealth.

The Center for Health Care Quality asserts that there are "numerous studies" documenting that even after holding constant income, education level, insurance status, and other socioeconomic details, there are disparities in the care delivered to white, African American, and Hispanic patients (Center for Health Care Quality, 2009, para. 2). The Center observes that unfortunately, "most hospitals, health systems, and providers deny such disparities exist within their organizations" (para. 2). The Center and the Robert Wood Johnson Foundation (RWJF) define *disparities* as unexplained variations in the delivery of care to minorities that are not explained by *differences* related to biology, preferences, insurance, access, or social/economic capital. Their program, *Expecting Excellence*, demonstrated that awareness of variations in care within a specific setting—sharing data—leads to improved quality of care and greater equity. Awareness of differences that are attributable to variables in the delivery system can be sobering to healthcare providers and prompt new strategies for equity.

Environmental factors specific to healthcare encounters that might play a role in sustaining disparities note persistent poorer chronic disease outcomes for minority patients and look at the environment of care (Varkey et al., 2009). To understand these differences from an ecological perspective—independent of illness and personality variables—they interviewed clinic managers, primary care physicians, and patients. There were two samples: clinics with at least 30% minority patients and clinics with less than 30% minority patients. In their report, entitled *Separate and Unequal*, the minority patients and physicians had less access to supplies, fewer exam rooms, fewer specialists, and many instances of language problems. In addition, the clinics with 30% minority patients had more chaotic work environments and fewer physicians with high work control or high job satisfaction. This case is illustrative of the imperative to look at individual variables and social conditions as only part of the wicked problem of health disparities. Physical environments and infrastructure leverage the everyday experience.

From an ecological perspective, both patient and staff well-being are compromised in poor delivery environments. A well-designed telehealth system could alleviate some of the problems. Specialist access could be improved with online videoconferencing, exam rooms freed up with virtual visits, and atmospheres calmed by systems that collect and trend data (sensors and messaging machines) for those consumers struggling with chronic conditions. Minority families are often stressed by the need to bring children and adults under their care to the appointment—adding to the general sense of chaos. Telehealth would allow consumers to interface without having to monitor the needs and wants of their family who are in a formal setting with rules and arrangements not compatible with their needs and wants.

It is important as new facilities are built that provisions are made for telehealth and participatory health. Regardless of the history of the population served, policy makers and planners who do not anticipate health technology are doing a disservice to their client base—both the health professionals and the consumers. This is particularly a risk in low-income areas where unwarranted assumptions may be made about client willingness to use technology and levels of experience. In Los Angeles, the Urban League has underway a project to bring computers and Internet access to every family in a defined low-income, high-minority area. Telehealth participation is a specific objective.

Telehealth is not a panacea. However, telehealth can be more than technology that replicates the medical model in a home setting. Online educational and support resources can be designed to equitable standards of quality and offer tailoring options to meet the needs of true differences. Telecare monitoring allows for quality improvement surveillance with minimal intrusion for the patient and diminished observer effects on the patient under scrutiny. Accountability can be established based on observations rather than subjective reports. Informed consent for all stakeholders is essential. Cultural competence can be developed. The Office of Minority Health provides one model of online education (available free at https://www.thinkculturalhealth.org/cccminfo.asp).

Everyone and Everything Is Connected: Ethical Dilemmas

Implementing telehealth in an equitable, consumer-centric fashion requires attention to risks and barriers as well as moral issues. Keeping in mind that everything and everyone is connected is key to creating policies and inventing innovations. An ecosystem or socioecological perspective takes into account the physical and social environments as well as the needs and characteristics of the individual.

Every stakeholder must be seen as a consumer (see Table 7.2). This table provides a context for appreciating the consumer perspective of various stakeholders. The goal is to provide productive and satisfying everyday experiences and acceptable outcomes for all stakeholders in a healthcare system organized around telehealth. Implementing telehealth creates complex ethical dilemmas at the social level.

Cultural Frame for Ethical Analysis: Global Collaborations

Many experts (European Network and Information Security Agency [ENISA], 2009; Gammon, Christiansen, & Wynn, 2009; Layman, 2003; Rigby, 2007; Staggers, McCasky, Brazelton, & Kennedy, 2008) have expressed overlapping concerns about the evolution of health technology applications without explicit attention to ethical aspects. As summarized earlier, they have raised a set of concerns and conundrums that get insufficient attention. In fact this is a global concern.

The European Network for Health Technology Assessment (EUNetHTA) is a working group that recently confirmed that ethical issues are rarely addressed (Saarni et al., 2008). This group consists of 25 of the 27 European Union countries (not Slovakia or Bulgaria); Norway, Iceland, and Switzerland; and four countries outside Europe: the United States, Canada, Australia, and Israel. In the United States, the Agency for Healthcare Quality and Research (AHRQ) and the private, nonprofit group Center for Medical Technology Policy send representatives. Their work was recently summarized by Saarni et al. (2008).

This group proposes that technology is very value laden in the cultural context where it is in place. They anticipate that as health technology becomes internationally transferable a global perspective will be critical. They campaign for not getting too wedded to outcomes such as mortality (the thin side of ethics) and propose that patient-centered outcomes and societal and organizational outcomes, although difficult to quantify (the thick side of ethics) be included. Their work is still in draft form and not to be cited, but the draft is posted at http://www.eunethta.net/Work_Packages/WP_4.

In a *World Health Bulletin* summary, Saarni et al. (2008) report that a set of 16 questions has been agreed on "to increase standardization, transparency, and the international transferability of the assessment"(p. 618). Engaging stakeholders in the ethical dialogues is emphasized. The analysis proposes to begin with exploring whether a new technology is likely to "challenge the religious, cultural, or moral convictions or beliefs of some groups or change current social arrangements." The model is organized to address issues of autonomy.

Beneficence is a central concern as to whether unwanted or harmful effects might unfold. One example is genetic tests that might interfere with family planning and social life of the individual but also the extended family. The other major focus is consistent with dilemmas raised earlier: the consequences of using or not using technology on justice. Closely related is the extent to which principles of fairness, justness, and solidarity are respected. "New interventions often require reallocation of resources" (Saarni et al., 2008, p. 619). The EUNetHTA collaborative reminds analysts that all stakeholders must be assessed in terms of consequences.

They suggest that there is risk of inequalities that may relate to religion, employment, geography, gender, insurance, and ethnicity. Although not included, political affiliations and sexual preferences are certainly implied as potential levers of inequity. The collaborative proposes that a variety of methods can be used. These include casuistry, coherence analysis, principlism, interactive participatory approaches, social shaping of technology, and a wide reflective equilibrium.

A summary of these approaches is presented in the Saarni et al. (2008) report. The core assumption is that all technology assessments should benefit public health and well-being. "A basic consideration of ethical issues is better than no consideration at all" (Saarni et al., 2008, p. 621). And finally, when resources are scarce, as in developing countries or economically devastated communities, early analysis of ethical, social, and organizational implications might take priority over effectiveness deliberations. Social values may take precedence over a desire to be cutting edge with respect to health technology.

Personal Experience as Frame for Ethical Analysis: Individual and Community Interface

Aggregation of data and pervasive monitoring are components of ethical dilemmas in personal experiences of telehealth. These dilemmas are of concern across a broad range of disciplinary experts (Demiris, Parker Oliver, & Courtney, 2006; ENISA, 2009; Gammon, Johannessen, Sorensen, Wynn, & Whitten, 2008; Layman, 2003; Rigby, 2007; Staggers et al., 2008). Taking a socioecological framework, a wide range of issues surface that vary by the structure of telehealth, the individual's and family's situation, and community resources.

Balancing Mistrust and Frustration with Fragmentation

Web-based health activities lend themselves to new opportunities to gather data in one place for health professional, consumer, and service provider access. In 2003, Layman concluded that the risks attendant on data aggregation were so high that consumers would not accept Web-based health records. Publicized occurrences of healthcare agencies that either post data on the

Internet inadvertently or lose data-laden electronic devices have bred mistrust. However, evidence is accumulating that individuals are so frustrated with the breakdown of the American healthcare system that they would now even be willing to pay for systems that aggregate data on themselves or loved ones. Moreover, families that have had negative experiences with the location-centered, episodic, provider-based healthcare system may embrace new technologies without thoroughly investigating the relative merits and risks. This creates vulnerability to system abuses.

Injustices of Allocation and Stereotypes: Disparities

Potential injustices are related to allocation of telehealth resources. Layman (2003) notes that equity will rapidly become an issue. There are issues of supply and demand and the problem of who will pay for the associated costs of telecare. Individuals living in poverty who already have access problems may be unlikely to receive telehealth-based access.

Aggregating data (Layman, 2003) based on geographic location can create a profile unflattering to a specific ethnic or geographic group because it is the dominant demographic. Justice may be compromised by analysts (professional or lay reviewers) assuming that a particular individual can be characterized by the data averages for the group. These assumptions may lead to a generalization that a particular group is at risk for noncompliance with telecare. This prejudice could be applied wholesale to justify denying telecare to an individual. Alternatively, political support for funding to a stigmatized group may be difficult to muster "in the face of the facts."

If there is a limit in the supply of required devices and personnel available to interpret and respond, how will decisions be made about allocation? By whom? And with what rubric? What devices and services will become the standard of care, and which will be considered exotic luxuries? In the United Kingdom (UK), consumer panels have been developed so that such decisions about standard of care for high-priced innovations are not the sole province of health professionals or politicians. These panels, in existence for 10 years, are commissioned by the National Institute for Clinical Excellence. Their charge is to weigh the evidence of cost-effectiveness of medications, treatments, and services. They advise on whether the cost is justified as a routine expense for the National Health Service. Details and reports are available at http://www.nice.org.uk.

Autonomy: Conflicts Related to Intrusive Oversight

Multiple scenarios are possible that create other ethical dilemmas. The telecare system may have the capacity to detect sexual liaisons, heavy drinking events, consumption of illegal drugs, or other "misbehavior" (Rigby, 2007). Rigby asks, "must monitored persons 'behave themselves' or be disqualified from health support?" (p. S352). If an individual circumvents the system frequently to maintain privacy, what are the liability issues?

There are also equity issues in terms of a scarce, expensive resource. As Rigby notes, to date, disqualification from health services is not a routine happening in unmonitored healthcare relationships. It is rare that a health professional denies service related to noncompliance.

Intergenerational Issues in Monitoring: Rights and Responsibilities

Rigby (2007) also proposes that family or health professionals may demand telecare when older adults or handicapped individuals are at risk for poor care. Some older adults or individuals with long-term health problems may believe they have little to lose and not desire to live a highly restricted healthy lifestyle. He speculates on those situations where the individual refuses to allow the system, ignores, or threatens to disrupt it; what are the responsibilities of family, the agency, or the care manager? Similarly, Staggers et al. (2008) warn that insurance companies might rule against reimbursement for advanced treatments if there is evidence from telecare records that warnings were not heeded.

Other dilemmas of monitoring across generations occur when parents want to monitor the health-related behaviors of their children. Gammon et al. (2009) describe emerging moral dilemmas for parents. They note that in the United States, the procedures for establishing health-specific value of technology are expensive and move slowly. This creates an undermarket for self-management systems that are not tethered to healthcare agents (Redman, 2007, as cited by Gammon et al.). The ethical issues that emerge can be contextualized, Gammon et al. argue, in traditional medical ethics (*thin* ethics) or a socioecological perspective (*thick*). Using Braunack-Mayers's (2006, as cited in Gammon et al.) thick–thin approach, thin medical ethics focuses on maximizing treatment outcome in a scientific evidence-based context of controlled trials. The thick accounts are contextualized by social and cultural norms and values of health, individualism, risk, privacy, and lifestyle (p. 425). Gammon et al. make the case that with respect to health technology, both approaches are best brought into play.

Blood glucose monitoring has been used as a heuristic for understanding the tension experienced within families with respect to digital monitoring. Parents struggle with wanting to trust their child to take responsibility but at the same time feel motivated and obligated to provide oversight. A common fear is that lack of parent oversight of child adherence could lead to irreversible damage (Gammon et al., 2009). The authors describe a dynamic tension between protecting privacy and sustaining the development of autonomy and the surveillance society imperative of monitoring as an indication of good parenting. The thin approach emphasizes the medical consequences, and a thick approach balances these concerns with attention to the parent–child relationship and implicit messages about trust and love. A thin account emphasizes outcomes of monitoring and weighs scientific clinical data heavily. A thick account appreciates the relational and political values at play.

Gammon et al. (2009) suggest it is useful to weigh the similarities between sharing blood glucose monitoring data and decisions to placing spyware on family members' computers' positioning systems to track movements of family members (p. 426). The tracking may be of elderly relatives who travel outside the home or teen drivers, or even using GPS on cell phones to track children's paths when they are away from home. For some families, it would be productive to turn the question around and request an analysis of the extent to which the child's health or the parent's peace of mind is protected by the technology. As Gammon et al. ask, "What is it worth to us to maintain recommended BG [blood glucose] levels in our family?" (p. 427). Or finding one's grandmother soon after a fall or a walk? Who gets to choose? This Norwegian telemedicine team advocates cocreation of arrangements within families (Gammon et al.).

Gammon et al. (2009) recommend setting up the expectation, through user instructions, that families will engage in a process of discussion of the relevant moral questions in the context of best practice knowledge and skills. Such discussions can be powerful and important to building and sustaining family cohesion at any age. However, families should not lose sight of the potential of arranging a contract (with child or aging parent) that engages a neutral third party as monitor with permission to sound an alert that goes simultaneously to the parent or adult child. This kind of arrangement with a trusted outsider, or even a trusted extended family member, can go a long way in minimizing stress on family bonds during the transition to adulthood for teens and the transition to end of life for older adults.

Risks Inherent in Everyday Experience of Telehealth Implementation

The ENISA group (2009) in their article, "Being Diabetic in 2011," detailed 14 risks specific to telehealth. The subsequent section closely follows their discussion of risk (pp. 17–20) with notes specific to implementation in the United States (Table 7.4). The ENISA list is supplemented with issues raised by other experts, particularly with respect to social networks and ethics. Recommendations for minimizing the occurrence or impact of such issues are added here to the ENISA presentation of risk issues.

Table 7.4   The Risk Side of Telehealth

Data access risks

- Informed consent?
- Noncompliance with data protection regulations
- Data breaches
- Repurposing or secondary use of data
- Misinterpretation of data by patient
- Misinterpretation, modification, or deletion of data by staff
- Data surveillance and profiling

Service and device-related risks

- Access denials
- Disruption of services
- Theft
- Access to services and response teams
- Human error in emergencies
- User interface errors

Social network and ethical issues linked to monitoring

- Adequate briefing for health professionals, patients, families
- Autonomy: conflicts related to intrusive oversight
- Liability issues related to device or algorithm failure

Sources: ENISA, 2009; Gammon et al., 2009; Layman, 2003; Rigby, 2007; Staggers et al., 2008.

The ENISA (2009) list begins with informed consent for data access. The ENISA paper raises concerns related to data issues—such as unauthorized access and interpretation problems. It also indicates other concerns related to the devices or complementary services. These concerns overlap those identified by Demiris et al. (2006) for nurse practitioners using telehealth in a hospice context. Taking a socioecological perspective, the aspect of social network engagement and medicalization of the environment as ethical or moral dilemmas are added to the discussion.

Informed Consent

Confusions abound. When should consent be obtained, and who should have access? Telehealth provides secondary data that could be important to policy planning and research. Obtaining consent for every use may be intrusive and difficult. If a patient has granted access to a caregiver or family member, when is their consent required with respect to data they input about their actions and reactions?

ENISA (2009) notes that governments and citizens often treat medical information differently than other forms of personal information. For some people, medical information is more private than economic or social information. Others argue that, especially within the healthcare community, any professional who provides treatment has an inherent right to all pertinent data in order to deliver quality care. Consumers sometimes do not see the necessity of open access for every member of the healthcare team. As electronic health records and personal health record extensions take hold, consumers may be more aware of the extent of data and information about them that is known to any healthcare professional with record access.

In the area of informed consent, there is also the dilemma of the consumer's right not to know. Staggers et al. (2008) highlight this as a new area specific to technology. However, this right, in the experience of the author, has been a common area of contention in cross-cultural health settings. The American healthcare system is built on an assumption that the patient not only has a right but an obligation to know. This is inconsistent with the values and practices of many cultural groups where disclosure is not an individual decision. The conflict has been intense around end-of-life issues (Frank et al., 1998, 2002). In some cases, a court order has had to be obtained to enjoin health professional staff from telling a family member information the family had declined to have the patient hear. Understanding the complex issues related to knowledge newly available about genes in the context of cultural differences can be informed by looking at end-of-life issues. See Crawley (2005) for a thoughtful exploration of the American dilemmas in sharing or withholding health information in end-of-life contexts.

Graber (2010) has also raised issues related to informed consent when avatars are created in online applications. As discussed under games (Chapter 6), the avatar is often presented as a representation of the self. In these cases, there are moral issues related to informed consent for using information created when the avatar is in play. There is great potential for using avatars to encourage trial of new health behaviors in telehealth applications. However, human rights, Graber reminds us, will need to be negotiated and relevant norms developed.

Noncompliance with Data Protection Regulations

In the United States, the Health Insurance Portability and Accountability Act (HIPAA) specifically did not cover electronic transmissions. As interoperability becomes a requirement, new protections will be in place. Confusion is likely to ensue as new programs come online and regulations are interpreted. Data can be posted in the interests of accountability at the program level that is actually harmful to individuals (Layman, 2003).

Data Breaches

"Evildoers might eavesdrop," steal personal data, and they might be "insiders" (ENISA, 2009, p. 19) Negligence or carelessness may result in making data available beyond necessary personnel. Clear penalties and a monitoring system for staff violations are increasingly in place. Electronic records actually make it easier to detect breaches and determine the responsible person. Leaving a screen open during conversation and storing files on personal equipment used by others are examples. Role modeling and monitoring of these habits will be important in minimizing these risks.

Repurposing or Secondary Use of Data: Mission Creep

Telehealth data is collected for purposes specific to the care of individuals or family groups. The real-time nature of inadvertent opportunities for data breaches, the engagement of a wide range of professionals, and even patients in variable settings make this information of great interest to a variety of groups. In the United States, there are already concerns over whether researchers will be locked out of critical databases by new privacy regulations. Consumers and healthcare providers have concerns that data on their behaviors will be available without their knowledge and consent. Transparency at the agency and national levels will become critical. Gaining the trust of patients and advocacy groups will be essential to having these new databases available under any circumstances for policy analysis and research.

Data Surveillance and Profiling

In telehealth, it is common for sensors to provide data that locates the individual (GPS coordinates, for example). This can be very useful when an alert is activated. However, this potentially provides information both to law enforcement or criminal elements as to when a house is empty. If the data protection is inadequate or access controls fail to filter out illegitimate viewers, a wide range of *superinterested* parties may gather data (ENISA, 2009).

This *dataveillance* could also be used by employers, insurance companies, credit-checking services, and researchers for subsequent profiling. Consumers would benefit by understanding and making a commitment to the extra steps required for secure connections and restricting password access. As personal health records become more common, and families wish to share data, this risk increases. Families should limit sharing to a need-to-know basis and use a system where each member has his or her own password. Password coaching minimizes risk. Changing passwords regularly and refusing to share passwords are important.

Inadequate Briefing of Health Professionals, Patients, and Families

As telehealth applications are installed and implemented, it is imperative that users all receive adequate training and briefing about effective use of the technology and the possible risks as described above with respect to data and services. Feedback loops that link the consumer/patient and designated members of the support system are key to long-term change (Sarasohn-Kahn, 2009).

In a traditional model of care, information travels one way. Information is often unavailable even to other members of the healthcare team if they did not order the tests. Unfortunately, feedback loops are not inherent in telehealth. Even the VHA comprehensive telehealth program is a one-way system (Hopp et al., 2006). Loops are easily built in and can operate automatically, but designers and consumers must be proactive in creating, maintaining, and monitoring the loops.

Systems that track changes in access and alert a care manager can prevent some of the problems and errors that occur with naïve users. Such a system may also function as an alert when an unknown user signs on and the person is not really authorized. The care manager or care sharer can connect with the patient and determine his or her wishes.

A tension in the telecare design is whether the data is passively recorded for expert clinician review or has a built in algorithm that triggers alerts and actions based on interpretation of observed patterns (Rigby, 2007). Rigby notes that unless there is direct video surveillance, sensors only signal patterns of daily living—such as doors opened at usual times and bathroom trips at average frequency. Devices embedded in clothing or the body may provide more accurate data on the status of the person. The presence of a camera or sensor may be interpreted as continuous monitoring by a live person. This difference needs to be transparent to consumers, their social support network, and all of those in their ecosystem.

Patient Might Misinterpret Data

Interfacing with a telehealth system requires a fair amount of overall literacy, visual literacy, computer literacy, and health literacy. Unfortunately, common sense, general intelligence, and a calm approach to healthcare issue management are not universal assets. The move to enhance self-management with access to one's electronic health record and a personal health record add-on can create great complexity. This shift can generate considerable anxiety. Ideally, adults with minimal computer experience, new diagnoses, or computer anxiety related to past problems with technology will be linked to technical assistance available around the clock.

Issues of interpretation are more urgent as nanotechnology applications become more common. Staggers et al. (2008) note that these novel bridges between health sciences and engineering will bring information to consumers first. They argue that this may lead to changes in the role of the expert clinician. "Nanotechnology may change the power base of health care, with consumers emerging at the center of the team in an era of highly individualized care" (p. 273).

Early intense "hand holding," on-site coaching, and peer partnerships can be very effective. Opportunities to learn skills in community centers with others also struggling to learn can be very motivating as well (Jordan-Marsh et al., 2006). The St. Barnabas group also found that clear, easily accessible cue sheets were reinforcing and reassuring.

Data Mismanagement by Healthcare Professional or Systems

Flaws in the system, user's lack of knowledge, complexity of the data, mistakes in the data, or outright distraction can create problems. Data might be modified or deleted inappropriately. Hand-entered data or information summarized to support a treatment decision might be entered on the wrong record. Problems with accuracy and completeness of the medical record in primary care are related to past history (Greenhalgh, Wood, Bratan, Stramer, & Hinder, 2008). The researchers note that common errors occur when a letter sent to a patient is not read carefully by the coder, or a provisional diagnosis is coded when a physician states it has been excluded. Greenlaugh et al. warn when patients move to a new practice, perpetuation of errors is likely if the health record is not reviewed. However, given the state of the healthcare system, this review by the former practice is unlikely. This is another example of how consumer access to his or her own records may minimize errors that lead to more tests or inappropriate treatment. An unempowered, ignorant patient may submit even if he or she feels confused.

Streams of data from telecare and telemedicine create special problems. Rigby (2007) notes that the volume of data from ubiquitous or continuous monitoring is so massive, only summated data may be transferred to the record. Details may be lost unless there is a structure to capture outliers for review.

System Access Denials

Circumstances might tempt or require a patient to access services in an unprotected environment over an unsecured channel. Lacking authentication, service would be denied when it seems urgent to the patient. Education on the role of authentication in protecting the client and strategies for moving to a secured environment should be reviewed periodically. Such issues often arise when the patient is traveling.

Disruption of Services

Flaws in the design or infrastructure could lead to breakdowns. Systems are most unstable when upgrades are offered. Natural catastrophes such as storms, fires, and earthquakes may damage the infrastructure. Power outages during peak demand times may disrupt service. Construction or utility workers may inadvertently cut cables. Healthcare providers can work with patients to plan for these contingencies. A plan for alerting the key members of the patient's support network that a technical error has occurred is important. Otherwise emergency services may be dispatched without cause (fire, police, or family members on standby).

Access to Services and Response Teams

Geographic mobility considerations arise when patients become linked to telehealth resources or are considered candidates for such resources. Some healthcare agencies are unwilling or ill-equipped to connect to telecare facilities that patients desire. Not all neighborhoods have the broadband capacity to sustain the service at optimal speeds. When an alert is activated, patients and families want to know the extent of available responses from emergency services.

As the global economic downturn unfolds, some communities are reducing or, in very small communities, eliminating core backup services. These can range from reduced police and fire services to visiting nurse and other specialists provided under government or grant funding. As layoffs occur, family incomes decrease sharply, making copayments more difficult. The insurance providing coverage may be lost with job termination. These issues are critical when families consider discharge plans, combining households to accommodate a family member, anticipate downsizing housing or using senior housing, or even plan vacations or career moves. Unfortunately, current healthcare reimbursement systems in the United States still favor episodic, hospital-based care over home-based, patient-centered models.

Just as agencies may not provide a service, or a community fail to support needed technology and adequate response teams, a consumer may choose not to bear the costs. These costs include funding, sacrificing space and ambience for equipment, and time required to install, learn, use, troubleshoot and maintain the devices, software, and interrelationships with the healthcare team.

Human Error in Emergencies

When catastrophes occur, whether they involve individuals or communities, the risk of errors escalates. These errors can be caused by not following the usual steps to protect privacy, correctly enter data, hook up cables, keep liquids away from equipment, and so on. These errors can result from anxiety, speed, and working in close, unfamiliar quarters.

If emergency workers respond to an alarm, it is useful to be prepared to quickly recognize the electronic resources to which the patient is connected. A common problem with telehealth is clutter of cables. This clutter can create a hazard zone for the patient and visitors and becomes truly risky as emergency crews go about their routines and spread their equipment in a small home space. Designing and monitoring a telecare environment requires attention to cable and equipment clutter. Work-arounds to accommodate patient preferences or the addition of new devices create special risks until an objective third party can assess the consequences of new arrangements.

User Interface Errors

Some errors will be almost built in because of poor design. A recurring problem is failure to engage consumers early in the process for technology innovations (Vanderheiden, 2007). A telehealth setup may have so many components installed at varying times with different conventions for operations and varying defaults that users and caregivers get confused. Sometimes a user or caregiver will turn off an alert and forget to take the required action. For example, a system is deactivated when guests are present or work is being done (cleaning and construction), and the user forgets to turn it back on. Developing a check or reminder system for planned interruptions can be helpful.

Negotiating System Check-Ins

Families may agree that inquiring about the operation of the system is *caring* and not *intruding*. Negotiating how often these inquiries may be made can be part of the social contract among family members. It is very conducive to feeling supported and not criticized if family members can agree on wording such inquiries as well. "Why is the monitor off?" can be very intimidating. "Mom, I am missing my link to your house" models the "I" statements that are a standby of effective relationships. Advance agreements avoid adding one more emotional burden when the family member may already be anxious about a technical problem.

Deliberate Interference

Someone with malicious or mischievous intent can interfere with the operation of the device. A visitor, family member, housekeeper, or child may inadvertently change defaults or turn off the system without appreciating the consequences. Again, a ritual of checking systems after interruptions or social events can avoid disruptions of service. Family members and other visitors can be advised that the telecare system is special even though it looks like an ordinary telephone, computer, PDA, or whatever.

Other issues may arise related to criminal intent as telehealth embraces creative interactions in virtual worlds to increase motivation, promote social networking, and allow for trial of new health behaviors. Graber (2010) has raised an alert related to avatar interaction in particular. He notes that some countries are already considering policies for dealing with theft of virtual assets and incidents of assault of one's avatar, such as rape.

Another user interface issue is when the telecare consumer chooses to ignore alerts. Both refusal to respond to alerts or resentment of the monitoring can create ethical dilemmas for families and health professionals. These are discussed in a subsequent section.

Nanotechnology Unknowns in Physical Materials

The microscopic nature of nanoparticles that make some technology possible make them hard to track and control. Staggers et al. (2008) note that more than 500 products are already available with healthcare application potential. The Nano-iPod, lotions, and biochips embedded for automated medication delivery are examples. Nanomaterials can be inadvertently inhaled. Existing protective clothing and barriers may not be adequate. New diseases or "mysterious symptoms" may result from embedded nanomaterials or "bugs" in the devices or software used in telecare (Staggers et al.). So little is known about the long-term effects of telecare, medical personnel must not be quick to dismiss reports of unusual signs and symptoms. Finally, both professionals and consumers may inappropriately assume that the availability of the products for human use means they are safe (Staggers et al.). This understanding may be faulty as applications may be experimental and that phase ill understood. In any case, the history of human use of nanomaterials is very brief, and long-term consequences with exposure accumulated over multiple exposures to treatments as a client, provider, or employee in an industrial setting is unknown (Staggers et al.).

Theft of Equipment

Patients using telehealth have a wide variety of items that may be attractive to thieves. The components at risk are the computer itself, sensors embedded in clothing, cameras, recording devices, specially adapted telephones, and other devices. One dilemma of theft is the disruption in access to services even if the cost of replacing the stolen item is low. The replacement process itself can be cumbersome. Patients should be encouraged to keep critical information about models and part numbers in a Web-based file for worldwide access.

There is limited merit to stockpiling replacement parts. Besides the cost and unlikely prospective reimbursement, obsolescence is a risk. Patients with insurance can be encouraged to explore whether their renter or homeowner policy covers replacement of components lost to theft. Although medical devices per se may be specifically excluded, ordinary consumer devices such as the computer itself may be covered for loss, theft, or damage. With respect to breakdowns independent of damage or theft, the cost of the warranty extensions can be balanced against the cost of a break in service. Costs include care-sharer lost wages and personal compromises required to arrange replacement and reinstallation.

Identity Theft

When a data storage device is lost or stolen, identity theft becomes an issue. New technology allows more comprehensive data with identifiers in huge databases to be stored on portable devices such as laptops. This creates great risk, especially if staff long accustomed to the limits of portable and handheld devices do not change their security practices. Policy setting, practice parameters, and persistent vigilance in a community of practice spirit are required to change behavior.

If the theft involves a device with embedded nanotechnology, the thief becomes exposed to all of the risks faced by the original owner. Even knowledgeable thieves may protect themselves and pass the items on to unsuspecting bargain hunters or scavengers. Consumers need to exercise new cautions with respect to their own habits of protecting devices, especially when they are mobile.

Risks Specific to Social Influence Aspects of Telehealth

A socioecological context for assessing risks brings attention to ways that the actions of groups and individuals may have consequences that consumers and health professionals do not anticipate. Vigilance from consumer advocates in the employment and community settings may be a useful strategy as telehealth applications spread. Attention during the design, implementation, and evaluation phases will be important.

Data Mining and Autonomy Compromises

As indicated above, *dataveillance* or data mining is a risk to the individual or family's autonomy. As Layman (2003) points out, in the past, the fragmentation of the episodic, location-based healthcare system with geographically distant filing systems provided some protection for privacy and autonomy. In fact, privacy was routinely breached in major medical centers without ability to trace breaks. Electronic systems leave a fingerprint that can be detected if monitoring is continual, information is reviewed systematically, or alerts triggered with unauthorized access.

Layman (2003) notes that aggregation of data may be used by employers to target workers who might become a liability. Subtle processes can be used over time, especially for the chronically ill so that demotions or dismissals seem like a logical consequence rather than discrimination. In a small community, Layman warns, posting health and vital statistics data in the name of accountability may create injustice. When the data breakdowns are sufficiently fine in a small community, for example, only one person in the geographic area may fit the demographic parameters and thus is easily identified as linked to the other data in a table. Justice might be served if software-based protections were installed so that outliers would be deleted in public presentations of health statistics.

Medicalization of Consumer Environments

When the devices and peripherals of telehealth become integral to the home, work, and leisure environment, the space may become medicalized (Demiris et al., 2006). This has potential for pervasive social consequences. Comprehensive, intrusive technology creates a pervasive reminder to the individual, his or her social supporters, and passers-through (repair people, salespeople, guests of other household members) that the consumer has a health problem. The individual and his or her family member may be treated differently depending on the perspective of the viewer. Ubiquitous and universal computing for well individuals committed to prevention and health promotion diminishes this risk. The presence of telehealth devices will become normalized and, for some consumers, desirable.

Ambivalence in Media

Americans in policy-influencing positions are not completely sold on technology as a health resource. For example, the Harris Interactive Poll group conducts an annual study of how many people are going online for health information. On the enlightening side, Humphrey (2002) notes that the numbers of people who have *ever* gone online has tripled in the past 10 years. On the dark side, the poll persists in calling those who go online for health information *cyberchondriacs*. This is a catchy, but highly pejorative term. Lewis (2006) suggests that Taylor (2002), who first used the term *cyberchondriac*, thought it was simply a descriptor. A definition more consistent with common use is suggested by White and Horvitz (2008). *Cyberchondria*, they propose, refers to "escalation of concern about what are likely to be common, innocuous symptoms to concerns about more serious illness" (White & Horvitz, p. 2). The concerns are recurrent and interrupt other activities of daily life. Lewis also suggests that searching for health information can be highly nuanced and not necessarily problematic.

One example of negative predispositions is how swiftly journalists leapt on the Cochrane database summary that showed some negative findings (Rada, 2005). The headline read "Click and Get Sick" implying that consumers who did interactive health programs not only failed to benefit, but got worse. The story was particularly interesting as even today, years later, the in-depth resources of the Cochrane Collaboration are not routinely cited in the lay press. So, to have this study appear and go *viral* (spinning around the information circuit to a wide variety of sources such as magazines, websites, blogs, and newspapers) was surprising. The Cochrane Collaboration later withdrew the review and apologized for the errors. Compared to the firestorm or viral response to the wrong report, little publicity was given to the retraction.

This built-in propensity of the media to promote near-pathologic levels in escalating the drama of health stories can also be a characteristic of algorithms built into search engines. White and Horvitz (2008) propose that search engine architects have a responsibility to consider the implications of page ranking, user modeling, and interface design for triggering fear and escalating concern. Perpetuating dark views of informatics and telecare may have long-term effects on politician, consumer, and professional willingness to make the changes needed for effective, efficient telecare that reduces costs and improves quality of life. Health professionals and consumer advocacy groups may have to take leadership in information mediation roles to preempt this leap to lurid headlines. Fledgling and unusual developments require enthusiastic support, thoughtful analysis, and evaluation to flourish and to set a culture of thoughtful experimentation.

BARRIERS TO IMPLEMENTATION: SOCIOECONOMIC AND POLITICAL CONTEXT

A consensus is emerging that the integration of telemedicine/telehealth and eHealth tools has moved beyond the demonstration stage (Doarn et al., 2008). For some time, there have been a few "mature and self-sustaining" telehealth systems (Shannon et al., 2002). Unfortunately, telehealth is still unfamiliar to the general public and health providers (Chang, 2007), despite government funding and enthusiasm from industries and businesses. Many projects fail once the start-up or grant funding is over (Mackert & Whitten, 2009). There are many barriers to its widespread implementation.

Economic Challenges

The equipment does have installation and maintenance costs for both the healthcare provider and the consumer. Broadband connections have at times proven prohibitively expensive, even in urban areas (Johnston & Solomon, 2008). The slowness of transmission and complexity requiring additional training time incur costs as well. It is not clear how these resources will be paid for. Few insurance companies or state Medicaid programs have arranged reimbursement, despite the "many benefits" and "so few down sides" (Leach, 2009, p. 1). The Medicare Telehealth Services Fact Sheet is an excellent resource: https://www.cms.gov/MLNproducts/downloads/TelehealthSrvcsfctsht.pdf.

Although savings to the healthcare system seem well documented, it is not clear that the provider or the individual patient and family will realize the financial benefits. The Centers for Medicare and Medicaid Services (CMS) reimbursement structure creates a formidable barrier (Bashshur et al., 2009). Leaders in national telemedicine and eHealth centers have highlighted this dilemma. Introduction of technology and new approaches that are more patient centered require initial-stage equipment and training costs that must be borne locally, while savings may only be realized at the governmental, insurance, or major employer level (Bashshur et al., 2009; CTECH, 2009; Wielawski, 2006). Wielawski (2006) has detailed the heavy burden on small private practices of telehealth installation and retraining costs—not only dollars and time but interpersonal stress. These costs need to be included when calculating total costs for a telehealth installation.

There remains considerable controversy in the literature as to whether the economic issue is cost savings or cost effectiveness (Kvedar, Hwang, Moorhead, Orlov & Ubel, 2009; Polisena, Coyle, Coyle, & McGill, 2009). Polisena et al. conducted a review of 22 studies on home health for chronic conditions (n = 4,871 patients). Given the limited quality of the studies, the reviewers observed that there seem to be savings in most studies. A persistent dilemma is the quality of studies (Polisena et al.). They called for careful attention to whether savings resulted from receiving fewer services or were tied to improved clinical outcomes. In a roundtable discussion, Kvedar et al. (2009) wondered if we could accomplish improved quality at current costs? Hwang, an expert in disruptive innovations, cautioned that we are struggling with a "guild mentality" as we attempt health care reform (Kvedar et al., p. 640). His goal would be to redefine workflows and workforce so that we no longer pay for a "one size fits all" centralized system of care (Kvedar et al., p. 640). Orlov (Kvedar et al.) made two points. One is that one study found patients were willing to monitor their health, but did not want to share their data, lest they be labeled as sick. She then pointed out the AARP study indicating 96% of patients wanted to participate in managing care along with the physician, "as long as the price for the necessary technology was below $50 a month" (p. 640). This set of findings underscores the value of a socioecological perspective. Telehealth cost savings dependent on shared observations of daily living and introduction of costly sensors and monitoring may not ever be realized for those "aging in place."

The thought leaders in the Roundtable (Kvedar et al., 2009) went on to note the dramatic decreases in costs for technology we now consider ubiquitous—video cameras and personal computers, for example. However inexpensive, they are still costs and require maintenance, updates, and replacements, and technical assistance. Adults in the future may have to recalibrate their expectations of the sustaining interdependence and trade-offs in disposable income. In subsequent sections, the complexity of reimbursement and return on investment as factors in cost are discussed.

Reimbursement Complexity

Reimbursement continues to be a major issue. The Spyglass executive summary (Spyglass Consulting, 2009) notes that a major issue is that the healthcare reimbursement system persists in providing incentives for the quantity of services provided and not the processes or outcomes of care. The Spyglass report notes that over 35,000 monitoring devices are in place for patients in the VA healthcare system. They conclude that telehealth works best for large systems like Kaiser Permanente or the VHA where they are both provider and payor or capitated systems needing to capture the highest return on investment. Medicare reimbursement continues to be problematic. Aspects that are covered include remote patient face-to-face services seen via live videoconferencing; non-face-to-face services that can be conducted either through live videoconferencing or via store-and-forward telecommunication services, and home telehealth services. A full report is available at the Center for Connected Health (http://www.centerforconnectedhealth.org).

As the Obama healthcare reform program evolves, the reimbursement model can be expected to change in unexpected ways. There are state and local variations that affect reimbursement. See the policy tab at the Center for Connected Health for updates (http://www.centerforconnectedhealth.org). Reimbursement will be advanced by studies where criteria for establishing necessary data are spelled out and validated over time (Tang, Black, & Young, 2006).

Reimbursement Shifts

The rate of reimbursement for telehealth in some instances was one-third that of an office visit. Lowes (2009) warns that physicians should not elect telecare options with the expectation of dramatic increases in revenue. However, he reports sufficient economic viability that medical companies have formed for the sole purpose of providing online or telephone consultations. These entrepreneurs do not have physical space constraints for equipment, parking, lobbies, and other amenities that more traditional medical practices must provide for patients and staff. They can operate in buildings where these costs are shared across a variety of tenants.

OVERVIEW OF THE RESEARCH ON TELECARE

Throughout the book research has been presented in the relevant context. This section provides overviews of three strong cases for telehealth that are organized around a conceptual framework if not a theory. First is a review of the evidence for the chronic care model (Coleman, Austin, Brach, & Wagner, 2009). Coleman et al. make the point that in complex models, it is difficult to parse out the components that are necessary but not sufficient to achieve the desired outcomes. Perhaps the next design imperative is a series of dismantling studies to determine which components are necessary. For example, composite measures of the chronic care model were significantly associated with favorable results, but across studies it is not clear which components are required minimums. The rigor of the designs was highly variable.

Another telehealth study (Reid et al., 2009) used a two-group evaluation model at baseline and at 12 months in a capitated practice (n = more than 3000 patients and 19 clinics). In this patient-centered medical home (PCMH) intervention adapted from the chronic care model (Wagner, 1998), an electronic medical record, patient portal, online medication refills and patient e-mails, and provider electronic alerts and reminders were core features. After 1 year, for no extra cost, the PCMH patients experienced more continuity of care, had 29% fewer emergent and urgent care visits, and different hospitalization rates than control patients. Patients were 62% women and 84% white with some college education (77%). Patients were more involved in their care, and providers in PCMH reported less burnout than those in control practices. Improvements in the primary care work environment are important, Reid et al. note, because of high attrition of physicians, complaints of hectic work environments, and low interest in primary care careers in contemporary trainee groups. The latter occurs for a variety of reasons, and huge debts and lower income streams in primary care cannot be discounted as factors. This study is notable in its lack of monitoring that Kibbe and Kvedar (2008) affirm is essential—results may have been far more dramatic. Also, nursing seemed to be limited to fielding calls for redirection to the care team. Adding a nurse and a social worker to this implementation, as is done in other applications of the chronic care model, might improve outcomes and escalate savings.

The largest, most rigorously articulated, and most intense telehealth model of care comes from the VA Care Coordination/Home Telehealth (CCHT) Program (Darkins et al., 2008). The VA used the chronic care model as the conceptual framework and incorporated elements consistent with the connected medical home criteria described by Kibbe and Kvedar (2008) and summarized in Table 1.6. The case outcomes of over 17,000 patients were compared from the year prior to enrollment to outcomes 6 months after enrollment. The cohort was 96.11% male, and ethnicity was not reported. The CCHT is unique in its translation to routine care on such a large scale. Costs were dramatically lower, there were fewer hospitalizations, fewer days in the hospital, and a carbon footprint benefit of reduced staff travel. Reduced travel may have been less stressful for staff. The model is notable in the leadership of the nurses (reflected in authorship) and flexibility in range of disciplines of care managers. The dilemma for other agencies is whether reduced costs also means reduced revenue.

Games as Telehealth Tools: Research Status

Although games are now recognized as inviting new tools for telehealth (Baranowski, Buday, Thompson, & Baranowski, 2008; Gotsis, 2009; Papastergiou, 2009), the research is limited and has issues similar to other aspects of telehealth. Papastergiou (2009) in her review notes that there is basically no data comparing electronic gaming to other means of reaching people to increase healthy behaviors. She concludes from the extant research that games "do have the power to help young people to adopt a healthy lifestyle and become physically active for life" (p. 613). There is little evidence with respect to individual differences in response to games; virtually no research exists on how games motivate collaborative activities or foster social support. Calls for building games to increase self-efficacy for health behaviors, capture data, and examine the impact on engagement in one's health care (Hawn, 2009) are equally relevant to telehealth in general. Some aspects of learning to use telehealth systems and the actual interaction may be so boring that games will be needed to encourage engagement.

Documenting Return on Investment: Limitations and Next Directions

There is considerable enthusiasm among diverse groups about tele-health. However, there is an emerging consensus that because of a lack of a solid evidence base, it is difficult to get key decision makers to commit to private investment and leadership (Currell, Urquhart, Wainwright, & Lewis, 2000; Doarn et al., 2008; Kobb, Chumbler, Brennan, & Rabinowitz, 2008; Miller, 2007). Many experts see a disjuncture between the enthusiasm and the research pattern. One of the dilemmas identified in bringing telehealth to the mainstream is the lack of convincing data. The dilemma is that although telemedicine has been in place for many years, there is no definitive research documenting its relative efficacy or cost-effectiveness (Leach, 2009). Martin, Kelly, Kernohan, McCreight, and Nugent (2008) in a Cochrane review, and later Polisena et al., (2009), concluded that although there are many studies, they are not conducted with sufficient rigor.

As summarized earlier, to some extent telehealth is in a vicious cycle where applications are many but consumer users few. This creates difficulty in designing rigorous studies. A major limitation is uneven distribution of studies across applications, demographic groups, and geographic locations. Miller (2007) cautions that researchers need to become proactive in assisting policy makers and funding groups to appreciate the potential return on investment. Lack of this foundation may continue to hinder reimbursement.

In their analysis of extant research, Grigsby and Bennett (2006) summarize that while programs have proliferated, the number of actual participants has been low. The low numbers of patients engaged in telehealth may have made administrators reluctant to divide available sites or clients in half in a randomized controlled trial. Blinding any of the participants is not possible without creating a risk of a Hawthorne effect. In addition, they observe that the novelty may change the interaction between client and provider. This may be negative in adding anxiety, or as Leach (2009) noted, positive if care is more likely with embarrassing health problems. This complex of factors may be one of the barriers to widespread adoption of the technology. The workshop summary on personal motion technology (McFarland-Horne & Li, 2010) validates that there are a wide range of research issues still unresolved with respect to telehealth.

Rethinking the RCT Gold Standard of Evidence

Multiple experts in the area of telehealth have expressed concern about the goal and methods chosen to study this innovation. One provocative note on telecare is an observation that the implicit assumption has been that in evaluating telehealth, the criterion is standard of care—without taking into account the quality of evidence for usual care (Martin et al., 2008).

The case against the current paradigm is also made by Leach (2009) who observes that the burden of proof, now required of telemedicine, should be reversed. Critical changes in reimbursement, he argues, would follow. His recommendation is that the default policy should be to reimburse for telemedicine, unless there was evidence of substandard outcomes.

Similarly, Kvedar (2009) has identified inappropriate research models as restraining the development of telehealth. Rosen (2007) in a letter to the editor reflected on the social network implications of obesity findings of Christakis and Fowler (2007). He expressed concern that a flaw in randomized controlled trials (RCTs) was the failure to take into account indirect social diffusion effects of changes in health behaviors. He observes that health technology assessments based on RCTs may underestimate the impact of an intervention. Other experts (Kobb et al., 2008) take a "get over it" approach. They admonish the RCT-bound reviewers that "rigorous statistical techniques aside from RCT are in extensive use, and are readily recognized and acceptable in research" (p. 979). Kobb et al. make the case that many practices in health care have no or minimal evidence but are accepted because of their obvious benefits.

Theory Limitations in Telehealth Research

Another barrier to solid research may be the lack of solid theories unique to telehealth and telemedicine. Researchers have a persistent consensus that theory-driven interventions are a "marker of success" (Duffett-Leger, Paterson, & Albert, 2008). However, as with other components of telehealth, building from theory to interactive learning or decision-making applications is rare in the literature. Gammon et al. (2008) reviewed literature twice and found few studies with any theoretical concepts. They observed that "interestingly, journals dedicated to telemedicine have the least proportion of articles that apply theory" (p. 265).

An explanation might be that these journals seem to have been established by and for enthusiasts who are crossing traditional boundaries. Their work is predominantly empirical and papers more cheerleading and cautionary than in traditional journals. Although no data can be supplied, it is not unreasonable to surmise that these boundary spanners found traditional scholarly methods very confining (see earlier discussion on limitations of randomized controlled trials). In fact, it would be fair to examine reports of clinical trials of innovations in treatments that are not technology based to validate the currency of a universal use of theory to drive design and documentation of healthcare innovations.

Throughout this book, a case has been made for using a socioecological framework of empowerment to guide thinking about telehealth. Given the recurring references to "ecosystems" across disciplines, such a framework appears to be transdisciplinary.

Recurring Theories in Telehealth Literature

One set of reviewers (Gammon et al., 2008) created seven categories of theories that they labeled as "borrowed" with a critical note that there was no reinterpretation to establish uniquely defining characteristics of telemedicine per se. The manuscript presents a detailed table noting concept and study clusters under the headings of:

- Diffusion and technology acceptance
- Organizational and systems analysis
- Interpersonal and group interaction
- Health interventions and measures
- Human factors and user-centered design
- Biomedicine and measures
- Engineering models and methods

However, in the Gammon et al. (2008) presentation, notably absent were the following, which are valuable frameworks for designing and evaluating telehealth research:

- The Unified Theory of Acceptance and Use of Technology (UTAUT), a theory of technology acceptance that is widely used in technology studies outside health
- Social networking theories that increasingly explain health outcomes and behaviors
- Empowerment, which is both a goal and outcome of telehealth
- Ecosystems: As noted earlier, this "ecosystem" label is commonly attached to telehealth and medical home approaches but rarely explicated to clarify design or outcomes.

Socioecological Framework as Theory Springboard

Although a socioecological perspective is not truly a theory, it can be very helpful in resolving issues related to telehealth with its essential information component. As suggested in the first chapter, a health habitat[1] (Jordan-Marsh, 2008) or *health habitus* (Lewis, 2006) focus can be a way to accommodate diverse views and behaviors of stakeholders. Socioecological thinking recognizes the various environments consumers navigate and assesses capital available that may be attributed to personal characteristics (socioeconomic

---

[1]Jordan-Marsh developed the concept of *health habitat* and promoted it as an alternative to medical home prior to encountering Lewis's presentation of *health habitus* to describe the context of health information-seeking behavior. The concepts overlap in useful ways.

status, gender, race/ethnicity, social capital, and human capital of literacy). Sources of influence are taken into account in terms of their charismatic power. (See Figure 7.6.) Engagement in health behaviors is "embedded in questions of social identity and the pressures and constraints of everyday life" (Lewis, 2006, pp. 536–537). A core health behavior for those engaged in participatory health is information seeking on the part of all stakeholders.

Information Seeking Behavior and Theory Issues

There are theory issues related to the information gathering behaviors of consumers and health professionals (Bawden & Robinson, 2009). Great concern has been generated with respect to information pathologies (Bawden & Robinson, 2009; Lewis, 2006). Issues include the consequences of unfettered access to information on making sound choices and potential of information overload generating feelings of powerless and anxiety. Although they do not use the term, the article by Bawden and Robinson suggests that Web 2.0 is the nexus for a wicked problem. They identify stakeholders who may be advantaged by promulgating negative views of the Internet. Some problems they suggest may be more work overload or literacy issues than Internet information overload. They caution against "one-node knee-jerk solutions proposed such as e-mail-free Fridays" (p. 187). This change made in isolation is truly inappropriate for a wicked problem (see Table 7.1). Unfortunately, they note, "there is no generally accepted detailed theoretical framework for explaining and predicting the variety of [human information] behavior" (p. 188). Bawden and Robinson imply a socioecological perspective in their summary that information behavior solutions must engage solutions related to "much wider issues of education, the nature of work, and individual responses to an increasingly complex and largely digital information environment" (p. 188). Health professionals, consumer advocates, and the social network members wishing to recommend resources to others will find that it is nearly impossible to have a stock list of Internet information resources. In fact, as consumers progress on their health illness journey, their information needs, skills, and habits will change. The same is likely to occur for other stakeholders as their experience in telehealth deepens.

DELICIOUS COLLABORATION OPPORTUNITIES

Tools for Building the Evidence Case

Standardized Outcome Instruments

Telehealth experts wishing to compare delivery models on outcomes can take advantage of a little known but significant federal undertaking. PROMIS is a federal initiative to quantify symptoms and experiences in a systematic way across a wide variety of conditions that affect quality of life (Chang, 2007). One of the PROMIS objectives is to develop a publicly available computerized adaptive test for assessment of clinical interventions. The PROMIS initiative seeks to develop ways to measure patient-reported symptoms such as pain and fatigue and aspects of health-related quality of life across a wide variety of chronic diseases and conditions. It is *delicious* in that some tools have been released for public use, have strong reliability and validity, and others are in various stages of execution.

The PROMIS website is rich in resources and has an alert to upcoming funding opportunities—great timing for telehealth applications (http://www .nihpromis.org/default.aspx). Multiple articles have been published and presentations have been made. For a list of manuscripts go to PROMIS publications; for a full list of presentations go to PROMIS presentations.

At one point, the plan was that any federally funded health researchers in the future would be required to incorporate the PROMIS tools as outcome measures. Whether or not this requirement will stand is unclear now. Many practitioners and researchers are unaware of this resource.

A paper prepared at the prestigious Northwestern University Feinberg School of Medicine makes a powerful case for patient-reported outcomes as a tool for optimizing both quality care and research (Chang, 2007). Chang introduces the PROMIS project as an interdisciplinary model. This publication in a quality-of-life journal may extend audiences to clinicians who are attracted to reading about outcomes and measurement specific to quality of life but do not attend measurement conferences.

Tools for Building the Practice Case: Minimizing Disparities

An educational video and PowerPoint presentation for providers from the Center for Health Care Quality at the George Washington University Medical Center and the Robert Wood Johnson Foundation (2009) assesses important problem disparities in health care and explores ways providers can identify and work to reduce them. It examines the definition of healthcare disparities and the academic evidence of the existence of disparities as well as the lessons that experience in the fields of quality improvement and cardiovascular care can provide in reducing such disparities.

Finally, the video presents tested solutions from *Expecting Success*, a previous RWJF-funded initiative to study and reduce healthcare disparities in diverse hospitals across the country (Center for Health Care Quality at the George Washington University & Robert Wood Johnson Foundation, 2009). Related RWJF resources include *Speaking Together*. This tool kit provides advice to hospitals on improving quality and accessibility of language services (available at http://www.rwjf.org/pr/product.jsp?id=29653) The *Expecting Success* video and PowerPoint highlights the improvements experienced by 10 hospitals that participated in the RWJF *Excellence in Cardiac Care Program* (http://www.rwjf.org/pr/product.jsp?id=28433).

Digital Age Partnerships for Telehealth: Spanning Boundaries

Telehealth and its partners, telecare and telemedicine, have created new formal and informal collaborations. Social workers and nurses and occupational therapists are increasingly highlighted as empowered members of the team (Adams, Grundy, Kohn, & Mounib, 2009; Scott, 2009; van Bronswijk et al., 2009; Wielawski, 2006) as well as emerging new roles for pharmacists and physicians in the coordination of telehealth care management (Darkins et al., 2008). Other roles may be emerging for volunteers, and for professions and other players not usually engaged in health care at the individual and family level.

Games and Volunteers for Wait Times

Even with telehealth, some waiting time may be required as systems are down or a visit to the clinic location is required. An implicit boundary has been that only children's waiting rooms provide fun and entertainment— beyond magazines and office-controlled television. As family members provide support in the form of technical assistance for telehealth or transportation to healthcare facilities, they may have extended waiting time. This waiting time has been seen as an opportunity to provide health education with limited success. Games may enhance the health visit experience for anyone who must sit and wait. Games could be introduced to provide simple distraction, stress management, social support, and learning opportunities for consumers and staff. Games could be played on site, at home, or in any "waiting situation." Teenagers or others wanting to volunteer in healthcare settings, might productively engage visitors in learning the potential of games and developing the skills to play. Crossing the boundary of the digital divide could be valuable for both groups.

Gerontechnology: An Interdisciplinary Boundary Spanner

The steady, steep increase in the population of community-dwelling older adults across the globe has led to collaborations for *gerontechnology*. The emergence of gerontechnology has brought engineers, industrial designers, and interdisciplinary gerontologists together (van Bronswijk et al., 2009). Gerontechnology is touted by van Bronswijk et al. as a means to achieve sustainable development and social sustainability with specific attention to the environment that consumers must either change or cope with. Environments described as experienced by adults (people from age 20 on) include housing, transport/mobility, and work/leisure. The healthcare environment at home and in formal healthcare settings are recommended here as an important addition to this model.

Designing a Habitat for Health and Quality of Life: Interior Design Consultation

However, one key player is continually ignored as technology drastically changes the space in which consumer/patients and professionals spend time. The missing player in managing this transition is the interior design consultant. Independent of age and ability, most humans prefer that their primary habitat—the place where they spend most of their time and establish their quality of life— is pleasant and has an ambience of comfort and inclusion.

Healthcare professionals do not always consider aesthetics when suggesting or planning home modifications for clients who wish to remain independent as they age. The result can be the medicalization of the home environment, previously discussed as a risk of telecare. The telecare team focus is most often on function and the clinical needs of their clients. Even the consumer and their family can get caught up in giving priority to the new equipment. The consequence is diminished sense of self, an image of invalidism and sickness. Interdependence is a healthier expectation than an environment arranged to convey dependence. Creating a safe, beautiful, accessible, and welcoming space calls on the expertise of a variety of team members (Kellett, 2009). (An overview is available at www.akinderspace.com. Another resource is the "Home Sweet Home: Aging in Place" video, with design tips to prevent falls, from Anne Kellett, a Certified Aging in Place Specialist, and Dr. Kimberley Bell from the San Diego Fall Prevention Task Force: http://www.sdhomerevisions.org/IdeaGallery/HomeSweetHomeAginginPlaceVideo/tabid/2580/Default.aspx.)

How these demedicalizing solutions look and how they are integrated into the overall design of the client's home is the realm of the interior designer. The ecosystem spirit of the integration is design that anticipates future needs and creates positive living spaces where people can age independently (Kellett, 2009).

Interior designers are uniquely qualified to create supportive, livable environ-ments for older persons that are functional, healthy, and safe. Including a qual-ified interior designer on the team often makes the final results seamlessly integrated into the client's living space. Two organizations are available to assist in locating just such a team member. The American Society of Interior Design-ers (ASID) provides a referral service to locate a designer in a specific geo-graphic area with healthcare or design for aging expertise (www.asid.org). The National Association of Home Builders (NAHB) Remodelers Council in collab-oration with AARP, the NAHB Research Center, and the NAHB Senior Housing Council developed a Certified Aging in Place Specialist training program. Inte-rior designers, contractors, and occupational therapists who complete this training can be located through their website at www.nahb.org.

Just as with any referral, consumers need to appreciate that charisma does matter in achieving the influence desired for a compatible design. A match between consumer and designer may not occur on the first try. As more *near-old* adults begin to plan for the later half of their lifetime, templates and online tutorials for interdependent habitat design may become available to assist in demedicalizing the home telecare process.

Boundary-Spanning: Naming Names

Individual Exemplars of Transdisciplinarity

Traditional point-of-care professionals are crossing boundaries and blend-ing areas of expertise to enhance design and evaluation of telehealth applica-tions, which require new human–environment interactions. These exemplars of transdisciplinarity were selected as being particularly *delicious* in their com-binations. Patti Brennan, for example, is a nurse engineer computer scientist expert in telehealth design (http://www.son.wisc.edu/news/brennan.html). She is the leading expert on personal health records for observations of daily life. She is about to embark on a new laboratory for health technology design in living environments. Margaret McLaughlin, a professor of health communica-tion at the University of Southern California, has also partnered with engineers. Her latest project will revolutionize how healthcare professionals and their clients from varying cradle languages communicate. Helen Osborne, an occu-pational therapist who established Health Literacy Month, has a practical hand-book (Osborne, 2004) and a website on health literacy strategies and tools (www.healthliteracy.com). Faith Hopp, a faculty member at the School of Social Work at Wayne State University has provided important insights based on the human–device interface for persons with chronic diseases in large healthcare systems such as the Veterans Health Administration (Hopp et al., 2006; see bio available at http://socialwork.wayne.edu/bio.php?id=852). Gerald Davison, Dean of the Davis School of Gerontology at USC, is a psychologist, long known for his work in clinical behavior therapy. He has become engaged in *gerontechnology*, a marriage of gerontology and technology that pays attention to the ways the physical environment of older adults can be designed to support independent living and improve quality of life (van Bronswijk et al., 2009). Marientina Gotsis (http://marientina.com) is an artist, designer, and technologist interested in interactive media and health applications who collaborates with the author on unique partnerships (nursing, cinema, dance, social work, engineering, medicine) to explore the interface among games, physical interfaces, and family-centered, intergenerational healthcare interventions (Gotsis, 2009). These exemplars of transdisciplinarity promote building new disruptive frameworks for solving the wicked problems attendant on living well with chronic illness and aging productively.

Pan-Industrial Exemplar: Promoting Interoperability and Credibility

The nonprofit, open-industry Continua Alliance is very notable in building a cluster of over 200 services and businesses that collaborate to promote interoperability (devices and programs connecting across designers and manufacturers). The alliance gives a stamp of approval to certify devices and services that meet standards set across international boundaries (see http://continuaalliance.org). Having a collective set of standards may do much to advance global priorities for sharing devices and programs across geographic and commercial boundaries. Data is needed to determine whether consumers or health professionals use this approval in making recommendations and selecting telehealth devices. At present, the Continua Alliance is not routinely featured in academic journals, news articles, or websites discussing telehealth. A similar invisibility is noted for Health on the Net—a worldwide plan for establishing credibility of health information.

Industry–Academic Exemplar: Wireless Monitoring of Sensors

CAST, the Center for Aging Services Technology, was developed in 2003 as an international collaborative base. The website notes "CAST is now an international coalition of more than 400 technology companies, aging-services organizations, businesses, research universities and government representatives working together under the auspices of the American Association of Homes and Services for the Aging (www.aahsa.org)" (CAST, 2004, para. 3).

Faculty at Dartmouth College have pulled together a collaboration with Google, Intel Labs, and the Veterans Affairs Medical Center in White River Junction, Vermont. The National Science Foundation provided $3 million to support the "next generation of wireless health monitoring tools" (RWJF, 2009, para. 1). Devices will facilitate health monitoring using mobile phones and wearable wireless medical sensors. It is not clear how the new collaboration between Intel and GE for Health Guide will interface with this effort. Developments in the United States are described by Weintraub (2009) in the context of a predicted $20 billion marked by 2020. Pilot testing is underway, she reports, with Aetna and other insurance companies. A suite of products is being designed to address older adults' preference for "aging in place" and to avoid the $2000 a month projected costs for institutionalizing dependent older adults. One related project is being carried out in conjunction with the government of Hungary. And a $30 million research center is planned with the Irish Development Agency (see press release available at http://www.intel.com/pressroom/archive/releases/20090402corp.htm). There is some evidence that Europe may be moving more quickly in the development of telehealth resources. A subscription to *eHealth News: The First European eHealth Portal* is useful in maintaining an overview (available at http://www.ehealthnews.eu).

Academic–Media Exemplar: Ranking Performance on Continuum of Care

An interactive hospital-ranking resource collaboration between *Dartmouth Atlas Project* and *Consumer Reports* is unusual in its conceptual framework. The new Web tool, available at www.ConsumerReportsHealth.org, ranks hospitals on how aggressively they treat chronic illnesses. The underlying philosophy is that consumers need help to navigate the healthcare system. The goal is to create greater transparency with respect to out-of-pocket costs and intensity of care activities for nine chronic conditions. The website www.ConsumerReportsHealth.org displays ranks for an agency in terms of its approach to care: *aggressive* or *conservative.* Aggressive care means frequent diagnostic tests and doctor visits, more reliance on specialists instead of primary care doctors, prolonged hospital stays, more days in the intensive care unit, and higher out-of-pocket expenditures. Conservative care represents the flip side of aggressive care—fewer tests, fewer hospital and ICU days, fewer doctor visits, and a lower out-of-pocket expenditure (Consumer Reports Health, 2008)

A resource like this would be even more valuable if it could be linked to at-home healthcare services. Consumers increasingly want to make their own choices about the style of care they prefer. In the current model of reimbursement, consumers are finding they are paying more out-of-pocket costs regardless of insurance plan. As these costs escalate, consumers want more information to make wise choices. The combined charisma or credibility of major universities and established advocates are very influential when choices are weighed.

Unfortunately, the *Consumer Reports* Web rankings are difficult to locate, and at this date they are not available for free. Individuals must subscribe. As with any online subscription, consumers must be vigilant to ensure that they are not charged automatically when the resource is no longer useful. Consumers are advised to ask if they can refuse the automatic renewal.

Other academic–media partnerships are likely to emerge as participatory health and telehealth applications become more effective. The CDC social media tool kit will be an excellent resource for maximizing information sharing between academic experts and consumers (http://www.cdc.gov/socialmedia; see also the SlideShare link on using social media).

DELICIOUS DEVICES AND SOFTWARE ON THE HORIZON

There is a strong happiness factor in learning the field of telehealth. Almost every online connection brings a ping or notice of some new development that seems more exciting than what is already available. Capturing these to present the most up-to-date perspective is the dark side. Throughout the book, tables of resources have been provided so that readers can stay current.

Devices in Play and on the Horizon

Readers who are device oriented are encouraged to seek out the two sources for Table 7.5 to see the illustrations and read the engaging text for themselves. The key message to take away is that there are new developments to explore and bring to the attention of professional and consumer networks. Clearly, it is becoming easier to share information in real time. Cameras on computers and on cell phones make diagnosing and monitoring the progress of conditions with visible signs more thorough and timely. There are multiple sides to each advance. For example, the prospect of dispensing grandmother's medications from your computer might be a nightmare for a family with small children. However, homebound adults may find it freeing as they no longer have to depend on others to get routine medications. One can conserve social capital for unexpected errands. A socioecological analysis of the context in which an innovation is introduced can minimize unanticipated negative consequences.

Table 7.5   Devices for Telehealth Applications

Devices in Use

Skype provides free computer-to-computer calls, chat, and videoconferencing. Medical professionals can use Skype for consultations and interactions between colleagues.

http://www.skype.com

Skype Attendant is a new test program that may provide doctors with a tool for patients with emergencies who are in remote areas. Services may include tools such as online medical support and access to medical records.

http://skypejournal.com/blog/archives/2006/03/skype_attendant.php

Webcam MD employs a handheld USB camera with a light, which patients would use to transmit images of their ailments to their doctors via the Internet.

http://www.webcammd.com

Robots can be controlled by doctors locally or remotely. Some strides have been made toward robots that could be used in the home, such as the Personal Robotic Assistants for the Elderly (PEARL) from Carnegie Mellon, although this project has been discontinued.

http://www.intuitivesurgical.com/products/davinci_surgicalsystem/index.aspx
http://www.ri.cmu.edu/research_project_detail.html?project_id=347&menu_id=261

eTime's Home Endoscope would involve patients using an endoscope with an attached USB and sending the scans to doctors without geographical constraints.

http://www.e-h-e.cn/en/index.asp

Vidyo is similar to Skype, but provides features such as HD video and multiple video window displays. It may be a good option for medical professionals who engage in a lot of videoconferencing.

http://www.vidyo.com

Radvision has developed a system for use on office or laptop computers that allows you to link different video sources together so that you can have a conference with several different people simultaneously.

http://www.radvision.com/Products/Video-Products/Desktop-Video-Communications/SCOPIA-Desktop-Video-Conferencing/default.htm

Telemedicine via cell phone would be an application in which patients use cell phone cameras to send pictures to doctors about medical conditions. This would be particularly useful in the areas where populations have greater access to cell phones than the Internet.

(continues)

Table 7.5   Devices for Telehealth Applications (*continued*)

http://portal.acs.org/portal/acs/corg/content?_nfpb=true&_pageLabel=PP_
ARTICLEMAIN&node_id=222&content_id=WPCP_008900&use_sec=true&sec_
url_var=region1&__uuid=12dcad3b-fa63-40f2-aac2-daa00faa5123

Telepresence for heart monitoring includes advances such as a Bluetooth that can monitor your heart and sends a text message to a local hospital if you are about to have a heart attack.

http://www.news-medical.net/news/2007/07/18/27774.aspx

Devices on the Horizon

Dietary intake on a mobile phone is an assessment tool that could measure a meal's nutritional content and give users more knowledge about what they are eating. The Food Intake Visualization and Voice Recognizer (FIVR) uses a combination of photographs and speech recognition to identify food and provide an estimate of the calories an individual will be consuming.

MediDome is a syringe-free medication applicator designed to eliminate needlestick injuries and speed up patient treatment. A MediDome unit, made of flexible plastic, is filled with a measured drug dose that is administered by pressing the device onto the skin until a small amount of resistance is felt. MediDome uses minimal packaging and a universal color-coding system to reduce production costs and prevent medication errors.

CellScope is an attachment that turns a mobile phone into a microscope. It can capture individual white and red blood cells, such that malaria or sickle-cell anemia could be identified, as well as infected skin, cancerous cells, or ulcerous lesions. This would allow people in developing countries and others to take blood samples, then transmit the images to a medical expert who can diagnose the problem remotely.

Drugstore in a box are units similar to computer printers that dispense different medications from cartridges, based on a prescription transmitted from your doctor's computer. The drug "tablets" would be printed on sheets resembling mailing labels that dissolve in a patient's mouth.

A cell phone-based breath analyzer would be a phone that contains breath analysis technology like breathalyzers and could detect a person's blood alcohol level. Other advancements could include breath analysis for diseases, chemical imbalances, or other problems, and the findings could be transmitted to a hospital or clinic for possible treatment.

The handheld psychiatrist would be a cell phone that could analyze rapid changes in a person's neurological state, with the ability to diagnose disorders such as Parkinson's or a lithium tremor through the phone's camera, microphone,

Table 7.5   Devices for Telehealth Applications (*continued*)

and custom software. Its purpose would be to help busy emergency room physicians assess patients before ordering a psych consult. The device could also include telemedicine-based counseling sessions.

Sources: Naditz, 2008; Winter, 2009.

Social Awareness: Devices and Interactive Options

Since 2004, the folks at Intel have intrigued us with potentially dramatic resources for social capital. In the chapter by Dishman, Matthews, and Dunbar-Jacob (2004) exciting developments like the presence lamp were mentioned. Searches found elusive website offers that were broken links. In 2009, an Intel team of social scientists tackled ubiquitous computing devices and software that would promote social engagement (Morris, Lundell, Dishongh, & Needham, 2009). They moved from their conviction that social capital was essential for successful aging—especially for preventing the onset and progression of dementia. They speculated that the mechanism was built around "emotional and instrumental support, the continuation of meaningful life activities, and the feeling of having a positive impact on others" (Morris et al., p. 336). There were four core propositions in their research:

- Many older adults have challenges in sustaining social engagement.
- Caregivers and older adults are stressed by cognitive overload and declines.
- Cognitive changes distort social identity (rooted in ability to influence and help others).
- Hopelessness about inability to change social circumstances impairs mental and physical health.

The Intel team set about to build tools for social self-efficacy that would create a perception that isolation was temporary and that declines could be managed with support from technology. In addition to the personal benefits, this attitude and new instrumental support could be a great relief to caregivers. Intel created a system that involves journaling, a social presence lamp, and data-driven displays of social networks and related interactions. Context cues were added to telephones based on journals so that conversation was not inhibited by memory issues. The social network display used a solar system model to portray potential contacts and actual engagement. This display could be shown in the constellation mode, as a line graph for overall contact, and a bar graph (see Figure 7.2). Friends and family were invited to see their position and activity.

Older adults are often concerned about being a burden and interrupting their friends and family. Caregivers at a distance wanted a simple reassurance that things were normal. The presence lamp developed at Interval provided cues for location awareness (Hindus et al., 2001, as cited in Morris et al., 2009). The older adult and the designated family member each had access to a switch that activated a light in the other's home. This application could provide great comfort to families as children head to independent living. Parents want to know a child has returned home safely after a late-night study date but don't want to be intrusive. The lamp says "I'm home, Mom—no need to keep calling!"

Another social support device addresses reluctance to make or receive phone calls for older adults with memory issues. The phone was adapted to display a photo and some notes from journals that were kept immediately after a previous call. This provided simple cues that were highly effective.

The Intel ethnographic studies revealed numerous positive outcomes:

- Display preferences varied by individual user.
- Variability in social activity data was welcomed as cue for interventions.
- Displays conveyed a need to shift contact habits.
- Social displays provoked conversation and gave permission to discuss sensitive issues.
- Online journals intended to validate sensor data became therapeutic outlets.
- Technology mastery was superior to researcher expectations.
- Caregivers recognized activity patterns and modulated to giving more or less care.

Figure 7.2   Mobile Applications for Remote Caregiving and Self-reflection

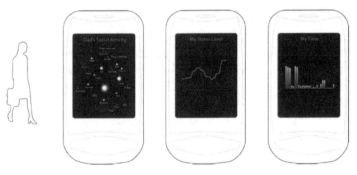

Source: Morris et al., 2009. Used with permission from Springer Science and Business Media.

- Presence lamps prompted feelings of connectedness without initiating phone calls.
- Active caregivers felt validated, and displays sparked sibling sharing.
- Caregiver reflection for some resulted from data showing neglect of self and overengagement in parent's lives (Morris et al., 2009, pp. 344–346).

Alternatives to Health-Specific Social Support and Massive Social Networking Sites

Caregiver support groups exist and are easily found by browsing. No support groups were found for those engaged in managing telehealth options in the caregiver role. Such groups will surely emerge over time. However, new models of social connection that operate differently from the frantic information posting of Facebook may be rich resources for socially isolated individuals whether caregivers or patients. The Comfort Café is such an alternative (available at http://www.comfortqueen.com/comfortcafe/about-the-cafe). It is moderated by a certified life coach, Jennifer Louden, and provides forums for inspiration, models for avoiding a sense of helplessness, and promotes a spirit of community. Retreats and other resources are offered for face-to-face encounters. Downloads of presentations for iPod and other resources built around art and literature enrich the experience (Figure 7.3 and Figure 7.4). Clearly this site is designed to meet the needs of women. Men are caregivers as well and their needs and preferences for online resources for social support are equally critical to sustaining their health and participation.

Devices for Cognitive Awareness and Adherence: Robots

This book has not dealt with robots as that is a very special technology with its own set of issues. However, two robots are worth mentioning as part of the larger literacy context. One is a therapeutic robot seal named Paro developed by Shibata at the National Institute of Advanced Industrial Science and Technology. In a small sample of older adults with cognition disorders, interaction with this animated creature was found to improve brain function based on real-time brain wave readings (National Institute of Advanced Industrial Science and Technology, 2005). There is little information available, although the AIST site indicated studies were done outside Japan. In 2009, this delightful robot was reintroduced on IEEE Spectrum (Guizzo, 2009). The press release noted that "artificial intelligence software changes the robot's behavior based on a host of sensors that monitor sound, light, temperature, and touch. Paro learns to respond to words its owner users frequently. And if it's not getting much petting time, it will cry" (Guizzo, p. 1). Shibata had hoped to diminish the need for institutionalizing older adults with cognitive declines. Given the promising results, the Danish Technological

Figure 7.3   Comfort Café

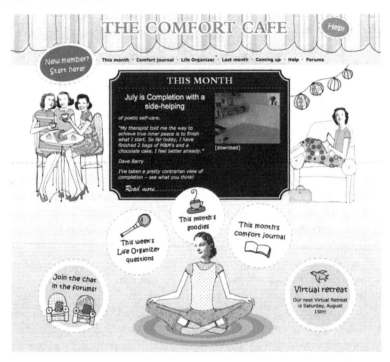

Source: Louden, 2009. Used with permission.

Institute's Centre for Robot Technology was reported to be launching long-term studies of outcomes in care of older adults. The Paro robot was announced as available in the United States in 2009, for about $5000. Other robots designed to improve medication adherence using face recognition are under development (Takacs & Hanak, 2008). Other toy or pet robots have been introduced that provide reminders. To keep the MIT AgeLab device "alive" users must report to the device—in a tamagotchi format. They were featured on the blog Align Map where the commenter raised concerns about emotional blackmail (Align Map Blog, 2007). Given the dearth of research to date, it is not clear what role these devices will play in the complex area of adherence.

Adherence as Telehealth Issue

Adherence is of concern in telehealth at two levels: adherence to recommended treatment regimens and adherence to partipating in the telehealth link. Experts

Figure 7.4 Comfort Café Forums

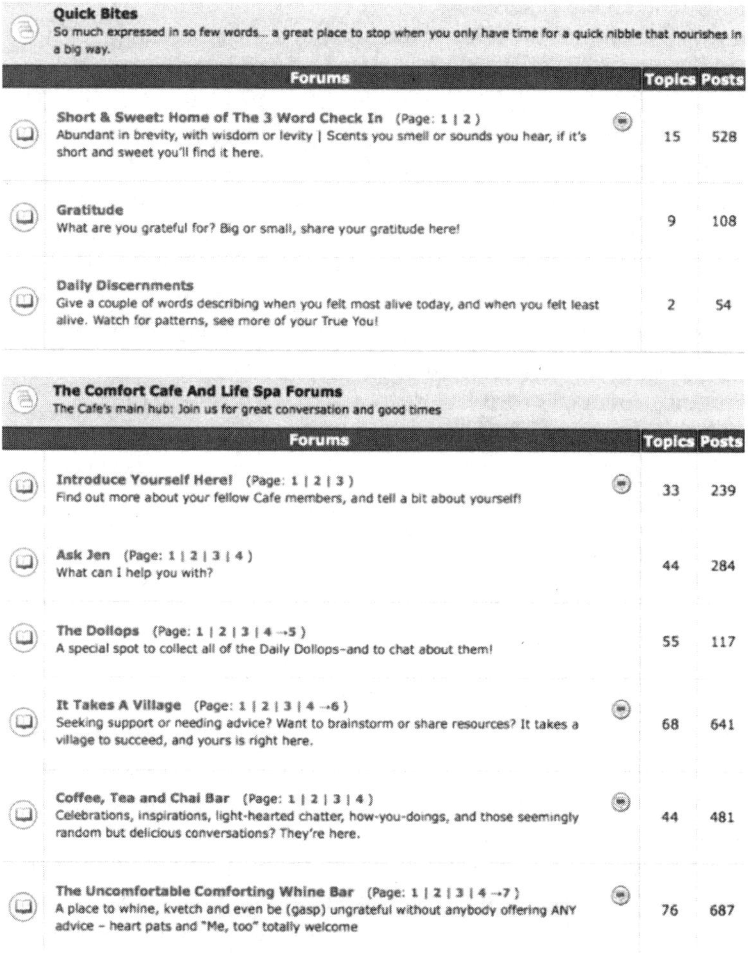

Quick Bites
So much expressed in so few words... a great place to stop when you only have time for a quick nibble that nourishes in a big way.

Forums	Topics	Posts
Short & Sweet: Home of The 3 Word Check In (Page: 1 | 2) Abundant in brevity, with wisdom or levity | Scents you smell or sounds you hear, if it's short and sweet you'll find it here.	15	528
Gratitude What are you grateful for? Big or small, share your gratitude here!	9	108
Daily Discernments Give a couple of words describing when you felt most alive today, and when you felt least alive. Watch for patterns, see more of your True You!	2	54

The Comfort Cafe And Life Spa Forums
The Cafe's main hub: Join us for great conversation and good times

Forums	Topics	Posts
Introduce Yourself Here! (Page: 1 | 2 | 3) Find out more about your fellow Cafe members, and tell a bit about yourself!	33	239
Ask Jen (Page: 1 | 2 | 3 | 4) What can I help you with?	44	284
The Dollops (Page: 1 | 2 | 3 | 4 →5) A special spot to collect all of the Daily Dollops–and to chat about them!	55	117
It Takes A Village (Page: 1 | 2 | 3 | 4 →6) Seeking support or needing advice? Want to brainstorm or share resources? It takes a village to succeed, and yours is right here.	68	641
Coffee, Tea and Chai Bar (Page: 1 | 2 | 3 | 4) Celebrations, inspirations, light-hearted chatter, how-you-doings, and those seemingly random but delicious conversations? They're here.	44	481
The Uncomfortable Comforting Whine Bar (Page: 1 | 2 | 3 | 4 →7) A place to whine, kvetch and even be (gasp) ungrateful without anybody offering ANY advice – heart pats and "Me, too" totally welcome	76	687

Source: Louden, 2009. Used with permission.

like Dunbar-Jacob, Gemmel, and Schlenk (2008) have found only modest effects for any single predictor of adherence to health recommendations. Self-efficacy, intentions, prior adherence and health literacy seem most promising. The advantage of participatory health linked to digital technology is the expectation that the consumer will be engaged in determining how to plan for adherence and the technology will facilitate collection of multifactorial data. The findings may be relevant to consumers who are not linked to telehealth programs as well.

THE FUTURE IS MOBILE AND CONNECTED: MHEALTH

The next steps are to make all these resources mobile and build in feedback so that the older adult, the adult child at a distance, and caregiver members of the network can develop awareness of their social interaction patterns. Mobility will allow contextually appropriate feedback as demonstrated in Figure 7.2. mHealth is considered a "revolution" by some (mHealth Initiative, 2009). Sarasohn-Kahn (2009) in her monograph on participatory health notes that health care management requires connectivity that is "continuous, tailored, and actionable" (p. 9). Mobile applications, or mHealth, she notes meet these criteria. Sarasohn-Kahn quotes experts who note that mobile devices level disparities as they are so widely available across the globe. The mHealth Initiative points out that mobile devices are characterized by interoperability and allow new 24/7 communication and observations of daily living recorded in real time. This nonprofit organization provides a resource site at http:www.mobih.org. On the site are multiple resources. A unique resource is labeled "The Observatory." On this page, mHealth players are invited to share their experiences with 12 different applications of mHealth.

Across the globe, in a report for the United Nations, it is projected that by 2012, "half of all individuals in remote areas of the world will have mobile phones" even where health infrastructure and technology are scarce (Vital Wave Consulting, 2009, p. 7). Mobile devices that deliver real-time health information and diagnoses are expected to improve health delivery on a "massive scale" (p. 7). Fox (2009, as cited in Sarasohn-Kahn, 2009, p. 9), noted that mobile health is a "game changer"—but only if people are willing to get engaged. Dr. Mechael is quoted (Vital Wave Consulting, p. 8) as calling for an ecosystems approach. This perspective is critical to bring new players into the mHealth game. All of the potential stakeholder groups must be consulted about this potentially disruptive innovation. Off-hours communication and sharing of personal information across a telephone network are a few of the challenges facing mHealth advocates. All of the risks and barriers of other aspects of telehealth apply. Insensitive, aggressive promotion may doom the implementation of mHealth whether in industrialized or remote populations. The Vital Wave Consulting report covers an array of applications that can be provided through mHealth: education and awareness, remote data collection, remote monitoring, communication and training for healthcare workers, disease and epidemic outbreak tracking, and diagnostic/treatment support. Forging strong partnerships is listed as one of the most crucial building blocks. A value chain model is proposed that highlights incentives for stakeholders and provides recommendations for working with each group. A compendium of 51 successful mHealth projects is provided.

Literacy as mHealth and Telehealth Constraint: Delicious Solutions

One of the biggest stumbling blocks identified is literacy. This is an issue around the globe. The mHealth report (Vital Wave Consulting, 2009) describes beta version speech recognition software from Microsoft. Also, Intel is launching Intel Reader in the UK to convert printed text to speech using a point-and-shoot, high-resolution camera. Perhaps the most exciting advance is a project underway at the University of Southern California that will translate spoken words into other languages for health applications (The doctor will understand you now, 2009). So, although the United Nations Vital Wave Consulting report is targeted to opportunities for health in the developing world, much of the content is relevant to mHealth anywhere.

DELICIOUS EVOLUTION OF THE WEB

What could be more delicious than a Web evolution that creates a personal assistant? Metz (2007) suggests that the next experience for Web users will be either reconfigured Web pages or built-in agents that make connections across pages. Four iterations are on the horizon. These include the semantic Web, 3D Web, media-centric Web, and the pervasive Web. Metz summarizes that the semantic Web first described by Berners-Lee actually reads sites and can check your calendar with calendars of doctors and dentists in a designated zip code—making appointment making easy. The 3-D Web will let you "walk through" the offices of those doctors to see if the style and equipment meet your expectations. Users could "walk" through Second Life, for example. The media-centric Web, Metz predicts, would let users present a photo of a painting and examples in the same school of art would be retrieved. The final prospect Metz projects is the pervasive Web, built into PC, cell phone, Windows, clothing, and jewelry—all around. Sensors would respond to changes in weather, schedule, even mood, then signal systems to take action on the user's behalf.

As Table 7.6 shows, consumer experience of the Web has metamorphosized from essentially a passive library under the control of experts to a decentralized conversation where users contribute original and borrowed content to the potential of a personal assistant (Strickland, n.d.). The priority setting has shifted from those of the technology developers to shifting with community standards to a very idiosyncratic personalized model. Strickland summarizes that filtering moves from upstream in Web 1.0 to an ongoing "midstream" or "pan stream" where multiple connections are being made to create a net of connections. The information is narrowly tailored to the user. The learning becomes exclusive in a new context—idiosyncratic to the user. Mash-ups that merge content from multiple sites with user-generated content are easily accomplished to create an "original" work. Credibility is simply user determined and tagged (see *folksonomy* in Chapter 2). One's tags become history and shape future searches. Strickland points out that the search will be shaped by the past and the preferences of the consumer. Each user with the same search parameters will thus have different results. Simply, the vision of Web 3.0 shapes up as an alternate and parallel universe unique to the individual.

Table 7.6   Comparison of Principles of Generations of the Web

Principle	Web 3.0	Web 2.0	Web 1.0 (Traditional)
Power	User-centric, interdependence	Decentralized (autonomy; information self-sufficiency)	Centralized (experts), dependence
Priorities	Guided by connecting information to user tastes and history	Guided by community perspectives/norms, bottom-up	Guided by technology developers
Filtering	Midstream, ongoing semantic	Downstream (e.g., user ranking)	Upstream
Consumption	Personal	Coproducers	Passive receivers— consumption
Learning	Idiosyncratic to user, mash-ups, and widgets	Collective— capacity building	Exclusive
Content	Based on consumer tags, experiential connections	Based on understandable language, experiential knowledge	Based on science
Culture	Personal assistant, interpretation	Enabling	Compliance

Sources: Metz, 2007; Kukafka, 2008, as cited in Institute of Medicine, 2009. Used with permission of the National Academies Press.

Smart Home Evolving to Wise Home

These new capacities of digital technology may be the key to previously unanticipated innovations. For example, the smart home may become a *wise home* (Charlie Hillman Speaks, 2009). At the 2009 UCLA Conference on Technology and Aging, Hillman speculated that the accumulation of wisdom with aging is probably a cultural universal. To propel the implementation of telehealth, he proposed that we advance from *smart* technology to *wise* technology. Examples he gave are that "a smart home detects a fall and summons help. A wise home embraces universal design and turns on a light to prevent that fall... . A smart home detects wandering patterns associated with dementia. A wise home encourages hydration, provides mental stimulation, and social connectivity to delay the onset of dementia" (Charlie Hillman Speaks, 2009, para. 4–6). The transcript of his speech provides the details of his prescription for social engineering. He calls for new standards of personal responsibility on the part of older adults and their social supporters. Hillman lays out five features of a wise house wellness system: physiological sensing, activity monitoring, social connectivity, cognitive assists, and home control for safety (Charlie Hillman Speaks, 2009).

DELICIOUSLY DISRUPTIVE INNOVATIONS ON THE PERSONNEL SIDE: CAREGIVERS AND PROFESSIONALS

Informal Caregivers or Care Sharers: Multitaskers Extraordinaire

Throughout the book, caregivers have been briefly mentioned. They are a critical component of aging in place and important partners in telehealth for well or chronically ill family members. These individuals have roles that cross staggering boundaries (Table 7.7).

The Institute of Medicine report *Retooling for an Aging America* estimates that as many as 31% of all Americans are unpaid caregivers (Institute of Medicine, 2008). These caregivers have been predominantly spouses or middle-aged daughters. In the UK, a commonly used expression is care sharers. Increasingly in the United States few caregivers receive help from others in their social network. Care is shared by paid workers and the health provider network. The Institute notes an alarming drop in the availability of informal, unpaid caregivers. Telehealth applications have great potential for relieving burdens of vigilance for caregivers, supplying social support that complements their engagement, and creating interdependence that allows respite and even pleasure in the caretaking. Attention to the experiences of caregivers is critical in the face of increases in chronic illness across age groups that require intense management outside institutional settings. A feedback loop has been identified as a critical aspect of self-care management (Sarasohn-Kahn, 2009). Feedback is equally central to sustaining caregiving engagement. Locating resources for engaging in telehealth as a caregiver (or patient) are difficult to locate. An iconographic symbol on websites, print matter, and devices might simplify browsing and targeted searching for consumers and providers. The icon features would include cues that digital links are a component, that data is shared, and that interaction is available. See Figure 7.5 as a potential example. As mHealth evolves, a mobile image will be more evocative for some groups. In the interim, any digitally connected consumer will recognize the significance.

Table 7.7   Health-Related Responsibilities Assumed by Informal Caregivers

Role	Function	Examples
Companion	Provide emotional support	Discuss ongoing life challenges, troubleshoot problems, facilitate and participate in leisure activities
Coach	Encourage patient self-care activities	Prompt patient's engagement in health care, encourage lifestyle (diet, exercise) and treatment adherence
Homemaker	Manage household activities	Inventory, purchase food and medications, prepare meals
Scheduler	Arrange medical care	Schedule tests, procedures, and services
Driver	Facilitate transportation	Provide transportation to medical appointments and emergency hospital visits
Patient extender	Facilitate provider understanding	Attend appointments; clarify and expand on patient history, symptoms, concerns; introduce topics to provider
Technical interpreter	Facilitate patient understanding	Clarify providers' explanations, technical terms, record and remember discussions with providers

Table 7.7 Health-Related Responsibilities Assumed by Informal Caregivers (*continued*)

Role	Function	Examples
Decision maker	Make medical decisions	Select among treatment alternatives; decide among settings of care
Coordinator	Coordinate care across providers and settings	Ensure flow of information among providers
Financial manager	Handle financial issues	Resolve issues relating to insurance claims, secondary coverage, copays, and benefit limits
Health provider	Deliver medical care	Administer medications, operate equipment
Attendant	Provide task assistance	Hands-on personal care task assistance
Monitor	Assess health status	Ensure that changes in health status are noted and properly addressed

Source: Wolff, 2007, as cited in Institute of Medicine, 2008. Used with permission of the National Academies Press.

Training Existing Staff and Preparing Next Generation

The World Health Organization (2005) and the Institute of Medicine (2003) both have laid out overlapping competencies that emphasize patient-centered care and the ability to use information and communication technology. Leaders in nursing and social work have endorsed the relevance of telehealth to practice and research. McCarty and Clancy (2002) see great promise for social work practice in the current openness about rules and regulations. They encourage social workers to thoughtfully enter the dialogue on telehealth.

Unfortunately, there seem to be significant gaps in professional curricula around this topic. McBride and others expressed concern that nursing faculty still do not know what to teach (Gassert, 2008; McBride & Detmer, 2008).

Figure 7.5   Proposed Icon for Telehealth Resources

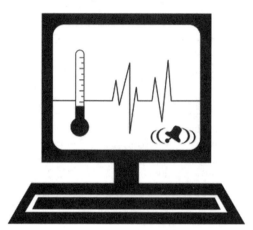

Gassert (2008) presented a detailed table of technology and informatics competencies based on previous work with Staggers et al. (2008). The list seems exclusively hospital and nurse focused. Patient empowerment competencies, telehealth monitoring, personal records, and games are not yet included.

The TIGER collaborative has over 100 organizations and 1000 independent nurse members dedicated to building excellence in informatics and telehealth. The TIGER collaborative has a summit website (www.tigersummit.com) that has wikis for each of the key components in telehealth, and provides a link to a state-of-the-practice summary report. The American Nurses Association provides a set of standards for nursing informatics, last updated in 2008 (American Nurses Association, 2008). Social work experts have begun to develop social work informatics (Parker-Oliver & Demiris, 2006). In social work, an extensive volume details educational implications of new technology initiatives for curriculum design (Vigilante, Beaulaurier, & Haffe, 2005).

If the health professions can agree on competencies for the next decade, games may be a way to rapidly advance development of students and current practitioners. A Cochrane collaboration review (Akl et al., 2008) found that a variety of games for health professionals are available. Games for teaching some surgical skills have been highly successful. However, even though health-related games for consumers are gaining acceptance and credibility, the research on games for professionals is still inconclusive. As the next generation comes to practice, well skilled in digital games, there may be more incentive to develop rigorously researched games to inculcate telehealth competencies.

Delicious Educational Resources

An amazing free resource is invaluable—each year—for designers of curriculum and instruction. The Horizon project is a collaboration on behalf of learning organizations that assembles an annual report. The group selects six emerging technologies or practices that will be major influences on curriculum and instruction in learning-focused organizations within the next 5 years. The report highlights both tools and trends. Although health technology is not a specific focus, the topics are relevant or might be with the right perspective. Topics for 2009 include mobiles, cloud computing, geo-everything, the personal Web, semantic-aware applications, and smart objects. Each is profiled in some detail with examples and URLs with a discussion of the projected relevance to teaching, learning, research, and creative expression. The report is available at http://wp.nmc.org/horizon2009.

Netiquette for Professionals and Consumers

New rules of engagement are not yet out in an etiquette book. The crescendo of voices would lead the naïve to believe that healthcare providers are eager to have informed patients. However, some consumers are experiencing resistance. In Chapter 1, reports show some physicians are handpicking patients who can use e-mail.

Consumers need to be thoughtful as they come to the provider encounter. Bringing stacks of printouts, even thoughtfully put in a tabbed notebook is not an auspicious start to a visit. For most practitioners, there is still a transition where respectful inquiry is expected. Most of the literature on health information seeking stated that even digitally dexterous consumers want their provider to be the core source of information and wisdom.

There is a whole new level of polite discourse. For example, what will agency policy be when patients want to be a friend on Facebook? Crawford (2009) lays out the multiple issues related to stress-relieving humor that turns up on YouTube and embarrasses patients, students, and agencies. Personal information on social networking sites available to all may give poor impressions of providers. Allowing views of group memberships may create dilemmas. Professionals and consumers alike are learning how easy it is to identify patients and providers when blogs appear. Posting stories of clinical encounters—from either perspective—is highly risky as true masking is difficult. Crawford suggests if photos or a teaching video are to be used, getting patient consent may be easier than expected and save a great deal of grief.

Engagement of New Patient-Centered Teams in Flow of Data, Information, Knowledge, and Wisdom

In the new paradigm, one can envision a cascade of inputs from persons and environments that both flows and requires energy and resources to be pumped through the system. In the premillennial healthcare system, many handmaidens and submissive participants were required to carry out the dictates of a network of policies and power brokers. The apparent expectation was to have individuals, employers, insurance companies, and governments dump seemingly unlimited resources (money, technological toys) into a river of wicked problems. As this flowed downstream, resources could be siphoned out as profits, salaries, money for offices, parking spaces, and fitful episodic care.

In the age of the empowered consumer of eHealth, a community-based, consumer-centric fountain provides a refreshing image. Figure 7.6 shows how the empowerment cycle works for consumer/patients and consumer/professionals. Empowerment means we can envision a new system no longer run exclusively by the wealthy and by powerful experts but by a transparent renewable resource where everyone can potentially contribute to keep the system flowing.

Figure 7.6   The Socioecology of Health Technology: The Empowerment Cycle

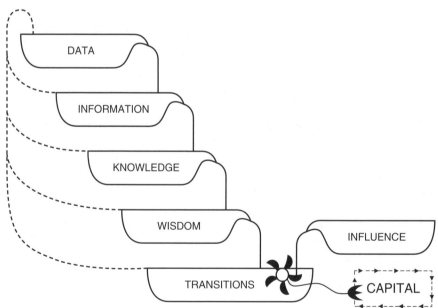

Illustration: Jin DePaul.

REPRISE OF SOCIOECOLOGICAL ANALYSIS IMPERATIVES

These themes support the system impact of small changes. Telehealth cheerleaders need to take equally seriously the wicked problem dilemma in a socioecological model. Everything and everyone is connected. A change at one point may have unintended consequences elsewhere. The changes may be serendipitous or catastrophic and that value may vary by the stakeholder caught in the consequences. As the Internet continues to support diversity, every introduction of a new feature can benefit from a cultural analysis with special attention to the ethical implications.

SUMMARY

In this book, major paradigm shifts have been presented in terms of telehealth in a digital age. The dominant change is in expectations and behaviors of consumers in their role as a well person, newly diagnosed, or coping with chronic illness. Consumers are increasingly empowered and obligated to engage in a lifestyle where they make decisions about their lifestyle, medical interactions, and the care of loved ones. The acceptance of this *participatory health* paradigm varies by consumer and provider. Although more and more Americans and citizens of the globe are going online, there will always be holdouts and people simply unable to connect.

Change and research happened much more slowly in the decades before the Internet (Doarn et al., 2008). Innovations like Facebook and Twitter appear and seemingly overnight are adopted and adapted across the globe. Many people choose not to use them, but increasingly the young to the near-old are confronted at the least with having to decide to use or hold out. This pace makes it extremely important to promote dialogue among diverse groups and to avoid rushing to embrace the latest technology without scoping out the socioecological repercussions. On the other hand, across the globe there is less tolerance for individuals and groups who persistently present barriers without alternate ways to optimize health and health care.

Acceptance of diversity as a human good is a value that can be respected more meaningfully with digital technology. To sustain this capacity, it is important that globally we take as universal values open architecture, interoperability, and neutrality of the Internet. Open architecture means that as new software and devices are envisioned, they can be produced without major outlays for patents, copyrights, and development agreements.[2]

[2]Engaging individuals with disabilities in commercial games is often prohibitive as quarter million dollar development kits are commonly required. Painstakingly adapted game devices lack interoperability with new devices, and there is currently no incentive for companies to cooperate in updates.

Network neutrality principles were released based on off-the-record discussions facilitated by the Annenberg Center for Communication (Aronson & Wilkie, 2006). They are summarized here. Informal agreements included investments where customers and operators win, and there is an option of unrestricted access to services and content on the global public Internet. Regulations should be formulated with a "light touch." Basic access broadband should be available to all. Transparency on conditions of service and use of personal information should become a hallmark of Internet services. Network operators should not give preferential treatment to their content or that of affiliates nor obstruct or divert network traffic flow. Universal agreement on these principles of neutrality would greatly advance global collaboration.

Innovation should be encouraged as context for solving the wicked problems of contemporary health care—in particular the mess of equity and access. National-level engagements such as health reform and the space program, and conflicts such as the wars in Iraq and Afghanistan should be overtly mined for civilian consumer services and new ways of organizing life. Serendipity and boundary blurring are values to be encouraged in multiple stakeholder dialogues. Promoting core values will enhance ethical and enjoyable telehealth:

- Everything and everyone is connected.
- Think globally, act locally.
- Cultivate engaged tolerance of multiple points of view.
- Balance high tech and high touch for a satisfying quality of life.
- Encourage innovation and minimize barriers.
- Cheer on mash-ups of user mixes of old and new content for unique results.
- Embrace empowerment as a flow of data to wisdom energized by charisma and capital across a range of stakeholders.

Telehealth is an extraordinarily disruptive innovation with potential to change daily life, established institutions, financial structures, and policies at every level of social life, government, and industry. A book cannot adequately catalogue the transitions, devices, software, or related changes. Each foray onto the Internet brings fresh data, information, and knowledge. Transforming these developments at key transitions into wise actions will require creative combinations of influence and capital. Transdisciplinary collaboration that empowers consumers in a socioecological framework will be a powerful lever for accomplishing healthy lifestyles in an uncertain but potentially delicious future.

REFERENCES

Ackoff, R. L. (1981). The art and science of mess management. *Interfaces*, *11*(1), 20–26. doi:10.1287/inte.11.1.20.

Adams, J., Grundy, P., Kohn, M. S., & Mounib, E. L. (2009). *Patient centered medical home: What, why and how?* Somers, NY: IBM Global Business Services. Retrieved July 9, 2010, from ftp://ftp.software.ibm.com/common/ssi/pm/xb/n/gbe03219usen/GBE03219USEN.PDF

Akl, E. A., Sackett, K., Erdley, S., Bhoopathi, P. S., Mustafa, R., & Schunemann, H. J. (2008). Educational games for health professionals [Review]. *Cochrane Database of Systematic Reviews, 1.* doi:10.1002/14651858.CD006411.pub2.

Align Map Blog. (2007, July 5). Cute, cuddly robots remind elderly to take pills. http://alignmap.com/2007/07/05/cute-cuddly-robot-pets-remind-elderly-to-take-pills

American Nurses Association (ANA). (2008). *Nursing informatics: Scope and standards of practice.* Silver Spring, MD: Author.

Aronson, J., & Wilkie, S. (2006). *The Annenberg Center principles for network neutrality.* Retrieved September 12, 2009, from http://www.benton.org/node/1877

Baranowski, T., Buday, R., Thompson, D. I., & Baranowski, J. (2008). Playing for real: Video games and stories for health-related behavior change. *American Journal of Preventive Medicine, 34*(1), 74–82.

Bashshur, R. L., Shannon, G. W., Krupinski, E. A., Grigsby, J., Kvedar, J. C., Weinstein, R. S., et al. (2009). National telemedicine initiatives: Essential to healthcare reform. *Telemedicine and E-Health, 15*(6), 600–610.

Bawden, D., & Robinson, L. (2009). The dark side of information: Overload, anxiety and other paradoxes and pathologies. *Journal of Information Science, 35*(2), 180–191. Retrieved September 12, 2009, from http://proquest.umi.com/pqdweb?did=1662929741&Fmt=7&clientId=5239&RQT=309&VName=PQD

Bos, L. (2007). Medical and care compunetics: The future of patient related ICT. In L. Bos & B. Blobel (Eds.), *Medical Care and Compunetics* (pp. 3–18). Amsterdam: IOS.

Carrier, E., & Reschovsky, J. D. (2009, December). *Expectations outpace reality: Physicians' use of care management tools for patients with chronic conditions* (Issue Brief No. 129). Washington, DC: Center for Studying Health System Change. Retrieved December 21, 2009, from http://www.hschange.com/CONTENT/1101/?words=chronic+illness

Center for Aging Services Technology (CAST). (2004). *CAST overview.* Retrieved December 27, 2009, from http://www.agingtech.org/about.aspx

Center for Health Care Quality at the George Washington University, & Robert Wood Johnson Foundation. (2009, June). *Educational video and presentation for addressing racial and ethnic disparities to improve quality.* Retrieved September 12, 2009, from http://www.rwjf.org/pr/product.jsp?id=44448

Chang, C. H. (2007). Patient-reported outcomes measurement and management with innovative methodologies and technologies. *Quality of Life Research, 16*(Suppl 1), 157–166.

Charlie Hillman speaks on the "WISE HOME": A transcript of Charlie's speech from UCLA Conference on Technology and Aging—September 30, 2009. (2009, November 3). *GrandCare Systems.* Retrieved July 20, 2010, from http://grandcare.wordpress.com/2009/11/03/charlie-hillman-speaks-on-the-wise-home

Christakis, N. A., & Fowler, J. H. (2007). The spread of obesity in a large social network over 32 years. *New England Journal of Medicine, 357*(4), 370–379.

Christensen, C. M., Bohmer, R., & Kenagy, J. (2001). Will disruptive innovations cure health care? *Harvard Business Review, 78*(5), 102–112.

Coleman, K., Austin, B. T., Brach, C., & Wagner, E. H. (2009). Evidence on the chronic care model in the new millennium. *Health Affairs, 28*(1), 75–85. doi:10.1377/hlthaff.28.1.75.

Consumer Reports Health. (2008). *About Consumer Reports Health: Our health ratings.* Retrieved December 21, 2009, from http://www.consumerreports.org/health/about/our-health-ratings.htm

Crawford, L. S. (2009, August 18). Doctors, patients and social networks. *Law Technology News.* Retrieved August 20, 2009, from http://www.law.com/jsp/lawtechnologynews/PubArticleLTN.jsp?id=1202433104233

Crawley, L. M. (2005). Racial, cultural, and ethnic factors influencing end-of-life care. *Journal of Palliative Medicine, 8*(Suppl 1), S58–S69.

CTECH: California Telemedicine and eHealth Center. (2009). *CTEC California Telemedicine and eHealth Center.* Retrieved August 23, 2009, from http://www.cteconline.org

Currell, R., Urquhart, C., Wainwright, P., & Lewis, R. (2000). Telemedicine versus face to face patient care: Effects on professional practice and health care outcomes. *Cochrane Database of Systematic Reviews, 2.* doi: 10.1002/14651858.CD002098.

Darkins, A., Ryan, P., Kobb, R., Foster, L., Edmonson, E., Wakefield, B., et al. (2008). Care coordination/home telehealth: The systematic implementation of health informatics, home telehealth, and disease management to support the care of veteran patients with chronic conditions. *Telemedicine Journal & E-Health, 14*(10), 1118–1126.

Demiris, G., Parker Oliver, D., & Courtney, K. L. (2006). Ethical considerations for the utilization of telehealth technologies in home and hospice care by the nursing profession. *Nursing Administration Quarterly, 30*(1), 56–66. Retrieved September 12, 2009, from http://ovidsp.ovid.com/ovidweb.cgi?T=JS&NEWS=N&PAGE=fulltext&AN=00006216-200601000-00009&D=ovfth

Disch, J. (2009, October). Participatory health care: Perspective from a nurse leader. *Journal of Participatory Medicine, 1* (1), e4. Retrieved August 20, 2009, from http://jopm.org/index.php/jpm/article/viewArticle/27/33

Dishman, E., Matthews, J., & Dunbar-Jacob, J. (2004). Everyday health: Technology for adaptive aging. In R. W. Pew, & S. B. Van Hemel (Eds.), *Technology for adaptive aging* (pp. 179–208). Washington, DC: National Academies Press.

Doarn, C. R., Yellowlees, P., Jeffries, D. A., Lordan, D., Davis, S., Hammack, G., et al. (2008). Societal drivers in the applications of telehealth. *Telemedicine Journal & E-Health, 14*(9), 998–1002.

Duffett-Leger, L., Paterson, B., & Albert, W. (2008). Optimizing health outcomes by integrating health behavior and communication theories in the development of e-health promotion interventions. *EHealth International Journal, 4*(2), 23–33.

Dunbar-Jacob, J., Gemmel, L. A., & Schlenk, E. A. (2008) Predictors of patient adherence: Patient characteristics. In S. A. Shumaker, E. Schron, J. Ockene, & W. L. McBee (Eds.), *Handbook of health behavior change* (3rd ed.). New York: Springer.

European Network and Information Security Agency (ENISA). (2009, March). *Being diabetic in 2011: Identifying emerging and future risks in remote health monitoring and treatment.* Retrieved December 21, 2009, from http://www.enisa.europa.eu/act/rm/files/deliverables/being-diabetic-2011?searchterm=being+diabetic+in+2011

Fox, S., & Jones, S. (2009). *The social life of health information.* Washington, DC: Pew Internet and American Life Project. Retrieved December 21, 2009, from http://www.pewinternet.org/Experts/~/link.aspx?_id=62F4D7EFB49C4F9FA384FDC9D3A4B49B&_z=z

Frank, G., Blackhall, L. J., Michel, V., Murphy, S. T., Azen, S. P., & Park, K. (1998). A discourse of relationships in bioethics: Patient autonomy and end-of-life decision making among elderly Korean Americans. *Medical Anthropology Quarterly, 12*(4), 403–423.

Frank, G., Blackhall, L. J., Murphy, S. T., Michel, V., Azen, S. P., Preloran, H. M., et al. (2002). Ambiguity and hope: Disclosure preferences of less acculturated elderly Mexican Americans concerning terminal cancer—A case story. *Cambridge Quarterly of Healthcare Ethics, 11*(2), 117–126.

Gammon, D., Christiansen, E. K., & Wynn, R. (2009). Exploring morally relevant issues facing families in their decisions to monitor the health-related behaviours of loved ones. *Journal of Medical Ethics, 35*(7), 424–428. doi:10.1136/jme.2008.027920.

Gammon, D., Johannessen, L. K., Sorensen, T., Wynn, R., & Whitten, P. (2008). An overview and analysis of theories employed in telemedicine studies: A field in search of an identity. *Methods of Information in Medicine, 47*(3), 260–269.

Gardner, A. (2009, June 18). Surging Internet use cutting into family time: Rise of Facebook, Twitter coincides with 30% drop in hours spent together, report finds. *HealthDay News.* Retrieved July 20, 2010, from http://health.allrefer.com/news/20090618628218/surging-internet-use-cutting-into-family-time.html

Gassert, C. A. (2008). Technology and informatics competencies. *Nursing Clinics of North America, 43*(4), 507–521.

Gotsis, M. (2009). Games, virtual reality, and the pursuit of happiness. *IEEE Computer Graphics and Applications, 29*(5), 14–19.

Graber, M. A. (2010). Get your paws off of my pixels: Personal identity and avatars as self. *Journal of Medical Internet Research, 12*(3), e28. Retrieved July 23, 2010, from http://www.jmir.org/2010/3/e28

Greenhalgh, T., Wood, G. W., Bratan, T., Stramer, K., & Hinder, S. (2008). Patients' attitudes to the summary care record and HealthSpace: Qualitative study. *British Medical Journal, 336*(7656), 1290–1295.

Grigsby, J., & Bennett, R. E. (2006). Alternatives to randomized controlled trials in telemedicine. *Journal of Telemedicine & Telecare, 12*(Suppl 2), S77–S84.

Guizzo, E. (2009). Paro the robotic seal could diminish dementia: First long-term study seeks to prove the benefits of a cybernetic pet. Retrieved December 27, 2009, from http://spectrum.ieee.org/robotics/home-robots/paro-the-robotic-seal-could-diminish-dementia

Hawn, C. (2009). Take two aspirin and tweet me in the morning: How Twitter, Facebook, and other social media are reshaping health care. *Health Affairs, 28*(2), 361–368. doi:10.1377/hlthaff.28.2.361.

Hopp, F., Whitten, P., Subramanian, U., Woodbridge, P., Mackert, M., & Lowery, J. (2006). Perspectives from the Veterans Health Administration about opportunities and barriers in telemedicine. *Journal of Telemedicine and Telecare, 12*, 404–409.

Humphrey, T. (2002). *Harris poll #21: Cyberchondriacs update.* Retrieved September 21, 2006, from http://www.harrisinteractive.com/harris_poll/index.asp?PID=299

Institute of Medicine. (2003). *Health professions education: A bridge to quality.* Washington, DC: National Academies Press.

Institute of Medicine. (2008). *Retooling for an aging America: Building the health care workforce.* Washington DC: National Academies Press.

Institute of Medicine. (2009). *Health literacy, eHealth, and communication: Putting the consumer first.* Washington, DC: National Academies Press.

Johnston, B., & Solomon, N. A. (2008). *Telemedicine in California: Progress, challenges, and opportunities.* Oakland, CA: California HealthCare Foundation. Retrieved December 21, 2009, from http://www.chcf.org/topics/view.cfm?itemid=133682

Jordan-Marsh, M. (2008). Health habitat aspects of software as a service (SAAS/WEB2.0) reinforcing diabetic self-confidence: The PHRddBRASIL case. *DESAFIO International Symposium: Diabetes, Health Education and Guided Physical Activities,* 39–42.

Jordan-Marsh, M., & May, K. A. (2008). *Nursing intelligence, technology, and the digital age: Shall we dance? University of Southern California, Los Angeles.* Unpublished manuscript.

Jordan-Marsh, M., McLaughlin, M., Chi, I., Brown, C., Moran, M., Jung, Y., et al. (2006). *St. Barnabas cyber café evaluation report 2004–2005.* Los Angeles, CA: University of Southern California, School of Social Work, Annenberg School of Communication, Davis School of Gerontology. Unpublished manuscript.

Kellett, A. (2009). *A Kinder Space.* Retrieved December 21, 2009, from http://www.asidsandiego.org/find_a_designer.php?d=10562_Anne_Kellett

Kibbe, D., & Kvedar, J. C. (2008, December 22). The health care blog: The connected medical home: Health 2.0 says "hello" to the medical home model. Retrieved December 21, 2009, from http://www.thehealthcareblog.com/the_health_care_blog/2008/12/the-connected-m.html

Kobb, R., Chumbler, N. R., Brennan, D. M., & Rabinowitz, T. (2008). Home telehealth: Mainstreaming what we do well. *Telemedicine Journal & E-Health, 14*(9), 977–981.

Kvedar, J., Hwang J., Moorhead, T., Orlov, L., & Ubel, P. A. (2009). Roundtable discussion. Up from crisis: Overhauling health care information, payment, and delivery in extraordinary times. *Telemedicine and e-Health, 15*(7), 634–641. doi: 10.1089/tmj.2009.9948.

Kvedar, J. C. (2009). The connected health evidence base. *Healthcare IT News.* Retrieved December 21, 2009, from http://www.healthcareitnews.com/blog/connected-health-evidence-base

Layman, E. (2003). Health informatics: Ethical issues. *Health Care Manager, 22*(1), 2–15.

Leach, W. D. (2009). *If you bill it, they will come: A literature review on clinical outcomes, cost-effectiveness, and reimbursement for telemedicine.* Sacramento, CA: California Telemedicine and eHealth Center. Retrieved December 21, 2009, from http://www.cteconline.org/_pdf/Literature-Review-Design.pdf

Lewis, T. (2006). Seeking health information on the Internet: Lifestyle choice or bad attack of cyberchondria? *Media, Culture & Society, 28*(4), 521–537. Retrieved December 21, 2009, from http://mcs.sagepub.com/cgi/content/abstract/28/4/521

Louden, J. (2009). *The comfort café.* Retrieved December 31, 2009, from http://www.comfortqueen.com/comfortcafe/about-the-cafe

Lowes, R. (2009). *Physicians practice articles: Getting paid for mouse calls.* Retrieved September 14, 2009, from http://www.physicianspractice.com/index/fuseaction/articles.details/articleID/1309.htm

Machlin, S., & Woodwell, D. (2009, April). Healthcare expenses for chronic conditions among nonelderly adults: Variations by insurance coverage, 2005–06 (average annual estimates). *Statistical Brief # 243.* Rockville, MD: Agency for Healthcare Research and Quality. Retrieved December 21, 2009, from http://www.meps.ahrq.gov/mepsweb/data_files/publications/st243/stat243.pdf

Mackert, M., & Whitten, P. (2009). Long term success of a telehealth network: A case study of the upper peninsula telehealth network. *International Journal of Healthcare Technology and Management, 10*(1–2), 66–81.

Martin, S., Kelly, G., Kernohan, W. G., McCreight, B., & Nugent, C. (2008). Smart home technologies for health and social care support. *Cochrane Database of Systematic Reviews, 4.* doi: 10.1002/14651858.CD006412.pub2.

McBride, A. B., & Detmer, D. E. (2008). Using informatics to go beyond technologic thinking. *Nursing Outlook, 56*(5), 195–196.

McCarty, D., & Clancy, C. (2002). Telehealth: Implications for social work practice. *Social Work, 47*(2), 153–161.

Metz, C. (2007, March 14). Web 3.0. Message posted to http://www.pcmag.com/article2/0,2817,2102852,00.asp.

McFarland-Horne, F., & Li, R. M. (2010). Personal motion technologies for healthy independent living: Workshop summary. *National Institute on Aging.* Retrieved July 22, 2010, from http://www.nibib.nih.gov/nibib/file/NewsandEvents/PreviousSymposiaandWorkshops/22June2010/Personal_Motion_Summary_Report.pdf

mHealth Initiative. (2009). Vision. Retrieved December 27, 2009, from http://www.mobih.org

Miller, E. A. (2007). Solving the disjuncture between research and practice: Telehealth trends in the 21st century. *Health Policy, 82*(2), 133–141.

Morris, M. E., Lundell, J., Dishongh, T., & Needham, B. (2009). Fostering social engagement and self-efficacy in later life: Studies with ubiquitous computing. In P. Markopoulos, B. De Ruyter, & W. Mackay (Eds.), *Awareness systems: Advances in theory, methodology, and design* (pp. 335–349). Berlin, Germany: Springer-Verlag.

Muennig, P., Fiscella, K., Tancredi, D., & Franks, P. (2009). The relative health burden of selected social and behavioral risk factors in the United States: Implications for policy. *American Journal of Public Health.* doi:10.2105/AJPH.2009.165019.

Naditz, A. (2008). New frontiers in telemedicine: Early-phase R & D promises exciting new telemedicine tools. *Telemedicine and e-Health, 14*(8), 747–752.

National Institute of Advanced Industrial Science and Technology (AIST). (2003). *Paro found to improve brain function in patients with cognition disorders.* Retrieved August 10, 2010, from http://www.aist.go.jp/aist_e/latest_research/2006/20060213/20060213.html

Osborne, H. (2004). *Health literacy from A to Z: Practical ways to communicate your health message.* Sudbury, MA: Jones and Bartlett.

Papastergiou, M. (2009). Exploring the potential of computer and video games for health and physical education: A literature review. *Computers & Education, 53,* 603–622.

Parker-Oliver, D., & Demiris, G. (2006). Social work informatics: A new specialty. *Social Work, 51*(2), 127.

Polisena, J., Coyle, D., Coyle, C., & McGill, S. (2009). Home telehealth for chronic disease management: A systematic review and an analysis of economic evaluations. *International Journal of Technology Assessment in Health Care, 25*(3), 339–349.

Rada, R. (2005). A case study of a retracted systematic review on interactive health communication applications: Impact on media, scientists, and patients [Electronic Resource]. *Journal of Medical Internet Research, 7*(2), e18. Retrieved December 21, 2009, from http://www.jmir.org/2005/2/e18

Reid, R. J., Fishman, P. A., Yu, O., Ross, T. R., Tufano, J. T., Soman, M. P., et al. (2009). Patient-centered medical home demonstration: A prospective, quasi-experimental, before and after evaluation. *American Journal of Managed Care, 15*(9), e71–e87.

Rigby, M. (2007). Applying emergent ubiquitous technologies in health: The need to respond to new challenges of opportunity, expectation, and responsibility. *International Journal of Medical Informatics, 76*(Suppl 3), S349–S352. doi:10.1016/j.ijmedinf.2007.03.002.

Rittel, H. W. J., & Webber, M. M. (1973). Dilemmas in a general theory of planning. *Policy Sciences, 4,* 155–169.

Robert Wood Johnson Foundation (RWJF). (2009, August 15). *Dartmouth College receives grant to develop health monitoring tools.* Retrieved July 20, 2010, from http://www.rwjf.org/qualityequality/digest.jsp?id=21468

Rosen, M. (2007). The spread of obesity in a social network [Comment]. *New England Journal of Medicine, 357*(18), 1867–1868.

Russo, A., Wier, L. M., & Elixhauser, A. (2009, August). *Hospital utilization among near-elderly adults, ages 55 to 64 years, 2007* (HCUP Statistical Brief No. 79). Rockville, MD: Agency for Healthcare Research and Quality. Retrieved December 21, 2009, from http://www.hcup-us.ahrq.gov/reports/statbriefs/sb79.jsp

Saarni, S. I., Hofmann, B., Lampe, K., Lühmann, D., Mäkelä, M., Velasco-Garrido, M., et al. (2008). Ethical analysis to improve decision-making on health technologies. *Bulletin of the World Health Organization, 86*(8), 617–623.

Sarasohn-Kahn, J. (2009). *Participatory health: Online and mobile tools help chronically ill manage their care.* Oakland, CA: California HealthCare Foundation. Retrieved July 20, 2010, from http://www.chcf.org/~/media/Files/PDF/P/ParticipatoryHealthTools.pdf

Schön, D. (1987). *The reflective practitioner.* San Francisco: Jossey-Bass.

Scott, R. (2009). Augmenting transitions: A unique and effective approach to securing fluid transitions. *Case in Point. Collaborative Practice Supplement,* 15–16. Retrieved December 21, 2009, from http://viewer.zmags.com/publication/b8e2b97d#/b8e2b97d/14

Shannon, G., Nesbitt, T., Bakalar, R., Kratochwill, E., Kvedar, J., & Vargas, L. (2002). Telemedicine/telehealth: An international perspective. Organizational models of telemedicine and regional telemedicine networks. *Telemedicine Journal & E-Health, 8*(1), 61–70.

Spyglass Consulting. (2009). Trends in remote patient monitoring 2009. Abstract available at http://www.spyglass-consulting.com/Abstracts/Spyglass_RPM2009_abstract.pdf

Staggers, N., McCasky, T., Brazelton, N., & Kennedy, R. (2008). Nanotechnology: The coming revolution and its implications for consumers, clinicians, and informatics. *Nursing Outlook, 56*(5), 268–274.

Strickland, J. (n.d.). How Web 3.0 will work. *HowStuffWorks*. Retrieved September 4, 2009, from http://computer.howstuffworks.com/web-30.htm#

Tang, P. C., Black, W., & Young, C. Y. (2006). Proposed criteria for reimbursing eVisits: Content analysis of secure patient messages in a personal health record system. *AMIA Annual Symposium Proceedings, 2006*, 764–768.

Taylor, H. (2002, May 1.). The Harris Poll #21: Cyberchondriacs update. *Harris Interactive*. Retrieved August 10, 2010, from http://www.harrisinteractive.com/vault/Harris-Interactive-Poll-Research-Cyberchondriacs-Update-2002-05.pdf

The doctor will understand you now. (2009). University of Southern California Viterbi School of Engineering. Retrieved December 27, 2009, from http://viterbi.usc.edu/news/news/2009/el-doctor-ya.htm

van Bronswijk, J. E. M. H., Bouma, H., Fozard, J. L., Kearns, W. D., Davison, G. C., & Tuan, P-C. (2009). Defining gerontechnology for R&D purposes. *Gerontechnology, 8*(1), 3–10.

Vanderheiden, G. C. (2007). Redefining assistive technology, accessibility and disability based on recent technical advances. *Journal of Technology in Human Services, 25*(1/2), 147–158.

Varkey, A. B., Manwell, L. B., Williams, E. S., Ibrahim, S. A., Brown, R. L., Bobula, J. A., et al. (2009). Separate and unequal: Clinics where minority and nonminority patients receive primary care. *Archives of Internal Medicine, 169*(3), 243–250.

Vigilante, F. W., Beaulaurier, R., & Haffe, M. (Eds.). (2005). *Technology in social work education and curriculum*. Philadelphia: Haworth Press.

Vital Wave Consulting. (2009). mHealth for development. The opportunity of mobile technology for health care in the developing world. Washington, DC and Berkshire, UK: UN Foundation-Vodafone Foundation Partnership. Retrieved December 27, 2009, from http://www.globalproblems-globalsolutions-files.org/unf_website/assets/publications/technology/mhealth/mHealth_for_Development_full.pdf

Wagner, E. H. (1998). Chronic disease management: What will it take to improve care for chronic illness? *Effective Clinical Practice, 1*(1), 2–4.

Weintraub, A. (2009, September 21). Intel wants you to age gracefully. *BusinessWeek*. Retrieved December 27, from http://www.businessweek.com/technology/content/sep2009/tc20090921_041069.htm

Westbrook, J. I., Braithwaite, J., Georgiou, A., Ampt, A., Creswick, N., Coiera, E., et al. (2007). Multimethod evaluation of information and communication technologies in health in the context of wicked problems and sociotechnical theory. *Journal of the American Medical Informatics Association, 14*(6), 746–755.

White, R. W., & Horvitz, E. (2008). *Cyberchondria: Studies of the escalation of medical concerns in web search* (No. MSR-TR-2008-177). Redmond, WA: Microsoft Research. Retrieved July 20, 2010, from http://www.chcf.org/~/media/Files/PDF/P/ParticipatoryHealthTools.pdf

Wielawski, I. M. (2006). Improving chronic illness care. *Robert Wood Johnson Foundation Anthology: To Improve Health and Health Care, 10*, 1–17.

Winter, R. (2009, July 21). *9 killer telemedicine apps that will revolutionize healthcare*. Retrieved December 21, 2009, from http://blog.soliant.com/healthcare-it/9-killer-apps-that-will-revolutionize-healthcare

World Health Organization. (2005). *Preparing a health care workforce for the 21st century: The challenge of chronic conditions*. Geneva, Switzerland: World Health Organization.

Index